Textbook of Allergen Tolerance

Vladimir V. Klimov

Textbook of Allergen Tolerance

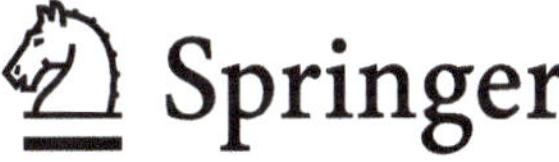

Vladimir V. Klimov
Clinical Immunology and Allergy Department
Siberian State Medical University
Tomsk, Russia

ISBN 978-3-031-04311-6 ISBN 978-3-031-04309-3 (eBook)
https://doi.org/10.1007/978-3-031-04309-3

This Springer imprint is published by the registered company Springer Nature Switzerland AG
The registered company address is: Gewerbestrasse 11, 6330 Cham, Switzerland

Werd ich zum Augenblicke sagen:
"Verweile doch! Du bist so schon!"
Dann magst du mich in Fesseln schlagen,
dann will ich gern zugrunde gehn!
Johann Wolfgang von Goethe
Faust I, 1699–1702
When, to the Moment then, I say:
"Ah, stay a while! You are so lovely!"
Then you can grasp me: then you may,
Then, to my ruin, I'll go gladly!

Johann Wolfgang von Goethe
Faust I, 1699–1702

The author dedicates this textbook to the memory of Dr. Leonard Noon (St. Mary's Hospital, Paddington/Imperial College London, United Kingdom), who helped millions of people with his revolutionary invention, allergen-specific immunotherapy.

Preface

The immune system is engaged in many fields related to health and illness, including allergy and nervous diseases, but can play both beneficial and harmful roles in the body. In many ways, it depends on the expression of either "good" or "bad" genes inherited from our ancestors. Such is the course of nature. Of course, our knowledge is still insufficient, but must respond to almost everyday attacks of allergens, microbes, tumor cells, and stress. These attacks continue to confront humans and well-being globally; in particular, a deep understanding of the immunologic mechanisms and processes will lead us to healthcare improvement.

This manual is written at the interface of allergy, basic immunology, and neuroscience. It may be helpful for postgraduate medical students, clinical allergists, and researchers in fundamental allergy and neuroscience fields. The textbook has been set out in a logical order to allow the reader to understand the basic principles of the subject.

Tomsk, Russia — Vladimir V. Klimov

Acknowledgments

The author wishes to express his gratitude to Professor Vladimir A. Kozlov, DSc, Research Supervisor, Academician, Novosibirsk Research Institute of Fundamental and Clinical Immunology (Russia) and Dr. Peter J. Mitchell, FCIL, CL, Founding Head, Department of Translation and Language Communication National Research Tomsk State University (United Kingdom, Russia).

Tomsk, Russia Vladimir V. Klimov

Contents

About the Author

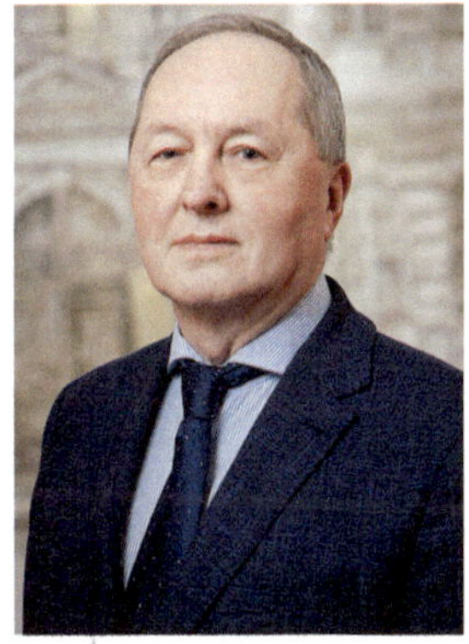

Vladimir V. Klimov, MD, PhD, DSc is the head of Siberian State Medical University's Immunology and Allergy Department. He is the author of the Multimedia Course "Basic Immunology Overview," which was published online in the late 1990s and became popular among students and physicians worldwide. For many years, Prof. Klimov has contributed to immunology education internationally with great enthusiasm. In 2019, he published the textbook *From Basic to Clinical Immunology*, which was an international success. This manual is written at the interface of fundamental immunology, neuroscience, and clinical allergology. Many people need clinical allergology today. It is a medical science about the allergies, breakdown and maintenance of allergen tolerance, and allergen-specific immunotherapy, says Prof. Klimov.

Abbreviations

5-HT1-5-HT7	Serotonin receptors
A1, A2A, A2B, A3	Adenosine receptors
a7nAchR	Nicotinic receptor
AAMP	Allergen-associated molecular patterns
ACE2	Angiotensin-converting enzyme 2 receptor
ACTH	Adrenocorticotropic hormone
AHR	Transcription factor
AIRE	Gene upregulating negative selection in the thymus
AIT	Allergen-specific immunotherapy
Akt/PI3-K	Signaling pathway
ALR	AIM-2-like receptor recognizing patterns
AP-1	Transcription factor
APC	Antigen-presenting cell
AR	Allergic (conventional) rhinitis
Ara h 1	Peanut's allergen
ATP	Adenosine triphosphate
B7	Costimulatory molecule
BALT	Bronchus-associated lymphoid tissue
BAT	Basophil activation test
BATF	Transcription factor
BAU	Bioequivalent allergen unit
Bcl6	Transcription factor
BCR	B-cell antigen-recognizing receptor
Bet v 1	Birch's allergen
Bos d 4	Milk's allergen
BRAK	Chemokine CXCL14
Breg	Regulatory B cells
BTLA	Coinhibitory molecule
C1-INH	C1 inhibitor
cAMP	Cyclic adenosine monophosphate
Can f 1	Dog's allergen
CB1, CB2	Cannabinoid receptors
CCR	Receptor to chemokine CC subfamily
CD28	Costimulatory molecule

cDNA	Complementary DNA
CFU	Colony-forming units
cGMP	Cyclic guanosine monophosphate
CGRP	Calcitonin-gene-related peptide
CL	Chemokine subfamily
CLC	Charcot–Leyden crystal protein (galectin-10)
CLR	CGRP's receptors
CLR	C-type lectin receptors
c-Maf	Transcription factor
c-Myc	Transcription factor
COPD	Chronic obstructive pulmonary disease
Cor a 9	Hazelnut's allergen
CpGs	Nonmethylated CG motifs in DNA
CR	Receptor to chemokine C subfamily
CRD	Carbohydrate recognition domain
CRD	Component resolved diagnosis
CRTH2	Chemoattractant receptor-homologous molecule expressed on Th2
CTACK	Chemokine CCL27
CTLA-4	Coinhibitory molecule
CX3CL	Chemokine subfamily
CX3CR	Receptor to chemokine CX3C subfamily
CXCL	Chemokine subfamily
CXCR	Receptor to chemokine CXC subfamily
Cyp c 1	Carp's allergen
D_1–D_5	Dopamine receptors
DAMP	Damage-associated molecular patterns
DC	Dendritic cells
DC-SIGN	C-type lectin receptor
DDC	DOPA decarboxylase gene
Der f 1	Allergen of *Dermatophagoides farinae*
Der p 1	Allergen of *Dermatophagoides pteronyssinus*
DPI	Dry powder inhaler
EAI	Epinephrine auto-injector
ENS	Enteric (autonomous) nervous system
ENT	Otorhinolaryngologist
Eotaxin-1	Chemokine CCL11
Eotaxin-2	Chemokine CCL24
Eotaxin-3	Chemokine CCL26
FasL/Fas	Molecules taking part in apoptosis
FcγR	Receptor to IgG
FcεRI	Type I receptor to IgE
fDCs	Follicular dendritic cells
Fel d	Cat's allergen
FeNO	Fractional exhaled nitric oxide

FEV1	1st second forced expiratory volume
FGF	Fibroblast growth factor
FoxP3+	Transcription factor (of Tregs)
FPIES	Food protein-induced enterocolitis syndrome (non-IgE-dependent)
FVC	Full vital capacity
GABA	γ Aminobutyric acid
$GABA_A$, $GABA_B$	GABA receptors
Gal d 2	Egg's allergen
GALT	Gut-associated lymphoid tissue
GATA1, GATA3	Transcription factors
GINA	Position paper on asthma
Gly m 4	Soybean's allergen
GlyRs	Glycine receptors
GM-CSF	Granulocyte-macrophage colony-stimulating factor
GROα	Chemokine CXCL1
H_1–H_4	Receptors to histamine
HDC	Histidine decarboxylase gene
HDM	House dust mites
HEP	Histamine equivalent prick test
HIV	Human immunodeficiency virus
HLA	Human histocompatibility system
HNMT	Histamine N-methyl transferase gene
HO-1	Heme oxygenase-1
HPA	Hypothalamic-pituitary-adrenal system
HPV	Human papilloma virus
ICOS	Costimulatory molecule
IDO	Indoleamin-2,3-dioxygenase
IELs	Interepithelial lymphocytes, γδT cells
IFN-γ	Interferon-γ
IgE-BF	IgE-blocking factor
IgE-FAB	IgE-facilitated antigen binding to B cells
IL	Interleukins
ILC	Innate lymphoid cells
IP-10	Chemokine CXCL10
IPEX	Polyendocrinopathy enteropathy X-linked syndrome
IR	Index of reactivity (of allergen)
IRF4	Transcription factor
ITAM	Immunoreceptor tyrosine-based activation motif
ITIM	Immunoreceptor tyrosine-based inhibition motif
iTreg	Induced T regulatory cell
Jak/STAT	Signaling pathway
JNK	Protein kinase
KIT gene	Gene encoded the tyrosine kinase receptor KIT
KLF4	Transcription factor

LAG-3	Coinhibitory molecule
LAP	Latency-associated peptide functionally linked with TGF-β
LAR	Local allergic rhinitis
Lep d 2	Allergen of *Lepidoglyphus destructor* (storage mite)
LRR	Leucine-rich repeat domains
LTB_4	Leukotriene B_4
LTC_4	Leukotriene C_4
M cells	"Multifold" cells
M1, M2	Types 1 and 2 macrophage
M1AchR, M2AchR	Muscarinic receptors
MAFB	Transcription factor
MAIT	Mucosal-associated invariant T cells
Mal d 1	Apple's allergen
MALT	Mucus-associated lymphoid tissue
MAPK	Signaling pathway
MBB	Mucosal brush biopsy
MCP-1	Chemokine CCL-2
MCP-2	Chemokine CCL8
MCP-3	Chemokine CCL7
MCP-4	Chemokine CCL13
MD-2	Molecule associated with TLR4
MDC	Chemokine CCL22
mDC	Myeloid (conventional) dendritic cell
MDI	Metered–dose inhaler
MEK	Protein kinase
Met e 1	A shrimp's allergen
mGluRs, iGluRs	L-glutamate receptors
MIG	Chemokine CXCL9
MIP-1α	Chemokine CCL3
MIP-1β	Chemokine CCL4
MIP-2α	Chemokine CXCL2
MIP-2β	Chemokine CXCL3
MIRACL-seq	Transcriptomic method
MRGPRX1-2	Human mas-related G-protein-coupled receptors X1-2
MW	Molecular weight
MyD88	Signaling molecule
NALT	Nasal-associated lymphoid tissue
NAPT	Nasal allergen provocation test
NFAT	Transcription factor
NF-κB	Transcription factor
NGF	Nerve growth factor
NK	Nature killer cells
NLR	NOD-like receptor recognizing patterns
NLRP	Inflammasome
NMUR1	Neuromedin U receptor1 gene

NMUR1, NMUR2	Neuromedin U receptors
NOS2	Inducible nitric oxidase synthase
nTregs	Natural regulatory T cells
OCT-3	Organic cation transporter-3 gene
OVA	Ovalbumin
PAF	Platelet-activating factor
PAMP	Pathogen-associated molecular patterns
PAR	Protease-activated receptors
PARC	Chemokine CCL18
PD-1	Coinhibitory molecule
pDC	Plasmacytoid dendritic cell
PDGF	Platelet-derived growth factor
PD-L1	Ligand to PD-1
Pen a 1	Shrimp's allergen
PGD_2	Prostaglandin D_2
PGM3	Gene of phosphoglucomutase 3
PI2-K, PI3-K	Molecules of Akt/PI3-K signaling pathway
PNU	Protein nitrogen unit
ppb	Parts per billion (FeNO measurement's units)
PRR	Pattern recognition z receptors
PSA	Prostate-specific antigen
pTregs	Peripheral (allergen-specific) regulatory T cells
PU.1	Transcription factor
RAISIN RNA-seq	Transcriptomic method
RANTES	Chemokine CCL5
RLR	RIG-1-like receptor recognizing patterns
RORα	Transcription factor
RORγt	Transcription factor
ROS	Reactive oxygen species
RunX	Transcription factor
SARS-CoV-2	Severe acute respiratory syndrome-related coronavirus 2
SBU	Standardized biological units
ScorAD	Index of clinical evaluation in atopic dermatitis
scRNA-seq	Single-cell RNA sequencing (transcriptomic method)
SERT	Serotonin transporter
sIgA	Secretory IgA
SMAD	Signaling pathway
SP	Substance P
SP-A, SP-D	Surfactant proteins
SPT	Skin prick testing
ssRNA	Single-stranded RNA
STAT	Molecules family of Jak/STAT signaling pathway
TAC1	Gene of substance P
TAM	Tumor-associated macrophages
TARC	Chemokine CCL17

Tbet	Transcription factor
TCR	T-cell antigen-recognizing receptor
tDCs	Tolerogenic dendritic cells
Tfh	Follicular helper T cell
Tfr	T follicular regulatory cell
TGF-β	Transforming growth factor-β
Th1	Type 1 helper T cell
Th17	Type 17 helper T cell
Th2	Type 2 helper T cell
Th22	Type 22 helper T cell
Th3	Type 3 helper T cell (a subset of pTregs)
Th9	Type 9 helper T cell
TIR	Toll/IL1 receptor domain
TLR	Toll-like receptors
TMPRSS2	Transmembrane serine protease-2
TNF-α	Tumor-necrosis factor-α
TNF-β	Tumor-necrosis factor-β
TPH2	5-tryptophan hydroxylase-2 gene
Tr1	Type 1 regulatory T cell
Treg	Regulatory T cell
Tri a 19	Wheat's allergen
TRIF	Signaling molecule
TSLP	Thymic stromal lymphopoietin
TSST	Trier social stress test
Tyk2	Tyrosine kinase of Jak/STAT signaling pathway
VAS	Visual analog scale
VIP	Gene of vasoactive intestinal peptide
VIP	Vasoactive intestinal peptide
VLP	Virus-like particles
VNS	Vegetative nervous system
VP	Vasopressin gene
VPAC1, VPAC2	Vasopressin receptors
ZAP70	Tyrosine kinase
α-Gal	Galactose-α-1,3-galactose
β_2AR	Adrenergic receptor
γδT	γδT cells, intraepithelial lymphocytes (IELs)

List of Videos

Antigens and Allergens

1

Contents

Didactics

Knowledge. Upon successful completion of this chapter, students should be able to:

1. Draw the role of the immune system in response to allergens.
2. Distinguish between immunogenicity and allergenicity.
3. List common environmental allergens.
4. List antigen properties.
5. Describe simple B cell-mediated responses.
6. Describe advanced B cell-mediated responses.
7. Describe the HLA II pathway of the T cell-mediated responses.
8. Describe the HLA I pathway of the T cell-mediated responses.
9. Briefly describe factors of allergen allergenicity.
10. Explain the concept of atopy in the context of an evolutionary vestige.
11. Explain principles of allergen nomenclature.
12. Describe the peculiarities of house dust mites (HDM).

Supplementary Information The online version contains supplementary material available at [https://doi.org/10.1007/978-3-031-04309-3_1].

V. V. Klimov, *Textbook of Allergen Tolerance*,
https://doi.org/10.1007/978-3-031-04309-3_1

Acquired Skills. Upon successful completion of this chapter, students should demonstrate the following skills, including:

1. Interpret the knowledge related to antigens and allergens.
2. Critically evaluate the scientific literature about antigens and allergens.
3. Discuss the scientific articles from the current research literature to criticize experimental data and formulate a new allergy hypothesis.
4. Have a clear perception of the presented allergy definitions expressed orally and in written form.
5. Formulate the presented allergy terms.
6. Correctly answer the quiz questions.

Attitude and Professional Behaviors. Students should be able to:

1. Have the readiness to be hard-working.
2. Behave professionally at all times.
3. Recognize the importance of studying and demonstrate a commitment.

1.1 Introduction

Antigens and allergens, molecules to which the immune system talks, differ by their number. Antigens present a "universe of antigens," about 10^{18} molecules, whereas allergens are only a small molecular group, less than 2% of all known protein families. However, allergens can cause sensitization, inflammation, and then clinical disease from skin rash through anaphylaxis that requires proper and emergency treatment. Atopy is a common and frequent form of allergy having polygenic inheritance and is linked with the IgE-mediated process.

Allergen sources are different. Environmental allergens include grass and tree pollens, fungal spores, house dust mites (HDM) and cockroach feces, animal scales and dander, food components, medications, latex, biologic products, and insect venoms and stings. Like antigens, allergens trigger an adaptive immune response leading to antibody production (in this case IgE) and allergen-specific memory B cells and T cells that survive a lifetime. Once an allergen enters the body, this memory remains in the person for a long time.

1.2 Antigens and Immune Responses

▶ **Definition** An adaptive immune response is an immunologic process of constituting protective effector cells and memory cells to antigen. Allergic IgE response, or sensitization, is a form of adaptive immune response caused by allergens that can come to allergic inflammation.

The *antigen* is a substance that triggers the adaptive immune responses to establish an effective defense against a pathogen containing this antigen and subsequent memory. If an antigen switches to a tolerogenic response, it is termed "tolerogen." In the enlarged sense, it is currently estimated that the amount of antigens makes up about 10^{18} molecules in the environment. The 1960 Nobel Laureate Sir F. MacFarlane Burnet called them the "universe of antigens."

All antigens may be divided into "non-self" (environmental proteins, phospholipids, glycolipids, and lipopolysaccharides), "self" (protein of the human body), "hidden self" (sequestrated or cryptic determinants of body's over-barrier organs), and "former self" (tumor proteins) [1].

Antigens have two features, immunogenicity and allergenicity. In other words, antigenicity is the capability of an antigen to specifically, beneficially, or harmfully, combine with the final products of the immune response, TCR, BCR, or antibodies [2]. In this sense, an *allergen* is an antigen with "harmful" antigenicity.

Immunogenicity is the potency of an antigen (immunogen) to develop an immunologic defense against pathogens, maintenance of immunologic homeostasis, and anti-tumor surveillance. High immunogenicity is inherent in vaccines and some microbial antigens.

Allergenicity is the allergen's ability to induce a non-adequate adaptive immune response, characterized by the overactivation of the immune system, absence of protective effect, and development of allergic inflammation and own tissue damage instead. Allergens with high allergenicity are called "major" allergens [3] and conversely. This division has gradually become outdated [4].

It is important to consider the adaptive and innate immunity function regarding antigens and allergens. *Adaptive immune responses* include antigen-specific defense mechanisms and may take days or weeks to develop. These responses are orchestrated by the complex interactions and activities of many various cell types involved in the processes. Adaptive immune responses establish effector cells, which fight against pathogens, and memory cells memorizing these pathogens. There are four pathways of adaptive immune responses depending on the type and location of the pathogen containing the antigen.

The *tolerogenic immune response* [3] is the opposite of adaptive responses because it constitutes immune tolerance [5] (see Chap. 2), including allergen tolerance [6] (see Chap. 3). *Tolergenicity* is the antigen property that, under certain conditions, can be tolerized, or the capacity of the immune system's cells to convert an antigen into tolerogen.

1. The *HLA II pathway of the T cell-mediated response* involves *naïve CD4+ T cells* that result in their clonal expansion and differentiation to effector CD4+ T cells with inflammatory potential. In the beginning, the same cells are type 1 helper CD4+ T (Th1) cells. This immune response is required to eliminate some intracellularly located exogenous antigens through immune inflammation. Long-term (lifelong) immunological memory CD4+ T cells are established in any case.
2. The *HLA I pathway of the T cell-mediated response* engages *naïve cytotoxic CD8+ T cells* activated with the aid of type 1 helper CD4+ T (Th1) cells. Subsequently, CD8+ T cell clonal expansion proceeds and the cells mature until they become effector cytotoxic CD8+ T cells to eliminate such endogenous (intracellular) pathogens like viruses. It is achieved via apoptosis in those target

cells, which contain the viruses. Besides, lifelong memory CD8+ T cells are always formed.

3. *Simple B cell-mediated responses* to T independent antigens and molecular patterns belonging to extracellularly located pathogens proceed with the involvement of *naïve B cells* but with no aid from helper T cells. However, such a response leads to the production of IgM only, whereas other isotypes of the antibodies and the long-term immunological memory do not occur.
4. *Advanced B cell-mediated responses* to antigens derived from extracellularly located pathogens and environmental allergens proceed with the participation of *naïve B cells* and type 2 helper CD4+ T (Th2) cells/follicular helper T (Tfh) cells. Such a response results in the maturation of plasma cells, antibody switching (continuously IgM, IgG, IgA, and IgE) by control of type 1 helper CD4+ T (Th1) cells in part, and producing long-term (lifelong) immunological memory to the antigen or allergen thanks to memory B cells, and a relatively short-term memory due to long-lived plasma cells.

1.2.1 Sensitization to Allergens

The type of advanced B cell Th2-dependent response to allergens involves innate immunity significantly [7, 8]. The process is called *sensitization*, resulting in IgE antibodies production and allergic diseases termed *atopy*, a common form of allergy.

In response to environmental allergens (see Fig. 1.1), epitheliocytes produce alarmins (danger signals), IL-25, IL-33, and thymic stromal lymphopoietin (TSLP), which upregulate group 2 innate lymphoid (ILC2) cells, dendritic (DCs) cells, and type 2 helper T (Th2) cells [9]. Pro-immunogenic neuropeptide neuromedin U also participates in this process, promoting ILC2 cells [10–12]. Conversely, endogenous neuropeptide calcitonin-gene-related peptide (CGRP) is a critical negative regulator of ILC2 responses in vivo [13, 14]. The alarmins are essential stimulators of type 2 immunity, as they lead to the production of IL-5, IL-9, and IL-13, but they can participate in the IgE-independent pathway of allergic inflammation [12, 15]. Allergens that pass the epithelial barriers are processed by allergen-presenting (APC) cells, DCs, which in turn migrate to draining lymph nodes, where they present allergen-derived peptides on HLA class II molecules to naïve T cells. The naïve T cells can differentiate into Th2 cells and follicular helper T (Tfh) cells.

Th2 cells produce type 2 cytokines such as IL-4, IL-5, IL-9, IL-13, IL-33 and drive allergic inflammation. Tfh cells produce IL-21, IL-4, IL-13, which promote IgE class switch recombination in B cells, plasma cell maturation, and allergen-specific IgE production. Simultaneously, the shaping of two types of allergen-specific memory cells, (1) memory T cells and (2) memory B cells, occurs. The allergen-specific IgE antibodies bind to FcεRI molecules on mast cells and basophils, resulting in their degranulation and allergic inflammation development due to histamine and other mediators [16, 17]. Toll-like receptors (TLRs) related to pattern recognition receptors (PRRs) bind to pathogen-associated molecular patterns (PAMP) or damage-associated molecular patterns (DAMP), and after signaling, promote the release of alarmins, the synthesis of cytokines, and development of pyroptosis, creating the link between adaptive and

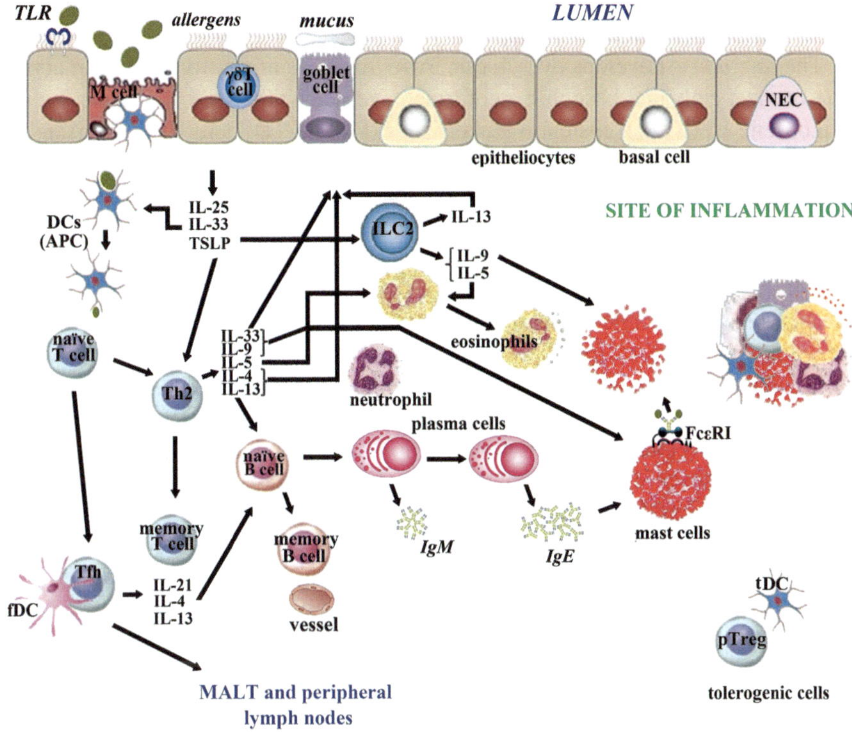

Fig. 1.1 Advanced B cell Th2-dependent response to allergens (sensitization). Penetrating through the epithelium using M cells and epithelium defects, an allergen occurs in the subepithelial region (submucosa). In the submucosa, there are eosinophils, neutrophils, dendritic cells (DCs), ILC2, mast cells, etc. Before the beginning of the immune response, ILC2, APC, and Th2 cells are upregulated by epithelium-derived alarmins, IL-25, IL-33, TSLP. Toll-like receptors (TLRs) can bind to allergens, and after signaling, also promote the release of alarmins. Activated ILC2 secrete IL-5, IL-9, and IL-13. Submucosal DCs are allergen-presenting cells required for allergen processing and type 2 helper T (Th2) cell proliferation. Th2 cells promote adaptive B cell response with IgE end-production and allergen-specific memory B and memory T cell establishment. Th2 cells produce type 2 cytokines such as IL-4, IL-5, IL-9, IL-13, and IL-33 and function as regulatory cells that drive allergic inflammation, including the activation of goblet cells and maturation of mast cells. Tfh secrete IL-21, IL-4, and IL-13, which are essential for promoting IgE class switch recombination in B cells, maturing plasma cells, and growing allergen-specific IgE affinity. TSLP thymic stromal lymphopoietin, ILC2 group 2 innate lymphoid cell, DCs dendritic cells, tDC tolerogenic dendritic cells, TLR toll-like receptors, Tfh follicular helper T cell, fDC follicular dendritic cell, APC allergen-presenting cell, NEC neuroendocrine cell

innate immunity. In addition, they sense house dust mites (HDMs), PAMPs, and allergens, and various allergens from distinct sources [18].

The effector stage of allergic response proceeds in three phases: (1) early phase, (2) late phase, and (3) chronic allergic inflammation [19, 20]. The *early phase* typically occurs within 10–20 min, or even seconds, following allergen exposure, caused by the release of preformed mediators of mast cells [21, 22] and basophils such as histamine, serotonin, chemotactic peptides for neutrophils and eosinophils, and enzymes (chymase and tryptase). These mediators affect the nerve cells causing an itch, smooth muscle contraction (e.g., asthmatic attack), mucus production by goblet cells, increased capillary permeability, subsequent tissue edema, and recruitment of neutrophils and eosinophils.

The *late phase* develops over 4–6 h. Two groups de novo produced after activation of mast cells and basophils neoformed and neosynthesized mediators include leukotriene B_4 (LTB_4), cysteinyl leukotrienes (LTC_4, LTD_4, and LTE_4), prostaglandin D_2 (PGD_2), platelet-activating factor (PAF), cytokines (IL-10, IL-8, IL-5, IL-3, IL-1, GM-CSF, TGF-β, TNF-α, etc.), chemokines, growth factors, nitric oxide, and components of complement (C3 and C5) [23, 24] as well as products of other inflammatory cells, in particular of degranulated eosinophils. However, a combination of different mediators in three phases is reported in a slightly contradictory manner [23, 24]. These biomolecules act on surrounding tissues promoting the inflammatory process. Endothelial cells express those adhesion molecules, which facilitate the recruitment and activation of neutrophils, eosinophils, dendritic cells, and monocytes from the blood into the site of the allergic inflammation. Commonly, the infiltrating cells contain a high proportion of eosinophils [25, 26]. The eosinophils release various inflammatory molecules, including major basic protein, eosinophilic cationic protein, IL-5, etc. The involved Th2 cells secrete cytokines among which Il-4, IL-13, and IL-33 are the most potent and affect plasma cells, promoting IgE isotype switching. So, the events acquire a long-term potential [1].

The process becomes *chronic allergic inflammation* after repeated exposures to allergens with the increased recruitment of immune cells, consequent elevated levels of Th2-related cytokines, substantial changes in the extracellular matrix, and alterations in the number, phenotype, and function of structural cells in the affected site [19].

There is accumulating evidence that the metabolic status of T cells, macrophages, and other immune cells is associated with phenotypes of chronic allergic inflammation. The metabolic pathways are closely tied to cells' differentiation, and this link between energy metabolism and inflammation can be assessed employing animal and cellular models and clinical studies in humans. Analytical approaches rank from classic immunological studies to integrated analysis of metabolomics, transcriptomics, and proteomics [27].

1.3 Allergenicity of Allergens

▶ **Definition** An allergen is an antigen triggering the sensitization in predisposed individuals. Allergenicity is the ability of an allergen to induce an allergic response and allergic inflammation. A major allergen is an allergen binding IgE antibodies in the serum of the most sensitized patients; a minor allergen is an allergen with weak binding properties concerning specific IgE antibodies.

Only a small number of proteins of plants, fungi, HDM, and animals, including human food, are known as allergens [28–31]. Although polysaccharides and low-molecular-weight substances may also be allergenic [32]. Allergens have been classified depending on their structural, biochemical, and functional features and allergenicity [7].

Table 1.1 Factors of allergenicity

Depending on allergen	Depending on biogenic cofactors	Depending on the immune system of the macroorganism itself
– Primary amino acid sequence of allergenic determinants	– Lack of bacterial homologs (with several exceptions)	– Predisposition to sensitization (atopy)
– Molecular weight and size	– Presence of molecular patterns	– Route of exposure (skin or sexual contact, inhalation, ingestion, and injection)
– Small isoelectric point (charge)	– Presence of adjuvants	– Involving of innate immunity
– Low hydrophobicity	– Pollens as allergen carriers	– Physiologic barriers defects
– High stability	– Environmental pollutants	– Sialylation of IgE
– Group of protein fold		
– Solubility		
– Oligomerization		
– Amount of determinants and their proximity to each other		
– Concentration, dose		
– Resistance to proteolysis and posttranslational glycosylation		
– Presence of intrinsic biologic activities		

Many limitations are relevant for allergens' allergenicity (see Table 1.1) [3, 7, 32–35]. The allergenicity of particular allergens, food proteins, will be considered in Chap. 7.

An allergenic protein's primary amino acid sequence displays its significant physicochemical properties, such as molecular weight, isoelectric point (charge), hydrophobicity, and stability. The optimal molecular weight of allergens varies from 5 to 100 kDa (with several exceptions) [7, 32]. Most allergens are grouped into four structural families when classified according to their protein folds [36] that influence allergenicity:

1. Antiparallel β-strands (some HDM' and grass allergens)
2. Antiparallel β-strands closely associated with one or more α-helices (tree allergens)
3. α- and β-structures not closely associated (some HDM's allergens)
4. α-helical structure (some pollen, insect, fish, and cat's allergens)

Allergens require at least two IgE-binding determinants to bind with IgE and provide cross-linking for activation of mast cells. IgE antibodies can either recognize "continuous epitopes" consisting of a row of consecutive amino acids or "discontinuous epitopes," composed of amino acids from different portions placed close together due to folding the allergen molecule. These epitopes must always be in proximity to each other as the optimal distance between two IgE sites is 92–102 Å [37].

Exposure to indoor allergens showed that allergen concentration could be different and impact allergenicity in a distinct manner [38]. For example, a measure of the major allergen *Der p 1* and *Der f 1* concentration displayed 400-fold lower than major cat and dog allergens (respectively, *Fel d 1* and *Can f 1*). There is a sample of the classical concept of low-dose and high-dose tolerance [5, 6].

Solubility of food allergens is now considered to decrease their allergenicity. However, for example, boiling and frying peanuts do not generate the hypoallergenic properties of *Ara h 1* and *Ara h 2* [39].

Some allergens have intrinsic biological activities thanks to the presence of proteases, pectate lyases, trypsin inhibitors, calcium-binding proteins, lipid transfer proteins, actin-binding proteins, etc. Allergens' intrinsic biologic properties due to posttranslational glycosylation and resistance to proteolysis enhance the stability and bioavailability of allergens [3]. They can contribute to allergenicity through an increase in the tissue distribution of the allergens. For example, allergens *Der p 1* and *Der f 1* have papain-like cysteine protease activity, which enables the recruitment of basophils to the area of the immune response, enhancement of production of IL-4 and thymic stromal lymphopoietin (TSLP), cleavage of CD25 on regulatory T (Treg) cells weakening the system of allergen tolerance maintenance [3]. Protease-activated receptors (PAR) are integral membrane G-coupled proteins that can be split by allergens causing allergic inflammation [40]. Besides, the intrinsic properties of allergens allow activating the innate immune system, inducing a more active allergic response [7].

Investigating homology showed that most allergens have no bacterial homologs [41], but some bacterial proteins as an exception may induce IgE-dependent response.

It has been found that such cofactors as pattern-associated molecular patterns (PAMP), allergen-associated molecular patterns (AAMP) [37], and biopolymer chitin can serve as adjuvants for allergens enhancing their allergenicity. PAMPs via Toll-like receptors (TLRs), and C-type lectin receptors (CLRs), result in the production of pro-inflammatory cytokines upregulating allergic inflammation, whereas AAMPs contribute to the natural or artificial oligomerization of allergens. Chitin is present in insects, HDM, mold, helminths, and crustaceans, upregulating the IgE response, production of IL-4 by eosinophils and basophils, and accumulation of ILCs in tissue [42].

Pollen particles between 20 and 60 μm in diameter may be carried by the wind and transfer other allergens and cause allergic symptoms in the unified airway [32]. In addition, traffic-derived pollutants cause the release of allergen-rich cytoplasmic granules from pollen, and, therefore, increase allergens' quantity [3].

The allergic response is dependent on the route of exposure to allergens. If the exposure is to an inhaled aeroallergen, allergic inflammation will develop in the unified airway. Ingested, dermal, or injected exposure lead to gastrointestinal, cutaneous, or anaphylactic reactions. Sexual exposure leads to genitourinary and extra organic allergies. Food allergens can evoke food allergies and respiratory and dermal manifestations [32, 43].

Physiological barriers of the body matter much. It is known that mutations of the *filaggrin gene*, a skin barrier protein, predispose to atopic dermatitis and psoriasis [44]. Typically, filaggrin is responsible for keratinization. For example, keratinized stratified squamous epithelium covering the glans penis in circumcised men plays a significant preventive role in both allergic and infectious inflammation (see Chap. 9) [45].

Sialylation of IgE occurs only in atopic individuals. Removing sialic acid from cell-bound IgE with a neuraminidase enzyme targeted toward the FcεRI, and administering asialylated IgE is a novel approach in the treatment of peanut allergies [46].

Eventually, the main point at which allergenicity of allergens depends at the whole body level is interaction with the innate immune cells via binding to pattern recognition receptors (PRRs), inducing group 2 innate lymphoid cells (ILC2), and contributing then to adaptive Th2-dependent IgE response [3, 7].

1.3.1 Allergen Nomenclature

Allergen nomenclature [3] is based on (1) the Linnaean binomial nomenclature identifying genus and species and (2) modern advances in both sequencing and bioinformatics. An abbreviation of the scientific name of the allergen source, including genus (3 letters) and species (1 letter), follows first. For example, *Der p* means an allergen from house dust mite *Dermatophagoides pteronyssinus.* Next, one Arabic numeral (the number when this allergen was described among other allergens of this species) follows. After a period (.), the first two digits designate isoallergens, defined as allergens from a single species with similar molecular masses and biochemical functions, and sequence identities >67%.

The following two digits denote different variants of the isoallergen, which are defined as proteins with more than 90% sequence identity. The full allergen's name may look like *Der p 1.0101*, which we will be able to see on allergen vials for allergen-specific immunotherapy (AIT) in the near future.

Historically, protein nitrogen units (PNU) were used when 1 PNU corresponded to 0.01 μg phosphotungstic acid-precipitable nitrogen, which stood for about 0.06 μg protein. Nowadays, various manufacturers use different allergen units, e.g., index of reactivity (IR), bioequivalent allergen units (BAU), standardized biological units (SBU), histamine equivalent prick test (HEP), etc. [47]. However, allergen standardization strategies should be uniform throughout the world to avoid confusion when estimating the potency of various allergen extracts and allergenic molecules. In the future, new technologies (e.g., mass spectrometry, etc.) makes an opportunity to redefine two main paths to allergen standardization, including product-specific standardization and comparability of products from different manufacturers and regulatory authorities. It is expected the process of innovative standardization will improve both the efficacy and safety of AIT [48].

Taken in a simplistic form, all allergens may be divided into *major* and *minor* allergens. Major allergens can induce a strong IgE response, whereas minor ones trigger only the weak formation of IgE-synthesizing plasma cells. The major allergen must preferentially be chosen for all routes of administration in AIT. However, this classification is already insufficient for the new chapter in the history of allergology, marking the molecular era's beginning [4].

Currently, there are two allergen generations, allergenic extracts, and allergenic molecules. Allergenic extracts are used for allergic skin tests and allergen-specific immunotherapy (AIT) for a long time, whereas allergenic molecules are recently made on the basis of a new biotechnology approach to be recruited in the new era of molecular allergology [49]. Allergens of different sources (plants, fungi, and animals) and routes of exposure capable of inducing an IgE response constitute the *Allergome database* based on the literature published since the early 1960s. Low-molecular substances causing non-type I hypersensitivity, pseudo allergic reactions, and intolerance are not a part of the Allergome database. Allergen-associated molecular patterns (AAMPs) are not included in the Allergome database yet. You can find information on any allergen at www.allergen.org if you know its biological source (i.e., the species' name). There are other databases of allergens [50]. Due to the omics revolution and development of artificial intelligence, new global databases are being created to facilitate precise diagnoses and therapy for the personalized medicine approaches in allergology [51].

Quiz A

Reading a question, please choose only one right answer.

Question 1

Sensitization is:

1. Natural cytotoxicity.
2. Simple B cell response with IgM production.
3. CD8+ T cell immune response.
4. Advanced B cell-mediated Th2-dependent response to an allergen.

Question 2

Antigen's antigenicity is characterized by:

1. Specificity of antigen.
2. Affinity and avidity.
3. Latent epitope.
4. Immunogenicity and allergenicity.

Question 3

The tolerogenic immune response is:

1. The capacity of upregulating clonal expansion of lymphocytes.
2. The ability to form immune tolerance.

3. The ability to promote the proliferation of Th2 cells.
4. The capacity of causing sensitization.

Question 4
Allergenicity is the allergen's ability to induce:

1. CD4+ T cell immune response.
2. Immune tolerance.
3. CD8+ T cell immune response.
4. Sensitization and allergic inflammation.

Question 5
CD8+ T cell immune response is directed against:

1. Intracellularly located pathogens like viruses.
2. Extracellularly located pathogens like bacteria.
3. Environmental allergens.
4. Pathogen-associated molecular patterns (PAMPs).

Question 6
Epithelial cells-derived alarmins are:

1. IFN-γ, IL-2, and TNF-β.
2. IL-10, TGF-β, and IL-27.
3. IL-25, IL-33, and thymic stromal lymphopoietin (TSLP).
4. IL-1β, IL-6, and TNF-α.

Question 7
Alarmins activate:

1. ILC2, dendritic cells, and Th2 cells.
2. Eosinophils and neutrophils.
3. Monocytes and macrophages.
4. Basophils and mast cells.

Question 8
The end-effect of sensitization is:

1. Forming allergen-specific memory B cells and T cells.
2. Eliminating the allergen.
3. Allergen tolerance.
4. Producing IgM.

Question 9
IgE-dependent allergic inflammation proceeds in:

1. One phase.
2. Early and late phases.
3. Three phases.
4. Constitent long-term phase.

Question 10
Environmental allergens include:

1. Timothy pollen.
2. Sagebrush pollen.
3. House dust mites feces.
4. All points.

Question 11
Environmental allergens include:

1. Ragweed pollen.
2. Peanuts.
3. All points.
4. Latex.

Question 12
Type 2 helper T cells secrete:

1. TNF-β, GM-CSF, and IL-1β.
2. IL-10, IL-35, and IL-27.
3. IFN-γ, TNF-β, and IL-2.
4. IL-4, IL-5, and IL-13.

Question 13
Allergen allergenicity depends on:

1. Primary amino acid sequence of allergenic epitopes.
2. Low hydrophobicity.
3. High stability.
4. All points.

Question 14
Allergen allergenicity also depends on:

1. Solubility.
2. Concentration and dose.

3. Presence of intrinsic biologic activities.
4. All points.

Question 15

Allergen nomenclature takes into account the following order of abbreviations related to allergens:

1. Genus, species, allergen identification number.
2. Allergen identification number, genus, species.
3. Species, sequence number, genus.
4. Species, genus, allergen identification number.

Question 16

IgE-independent pathway of allergic inflammation is promoted by:

1. Macrophages.
2. Th2 cells.
3. ILC2 cells.
4. Eosinophils.

1.4 Concept of Atopy

▶ **Definition** Atopy, a common form of allergy, is based on polygenic inheritance and developed by type I hypersensitivity.

In the past, the term "*atopy*" was denoted as "out of place" and "strange disease" by Coca and Cooke in 1923 in their seminal article [52, 53] when IgE was not yet discovered by Ishizaka et al. [54]. In 1963, Gell and Coombs [55] proposed an updated classification of known allergic phenomena where atopy was grouped as type I immediate hypersensitivity. This nomenclature remains in use today. Nowadays, there is the rising prevalence of many types of allergies in modern human populations and widely discussed but not yet proven hygiene hypothesis and toxin hypothesis [2, 56]. In particular, allergic reactions can be considered maladaptive IgE immune responses toward environmental antigens [57]. Intriguingly, these mechanisms are very similar to those implicated in acquiring an important degree of immunity against helminths and arthropods in human bodies. Based on the hypothesis that IgE-mediated immune responses evolved in humans and other mammals to provide extra protection against metazoan parasites rather than cause an allergy, the environmental allergens might share essential properties with the metazoan parasite antigens, which are specifically targeted by IgE in infected human populations [57].

The analyses conclusively demonstrate that house dust mites *Dermatophagoides* have abandoned a parasitic lifestyle, secondarily becoming free-living, and then speciated in several habitats, including human homes. On the phylogenetic tree they produced, house dust mites appear within a large lineage of parasitic mites, the

Psoroptidia. The *Psoroptidia* remain full-time parasites of birds and mammals that never leave the bodies of their hosts [58, 59].

On the other hand, type I, immediate hypersensitivity, or atopy, occurs in selected populations of *Homo sapiens*. It appears to be a polygeneously inherited disorder, as genome-wide association studies have convincingly detected many loci associated with allergic diseases [60], but there are probably so-called primary atopic conditions based on monogenous inheritance [61, 62]. In addition to that, epigenetics has recently been considered a potential mechanism involved in developing many disorders, including atopic diseases [63]. The atopy appears to show a solid hereditary component due to the evolution vestige (see Fig. 1.2). From an evolutionary point of view, house dust mites, *Dermatophagoides pteronyssinus* (European species) and *Dermatophagoides farinae* (American species) are the "kings of allergens" or panallergens [64, 65]. They probably used to be skin parasites in ancient humans in the Stone Age [1].

The term "atopy" is currently used by allergists and researchers for any hyper-IgE-mediated reaction induced by a B cell-mediated Th2-dependent response to various allergens like house dust mites, etc. [1]. There are also oligomeric components of allergen molecules, allergen-associated molecular patterns (AAMP), which may be responsible for effective cross-linking of an allergen by BCR/IgE [37]. Supposedly, a deficit of AAMPs leads to allergen tolerance maintenance, whereas an excess of them results in tolerance breakdown. Exposure to allergens may be by inhalation, ingestion, injection, or direct contact. In the course of a B cell-mediated immune response, plasma cells are stimulated by type 2 helper CD4+ T cells to produce IgE antibodies specific to one allergen or allergen group. The difference between a normal B cell-mediated response and a type I hypersensitivity response is that in type I hypersensitivity, IgE antibodies predominate over IgM, IgG, or IgA immunoglobulins instead. The IgE antibodies bind to type I Fcε (FcεRI) receptors on the surface of mast cells and circulating basophils. After exposure to the same allergen, the allergen cross-links the bound IgE on target cells resulting in the degranulation and secretion of inflammatory mediators.

Pathogenically, the atopic process proceeds in three phases, early phase, late phase, and chronic allergic inflammation, and leads to the particular group of allergic diseases: allergic rhinitis (perennial and seasonal), allergic asthma, atopic dermatitis, food allergies, urticaria, angioedema, and anaphylaxis (see Chaps. 5–7). Some rare atopic reactions are described such as allergy to sperm, allergic vulvovaginitis, and balanoposthitis (see Chap. 9).

House dust mites used to be skin parasites in ancient humans in the Stone Age, and IgE production in 100% of people was a defense tool against them. Later, they became free-living and speciated in several habitats, including human homes [58, 59]. Currently, IgE remains in limited human populations (7–10%) as an evolutionary vestige.

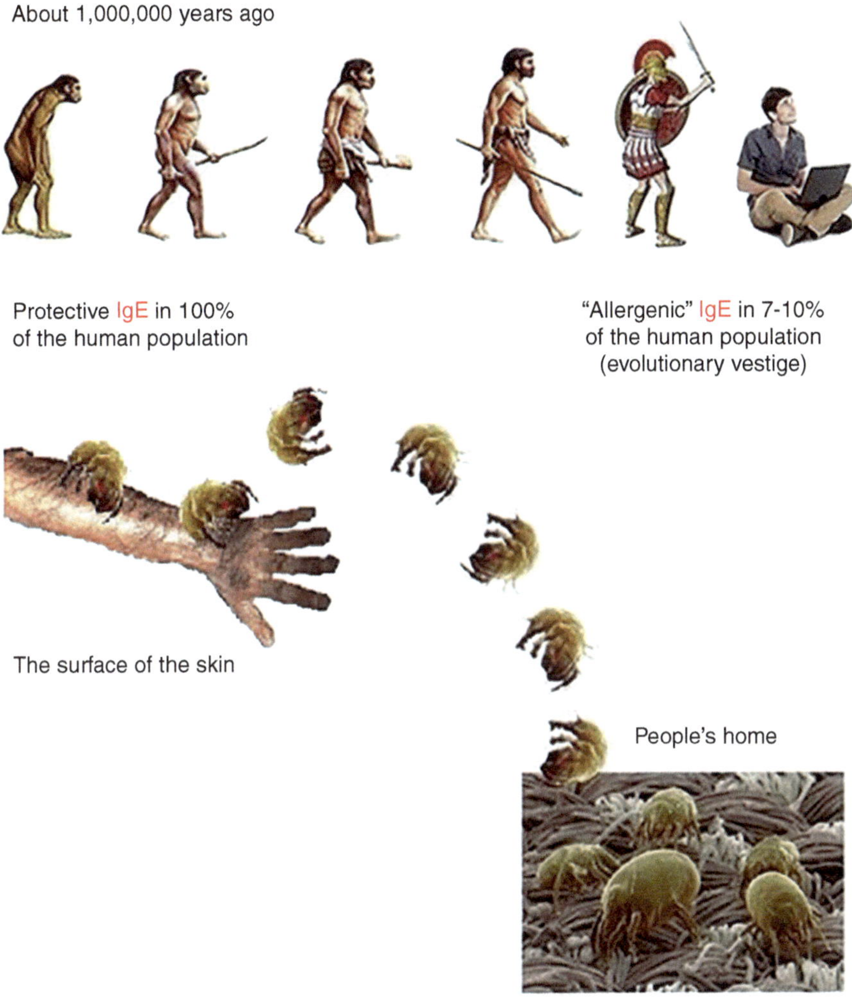

Fig. 1.2 Concept of atopy in the context of an evolutionary vestige. House dust mites used to be skin parasites in ancient humans in the Stone Age and IgE production in 100% of people was a defense tool against them. Currently, IgE remains in limited human populations as an evolutionary vestige

Eventually, it is clear atopy coexists with different allergic phenotypes and endotypes requiring distinct identification methods [66]. Apart from Th2-high (IgE-dependent) allergy phenotypes, some Th2-low, IgE-independent, and immune system-independent phenotypes of allergies exist.

1.5 House Dust Mites (HDM), "Masters of Allergenicity"

▶ **Definition** House dust mites are the source of the main allergens causing atopic sensitization and clinical symptoms worldwide.

Voorhorst et al. identified in 1967 *Dermatophagoides pteronyssinus* as the source of culprit allergens contained in household dust. The first allergen, *Der p 1*, was revealed in 1980 [67]. This allergen serves as the "maestro" in the maturation of the different HDM allergens of serine protease families (*Der p 3, Der p 6,* and *Der p 9*). High levels of IgE specific for *Der p 1* have been developed by more than 80% of patients sensitized to HDMs [68]. The role of HDM allergens is critical in the sensitization and manifestation of all atopic conditions worldwide when they promote IgE-dependent Th2 response and allergic inflammation in target organs. But systemic allergy symptoms from the ingestion of cross-reacting crustaceans and some plant food and the transformation of silent sensitization into the symptomatic disease are still incompletely explored. Therefore, mites are the masters of allergenicity [69] and "kings of allergens" or panallergens [1].

Proteolytically active HDM allergens play a critical role in initiating innate immunity and adaptive allergic response. Different mechanisms influence the proteolytic activity of HDM allergens, including cleavage of lung epithelium surfactant proteins (SP-A, SP-D), involvement of pathogen-associated molecular patterns (PAMPs) and damage-associated molecular patterns (DAMPs), upregulation of protease-activated receptors (PARs) expressed on airway epithelial cells, downregulation of Th1/Tregs differentiation, and inactivation of protease inhibitors such as α_1-antitrypsin [68]. The new mechanism linking atopy and *pseudo allergy* (the old term related to nonimmune allergic reactions) was recently revealed. It was found that *Der p 1* could activate human mas-related G-protein-coupled receptor X1 (MRGPRX1) that resulted in the production of pro-inflammatory IL-6, mast cell degranulation, and "neurogenic inflammation" [70, 71].

HDMs are related to the Phylum arthropods and are divided into three Genera: Dermatophagoides, Euroglyphus, and Blonia. The main allergenic HDM include *Dermatophagoides pteronyssinus*, *Dermatophagoides farinae*, and *Euroglyphus maynei* [69]. Mites are ancient organisms, former skin parasites and now free-living beings, which have unexpectedly become the main source of allergens for people and the problem for allergists [58, 59].

All HDM species reach adulthood within 4 weeks. They make up about one-fourth to one-third of a millimeter in size (250–350 μm in length), being at the threshold of visibility. Once mature, adult mites have a lifespan of 1.5–3 months, during which time HDM's females can lay between 40 and 80 eggs. With this fast reproductive turnover, mites can colonize new homes for a year [65, 69]. *Der p 1* and *Der f 1* were explored during typical domestic activity using an ion-charging device and a filter run in parallel and assessed inhaled by 1 ng/day [38]. The reproduction progresses more rapidly at higher temperatures and more constant humidity. According to the hygiene hypothesis, HDM allergen avoidance benefits the immune system, but excess apartment cleaning would promote HDM reproduction and it follows peoples sensitization to HDM in this apartment [2].

HDM use three key macromolecules serving as the food source:

- Keratin (shed scales from the human skin)
- Cellulose (textile fibers)
- Chitin (fungal hyphae and mite cuticles)

The other sources are fungi and yeast, bacteria and the spores of bacteria, and pollen.

Allergens from dust mites are associated with HDM's secretions (chitinase), feces (enzymes), and body (muscle tropomyosin and paramyosin). The allergenic digestive enzymes are small to reach nasal mucosa and deep down into the lung [65]. After contact with the epithelium, HDM allergens with proteolytic activity degrade epithelial junctions, get inside allergen-presenting cells, and promote Th2 response. Some components of HDMs are related to pathogen-associated molecular patterns (PAMPS): chitin, mite DNA, bacterial DNA, and endotoxin. These PAMPsS (e.g., endotoxin and *Der p 2*, ligands for TLR4) bind to pattern recognition receptors (PRRs) like TLR on the host epithelium [69]. Epithelium activation leads to a release of alarmins by epitheliocytes: IL-25, IL-33, and thymic stromal lymphopoietin (TSP) that upregulate ILC2, DCs, and Th2 cells (see Fig. 1.1) [18].

2.6% of the *D. pteronyssinus* proteins from 12,530 studied proteins have been identified as a possible unknown cause of an allergic response [72].

Allergenic products of various species incompletely cross-react, exhibiting both common and species-specific epitopes [73]. The recently updated list, available at www.allergen.org, shows 36 allergens for *D. farinae*, 30 allergens for *D. pteronyssinus*, and 5 allergens for *E. maynei*, with additions resulting from new techniques of transcriptome and proteome analysis [69]. Chitinases are an allergenic group of HDMs and have also been identified in silkworms, plant food, and plants (including the rubber tree, the latex source), causing cross-reactions [74]. Other HDM allergens like tropomyosin are present in crustaceans and fish. You can see the major allergens of *D. pteronyssinus* in Table 1.2.

Despite existing pharmacotherapy, those cases in which an HDM allergy plays a significant role may be treated explicitly with subcutaneous or sublingual allergen-specific immunotherapy (AIT). The preparation of HDM allergen extracts for AIT includes culturing, harvesting, inactivation, drying, purification, fractionation, characterization, and standardization, all of which have recently been reviewed by experts involved in these commercial processes [76]. The existing problem of severe

Table 1.2 Major allergens of *Dermatophagoides pteronissinus* [69, 75]

Allergen name	Biological properties	MW (kDa)	Role in allergy
Der p 1	Cysteine protease	25	Human allergy
Der p 2[a]	MD-2-like fatty acid-binding protein	14	Human allergy
Der p 5	Lipid/fatty acid-binding proteins	14	Human allergy
Der p 10[b]	Tropomyosin	33	Human allergy, cross-reactivity with crustaceans
Der p 11	Paramyosin	102	Human allergy, cross-reactivity with crustaceans
Der p 15	Chitinase	59	Human allergy, cross-reactivity with plant food
Der p 23	Peritrophin-like protein domain	8	Human allergy

[a] *MD-2* myeloid differentiation factor 2 (associated with TLR4)

[b] In some research, *Der p 10* is defined as a minor allergen

adverse reactions during AIT may be linked to the cosensitization to some different species of mites and the heterogeneous AIT's extracts [77]. Nowadays, used allergens for AIT are still natural extracts not meeting the current international standards regarding purity, biological activity, safety, sensitivity, and specificity, but this challenge has yet to be overcome [78, 79] (see Chap. 8).

Key Points

1. Allergens represent a small part of antigens and cause sensitization in the body leading to allergic inflammation and the manifestation of allergic diseases. The sensitization is based on an abnormal non-protective adaptive immune IgE response controlled by type 2 helper T cells.
2. Allergens may be major and minor and have a high or low level of allergenicity, depending on the allergen's structure and properties, biogenic environmental factors (adjuvants), and the body's immune system. The new division of allergens will be recruited when allergenic molecules, not allergen extracts, are used by allergists worldwide.
3. The main point at which allergenicity of allergens depends at the whole body level is interaction with the innate immune cells via binding to PRRs, inducing ILC2, and contributing to an adaptive Th2-dependent IgE response.
4. The suggested concept of atopy, a common form of allergy, is exciting and intriguing from an evolutionary viewpoint.

Take-Home Messages

1. Write a paragraph about antigenicity.
2. Write a paragraph about allergenicity.
3. Write an essay about B cell-mediated adaptive immune responses.
4. Write an essay about T cell-mediated adaptive immune responses.
5. Write an essay about the atopic allergic immune response.
6. List common environmental allergens.
7. List factors depending on allergen, which impact allergenicity.
8. List factors depending on biogenic cofactors, which impact allergenicity.
9. List factors depending on the immune system, which impact allergenicity.
10. Write an essay about atopy.
11. Describe how allergens interact with innate immunity.
12. List the major allergens of *Dermatophagoides pteronissinus.*

Quiz B

Reading a question, please choose only one right answer.

Question 1

Allergen allergenicity depends on:

1. Molecular weight and size of allergen.
2. Resistance to proteolysis and posttranslational glycosylation.

3. All points.
4. High stability.

Question 2
Mutations of the filaggrin gene are important for:

1. Blood-brain barrier.
2. Skin barrier.
3. The gut.
4. The endocrine system.

Question 3
Alarmins are produced by:

1. Epithelial cells.
2. Dendritic cells.
3. Macrophages.
4. Eosinophils.

Question 4
Sensitization is:

1. Reaction of innate immunity.
2. CD8+ T cell immune response.
3. Simple B cell response with IgM production.
4. Advanced B cell-mediated Th2-dependent response.

Question 5
Antigenicity has two features of antigen:

1. Immunogenicity and allergenicity.
2. Affinity and hypermutations.
3. Avidity and allotypy.
4. Immunogenicity and affinity.

Question 6
Allergenicity is the allergen's ability to induce:

1. CD8+ T cell immune response.
2. Sensitization and allergic inflammation.
3. Immune tolerance.
4. CD4+ T cell immune response.

Question 7
The tolerogenic immune response is:

1. The ability to promote the proliferation of plasma cells.
2. The ability to establish immune tolerance.

3. The capacity of upregulating clonal expansion of lymphocytes.
4. The capacity of causing sensitization.

Question 8
Environmental allergens include:

1. House dust mites and cockroach feces.
2. Birch pollen.
3. Insect venoms.
4. All points.

Question 9
The end-effect of sensitization is:

1. Establishing memory B cells to the allergen.
2. Producing IgM.
3. Immune tolerance.
4. Eliminating the allergen.

Question 10
Type 2 helper T cells secrete:

1. TNF-β, IL-1β, GM-CSF.
2. IL-4, IL-5, IL-13.
3. IFN-γ, TNF-β, IL-2.
4. TGF-β, IL-35, IL-27.

Question 11
The mast cell is the main cell participating in:

1. Early phase of allergic inflammation.
2. Immune inflammation based on type IV hypersensitivity.
3. Late phase of allergic inflammation.
4. Immune inflammation based on type III hypersensitivity.

Question 12
In allergic inflammation, histamine is released from:

1. Eosinophils.
2. Neutrophils.
3. Mast cells.
4. Lymphocytes.

Question 13

Atopy denotes:

1. Type IV hypersensitivity.
2. Type I hypersensitivity.
3. Type III hypersensitivity.
4. Type II hypersensitivity.

Question 14

"Masters of allergenicity" are the following allergens:

1. Birch pollen.
2. Timothy pollen.
3. Latex.
4. House dust mites.

Question 15

House dust mites' allergens promote:

1. Th2-dependent immune response.
2. Th1-dependent immune response.
3. CD4+ T cell immune response.
4. CD8+ T cell immune response.

Question 16

Major allergens can induce:

1. Strong IgE response.
2. Strong IgM response.
3. Weak IgE response.
4. No IgE response.

References

1. Klimov VV. Functional organization of the immune system. In: From basic to clinical immunology. Cham: Springer; 2019. https://doi.org/10.1007/978-3-030-0332301_1.
2. Zhang J, Tao A. Antigenicity, immunogenicity, allergenicity. In: Tao A, Raz E, editors. Allergy bioinformatics, Chapter 11. Cham: Springer; 2015. https://doi.org/10.1007/978-94-017-7444-4_11.
3. Traidl-Hoffmann C, Jakob T, Behrendt H. Determinants of allergenicity. J Allergy Clin Immunol. 2009;123:558–66. https://doi.org/10.1016/j.jaci.2008.12.003.
4. Caraballo L, Valenta R, Acevedo N, Zakzuk J. Are the terms major and minor allergens useful for precision allergology? Front Immunol. 2021;12:651500. https://doi.org/10.3389/fimmu.2021.651500.

5. Zouali M. Immunological tolerance: mechanisms. In: eLS. Paris: Wiley; 2007. p. 1–9. https://doi.org/10.1002/9780470015902.a0000950.pub2.
6. Wisniewski J, Agrawal R, Woodfolk JA. Mechanisms of tolerance induction in allergic disease: integrating current and emerging concepts. Clin Exp Allergy. 2013;43(2):164–76. https://doi.org/10.1111/cea.12016.
7. Scheurer S, Toda M, Vieths S. What makes an allergen? Clin Exp Allergy. 2015;45(7):1150–61. https://doi.org/10.1111/cea.12571.
8. Thomas WR. Allergen ligands in the initiation of allergic sensitization. Curr Allergy Asthma Rep. 2014;14(5):432–54. https://doi.org/10.1007/s11882-014-0432-x.
9. Lambrecht BN, Hammad H. Allergens and the airway epithelium response: gateway to allergic sensitization. J Allergy Clin Immunol. 2014;134(3):499–507. https://doi.org/10.1016/j.jaci.2014.06.036.
10. Zheng H, Zhang Y, Pan J, Liu N, Qin L, Liu M, Wang T. The role of type 2 innate lymphoid cells in allergic diseases. Front Immunol. 2021;12:586078. https://doi.org/10.3389/fimmu.2021.586078.
11. Wallrapp A, Riesenfeld SJ, Burkett PR, Abdulnour RE, Nyman J, Dionne D, et al. The neuropeptide NMU amplifies ILC2-driven allergic lung inflammation. Nature. 2017;549:351–6. https://doi.org/10.1038/nature24029.
12. Pasha MA, Patel G, Hopp R, Yang Q. Role of innate lymphoid cells in allergic diseases. Allergy Asthma Proc. 2019;40:138–45. https://doi.org/10.2500/aap.2019.40.4217.
13. Wallrapp A, Burkett PR, Riesenfeld SJ, Kim SJ, Christian E, Abdulnour RE, et al. Calcitonin gene-related peptide negatively regulates alarmin-driven type 2 innate lymphoid cell responses. Immunity. 2019;51:709–23.e6. https://doi.org/10.1016/j.immuni.2019.09.005.
14. Nagashima H, Mahlakoiv T, Shih HY, Davis FP, Meylan F, Huang Y, et al. Neuropeptide CGRP limits group 2 innate lymphoid cell responses and constrains type 2 inflammation. Immunity. 2019;51:682–95.e6. https://doi.org/10.1016/j.immuni.2019.06.009.
15. Yamauchi K, Ogasawara M. The role of histamine in the pathophysiology of asthma and the clinical efficacy of antihistamines in asthma therapy. Int J Mol Sci. 2019;20:1733. https://doi.org/10.3390/ijms20071733.
16. Drazdauskaitė G, Layhadi JA, Shamji MH. Mechanisms of allergen immunotherapy in allergic rhinitis. Curr Allergy Asthma Rep. 2021;21:2. https://doi.org/10.1007/s11882-020-00977-7.
17. Schoos A-MM, Bullens D, Chawes BL, De Vlieger L, DunnGalvin A, Epstein MM, et al. Immunological outcomes of allergen-specific immunotherapy in food allergy. Front Immunol. 2020;11:568598. https://doi.org/10.3389/fimmu.2020.568598.
18. Jacquet A. Characterization of innate immune responses to house dust mite allergens: pitfalls and limitations. Front Allergy. 2021;2:662378. https://doi.org/10.3389/falgy.2021.662378.
19. Galli SJ, Tsai M, Piliponsky AM. The development of allergic inflammation. Nature. 2008;454(7203):445–54. https://doi.org/10.1038/nature07204.
20. Abbas M, Moussa M, Akel H. Type I hypersensitivity reaction. In: StatPearls. Treasure Island: StatPearls Publishing; 2021. Access at: https://www.ncbi.nlm.nih.gov/books/NBK560561/
21. Krystel-Whittemore M, Dileepan KN, Wood JG. Mast cell: a multi-functional master cell. Front Immunol. 2016;6:620. https://doi.org/10.3389/fimmu.2015.00620.
22. Varricchi G, Rossi FW, Galdiero MR, Granata F, Criscuolo G, Spadaro G, et al. Physiological roles of mast cells: Collegium Internationale Allergologicum Update 2019. Int Arch Allergy Immunol. 2019;179:247–61. https://doi.org/10.1159/000500088.
23. Komi DEA, Wohrl S, Bielory L. Mast cell biology at molecular level: a comprehensive review. Clin Rev Allergy Immunol. 2020;58(3):342–65. https://doi.org/10.1007/s12016-019-08769-2.
24. da Silva EZM, Jamur MC, Oliver C. Mast cell function: a new vision of an old cell. J Histochem Cytochem. 2014;62(10):698–738. https://doi.org/10.1369/0022155414545334.
25. Nadif R, Zerimech F, Bouzigon E, Matran R. The role of eosinophils and basophils in allergic diseases considering genetic findings. Curr Opin Allergy Clin Immunol. 2013;13(5):507–13. https://doi.org/10.1097/ACI.0b013e328364e9c0.
26. Bochner BS. The eosinophil: for better or worse, in sickness and in health. Ann Allergy Asthma Immunol. 2018;121(2):150–5. https://doi.org/10.1016/j.anai.2018.02.031.

27. Rodriguez-Coira J, Villaseñor A, Izquierdo E, Huang M, Barker-Tejeda TC, Radzikowska U, Sokolowska M, Barber D. The importance of metabolism for immune homeostasis in allergic diseases. Front Immunol. 2021;12:692004. https://doi.org/10.3389/fimmu.2021.692004.
28. Stewart FA, Robinson C. Indoor and outdoor allergens and pollutants. In: O'Hehir RE, Holgate ST, Sheikh A, editors. Middleton's allergy essentials, Chapter 4. Amsterdam: Elsevier; 2017. p. 73-116. https://doi.org/10.1016/B978-0-323-37579-5.00004-0.
29. Costa J, Villa C, Verhoeckx K, Circovic-Velickovic T, Schrama D, Roncada P, Rodriguez PM. Are physicochemical properties shaping the allergenic potency of animal allergens? Clin Rev Allergy Immunol. 2022;62(1):1–36. https://doi.org/10.1007/s12016-020-08826-1.
30. Kuehn A, Swoboda I, Arumugam K, Hilger C, Hentges F. Fish allergens at a glance: variable allergenicity of parvalbumins, the major fish allergens. Front Immunol. 2014;5:179. https://doi.org/10.3389/fimmu.2014.00179.
31. Waserman S, Beegin P, Watson W. IgE-mediated food allergy. Allergy Asthma Clin Immunol. 2018;14(2):71–81. https://doi.org/10.1186/s13223-018-0284-3.
32. Lei D, Grammer LC. An overview of allergens. Allergy Asthma Proc. 2019;40(6):362–5. https://doi.org/10.2500/aap.2019.40.4247.
33. Huby RDJ, Dearman RJ, Kimber I. Why are some proteins allergens? Toxicol Sci. 2000;55:235–46. https://doi.org/10.1093/toxsci/55.2.235.
34. Fu L, Cherayil BJ, Shi H, Wang Y, Zhu Y. Allergenicity evaluation of food proteins. In: Food allergy. Singapore: Springer; 2019. p. 93–122. https://doi.org/10.1007/978-981-13-6928-5_5.
35. Hayes M. Allergenicity of food proteins. In: Hayes M, editor. Novel proteins for food, pharmaceuticals and agriculture: sources, applications and advances, Chapter 14. Chichester: Wiley; 2018. https://doi.org/10.1002/9781119385332.ch14.
36. Aalberse RC. Structural biology of allergens. J Allergy Clin Immunol. 2000;106(2):228–38. https://doi.org/10.1067/mai.2000.108434.
37. Pali-Schöll I, Jensen-Jarolim E. The concept of allergen-associated molecular patterns (AAMP). Curr Opin Immunol. 2016;42:113–8. https://doi.org/10.1016/j.coi.2016.08.004.
38. Custis NJ, Woodfolk JA, Vaughan JW, Platts-Mills TAE. Quantitative measurement of airborne allergens from dust mites, dogs, and cats using an ion-charging device. Clin Exp Allergy. 2003;33(7):986–91. https://doi.org/10.1046/j.1365-2222.2003.01706.x.
39. Comstock SS, Maleki SJ, Teuber SS. Boiling and frying peanuts decreases soluble peanut (*Arachis Hypogaea*) allergens *Ara h 1* and *Ara h 2* but does not generate hypoallergenic peanuts. PLoS One. 2016;11(6):e0157849. https://doi.org/10.1371/journal.pone.0157849.
40. Heuberger DM, Schepbach RA. Protease-activated receptors (PARs): mechanisms of action and potential therapeutic modulators in PAR-driven inflammatory diseases. Thromb J. 2019;17(4):1–24. https://doi.org/10.1186/s12959-019-0194-8.
41. Emanuelsson C, Spangfort MD. Allergens as eukaryotic proteins lacking bacterial homologues. Mol Immunol. 2007;44(12):3256–60. https://doi.org/10.1016/j.molimm.2007.01.019.
42. Reese TA, Liang HE, Tager ANM, Luster AD, Van Rooijen N, Voehringer D, Locksley RM. Chitin induces accumulation in tissue of innate immune cells associated with allergy. Nature. 2007;447:92–6. https://doi.org/10.1038/nature05746.
43. Valenta R, Hochwallner H, Linhart B, Pahr S. Food allergies: the basics. Gastroenterology. 2015;148(6):1120–31. https://doi.org/10.1053/j.gastro.2015.02.006.
44. Banks TA, Gada SM. Filaggrin mutations as an archetype for understanding the pathophysiology of atopic dermatitis. J Am Acad Dermatol. 2014;71(3):592–3. https://doi.org/10.1016/j.jaad.2014.04.075.
45. Pintye J, Baeten JM. Benefits of male circumcision for MSM: evidence for action. Lancet Glob Health. 2019;7:e388–9. https://doi.org/10.1016/S2214-109X(19)30038-5.
46. Shade KTC, Conroy ME, Washburn N, Kitaoka M, Huynh DJ, Laprise E, et al. Sialylation of immunoglobulin E is a determinant of allergic pathogenicity. Nature. 2020;582:265–70. https://doi.org/10.1038/s41586-020-2311-z.
47. Jeong KY, Hong C-S, Lee J-S, Park J-W. Optimization of allergen standardization. Yonsei Med J. 2011;52(3):393–400. https://doi.org/10.3349/ymj.2011.52.3.393.

48. Zimmer J, Bridgewater J, Ferreira F, van Ree R, Rabin RL, Vieths S. The history, present and future of allergen standardization in the United States and Europe. Front Immunol. 2021;12:725831. https://doi.org/10.3389/fimmu.2021.725831.
49. Brusca I, Barrale M, Onida R, La Chiusa SM, Gjomarkaj M, Uasuf CG. The extract, the molecular allergen or both for the in vitro diagnosis of peach and peanut sensitization? Clin Chim Acta. 2019;493:25–30. https://doi.org/10.1016/j.cca.2019.01.016.
50. Kadam K, Sawant S, Jayaraman VK, Kulkarni-Kale U. Databases and algorithms in allergen informatics. In: Abdurakhmonov IY, editor. Bioinformatics. London: IntechOpen; 2016. https://doi.org/10.5772/63083.
51. Breiteneder H, Diamant Z, Eiwegger T, Fokkens WJ, Traidl-Hoffmann C, Nadeau K, et al. Future research trends in understanding the mechanisms underlying allergic diseases for improved patient care. Allergy. 2019;74:2293–311. https://doi.org/10.1111/all.13851.
52. Coca AF, Cooke RA. On the classification of the phenomenon of hypersensitiveness. J Immunol. 1923;8:163–82.
53. Bellanti JA, Settipane RA. The atopic disorders and atopy... "strange diseases" now better defined! Allergy Asthma Proc. 2017;38(4):241–2. https://doi.org/10.2500/aap.2017.38.4074.
54. Ishizaka K, Ishizaka T, Hornbrook MM. Physico-chemical properties of human reaginic antibody. IV. Presence of a unique immunoglobulin as a carrier of reaginic activity. J Immunol. 1966;97(1):75–85.
55. Gell PGH, Coombs RRA. Clinical aspects of immunology. London: Blackwell; 1963.
56. Gross M. Why did evolution give us allergies? Curr Biol. 2015;25(2):53–5. https://doi.org/10.1016/j.cub.2015.01.002.
57. Tyagi N, Farnell EJ, Fitzsimmons CM, et al. Comparisons of allergenic and metazoan parasite proteins: allergy the price of immunity. PLoS Comput Biol. 2015;11:e1004546. https://doi.org/10.1371/journal.pcbi.1004546.
58. Klimov PB, O'Connor B. Is permanent parasitism reversible? - critical evidence from early evolution of house dust mites. Syst Biol. 2013;62(3):411–23. https://doi.org/10.1093/sysbio/syt008.
59. Mondal M, Klimov P, Flynt AS. Rewired RNAi-mediated genome surveillance in house dust mites. PLoS Genet. 2018;14(1):e1007183. https://doi.org/10.1371/journal.pgen.1007183.
60. Tamari M, Tanaka S, Hirota T. Genome-wide association studies of allergic diseases. Allergol Int. 2013;62(1):21–8. https://doi.org/10.2332/allergolint.13-RAI-0539.
61. Lyons JJ, Milner JD. Primary atopic disorders. J Exp Med. 2018;215(4):1009–22. https://doi.org/10.1084/jem.20172306.
62. Castagnoli R, Lougaris V, Giardino G, Volpi S, Leonardi L, La Torre F, et al. Inborn errors of immunity with atopic phenotypes: a practical guide for allergists. World Allergy Organ J. 2021;14(2):100513. https://doi.org/10.1016/j.waojou.2021.100513.
63. Tezza G, Mazzei F, Boner A. Epigenetics of allergy. Early Hum Dev. 2013;89(Suppl 1):S20–1. https://doi.org/10.1016/S0378-3782(13)70007-0.
64. Thomas WR. Hierarchy and molecular properties of house dust mite allergens. Allergol Int. 2015;64:304–11. https://doi.org/10.1016/j.alit.2015.05.004.
65. Calderón MA, Linnberg A, Kleine-Tebble J, De Bay F, de Rojas DHF, Virchow JC. Respiratory allergy caused by house dust mites: what do we really know? J Allergy Clin Immunol. 2015;136(1):38–48. https://doi.org/10.1016/j.jaci.2014.10.012.
66. Testera-Montes A, Salas M, Palomares F, Ariza A, Torres MJ, Rondón C, Eguiluz-Gracia I. Local respiratory allergy: from rhinitis phenotype to disease spectrum. Front Immunol. 2021;12:691964. https://doi.org/10.3389/fimmu.2021.691964.
67. Aggarwal P, Senthikumaran S. Dust mite allergy. In: StatPearls. Treasure Island: StatPearls Publishing; 2021. Access at: https://www.ncbi.nlm.nih.gov/books/NBK560718/
68. d'Alessandro M, Bergantini L, Perrone A, Cameli P, Beltrami V, Alderighi L, et al. House dust mite allergy and the Der p1 conundrum: a literature review and case series. Allergie. 2021;1:108–14. https://doi.org/10.3390/allergies1020008.
69. Miller JD. The role of dust mites in allergy. Clin Rev Allergy Immunol. 2019;57(3):312–29. https://doi.org/10.1007/s12016-018-8693-0.

70. Reddy VB, Lerner EA. Activation of mas-related G-protein–coupled receptors by the house dust mite cysteine protease Der p1 provides a new mechanism linking allergy and inflammation. J Biol Chem. 2017;292(42):P17399–406. https://doi.org/10.1074/jbc.M117.787887.
71. Carlton SM. Nociceptive primary afferents: they have a mind of their own. J Physiol. 2014;592(16):3403–11. https://doi.org/10.1113/jphysiol.2013.269654.
72. Waldron R, McGowan J, Gordon N, McCarthy C, Mitchell EB, Fitzpatrick DA. Proteome and allergenome of the European house dust mite *Dermatophagoides pteronyssinus*. PLoS One. 2019;14(5):e0216171. https://doi.org/10.1371/journal.pone.0216171.
73. Sarwar M. House dust mites: ecology, biology, prevalence, epidemiology and elimination. In: Pacheco GAB, Kamboh AA, editors. Parasitology and microbiology research. London: IntechOpen; 2020. https://doi.org/10.5772/intechopen.91891.
74. Leoni C, Volpicella M, Dileo MCD, Gattulli BAR, Ceci LR. Chitinases as food allergens. Molecules. 2019;24(11):2087. https://doi.org/10.3390/molecules24112087.
75. Stranzl T, Ipsen H, Christensen LH, Eiwegger T, Johansen N, Lund K, Andersen PS. Limited impact of Der p 23 IgE on treatment outcomes in tablet allergy immunotherapy phase III study. Allergy. 2020;76(4):1235–8. https://doi.org/10.1111/all.14200.
76. Carnés J, Iraola V, Cho SH, Esch RE. Mite allergen extracts and clinical practice. Ann Allergy Asthma Immunol. 2017;118:249–56. https://doi.org/10.1016/j.anai.2016.08.018.
77. Arroabarren E, Echechipía S, Galbete A, Lizaso MT, Olaguibel JM, Tabar AI. Association between component-resolved diagnosis of house dust mite allergy and efficacy and safety of specific immunotherapy. J Investig Allergol Clin Immunol. 2019;29(2):164–7. https://doi.org/10.18176/jiaci.0359.
78. Pfaar O, Lou H, Zhang Y, Klimek L, Zhang L. Recent developments and highlights in allergen immunotherapy. Allergy. 2018;73:2274–89. https://doi.org/10.1111/all/13652.
79. Valenta R, Karaulov A, Niederberger V, Zhernov Y, Elisyutina O, Campana R, et al. Allergen extracts for *in vivo* diagnosis and treatment of allergy: is there a future? J Allergy Clin Immunol Pract. 2018;6(6):1845–55.e2. https://doi.org/10.1016/j.jaip.2018.08.032.

Immune Tolerance at a Glance

2

Contents

Didactics
Knowledge. Upon successful completion of this chapter, students should be able to:

1. Draw the immune tolerance.
2. Distinguish between the adaptive response and tolerogenic response.
3. Name and describe two levels of immune tolerance.
4. List mechanisms of central tolerance.
5. List mechanisms of peripheral tolerance.
6. Describe peripheral regulatory T (pTregs) cells.
7. Characterize molecules to which the immune system is tolerant.
8. Characterize artificial and pathologic tolerance.
9. Briefly describe cells that maintain immune tolerance in the periphery.
10. List immunosuppressive cytokines.
11. Describe the role of coinhibitory molecules CTLA-4 and PD-1.

Supplementary Information The online version contains supplementary material available at [https://doi.org/10.1007/978-3-031-04309-3_2].

V. V. Klimov, *Textbook of Allergen Tolerance*,
https://doi.org/10.1007/978-3-031-04309-3_2

Acquired Skills. Upon successful completion of this chapter, students should demonstrate the following skills, including:

1. Interpret the knowledge related to immune tolerance.
2. Critically evaluate the scientific literature about immune tolerance.
3. Discuss the scientific articles from the current research literature to criticize experimental data and formulate new hypotheses on tolerance.
4. Have a clear perception of the presented immune tolerance definitions expressed orally and in written form.
5. Formulate the presented immunology terms.
6. Correctly answer the quiz questions.

Attitude and Professional Behaviors. Students should be able to:

1. Have the readiness to be hard-working.
2. Behave professionally at all times.
3. Recognize the importance of studying and demonstrate a commitment.

2.1 Introduction

In the narrow sense, immune tolerance can be considered a nonpathogenic immune response to a self-antigen, which has appeared through an active process. If immune tolerance is taken into account in the wider sense, it is the unresponsiveness to all undesirable antigens, including allergens. The specific antigen in tolerance may be called the *tolerogen*. An allergist dreams about allergens converting into tolerogens. The development of tolerance engages regulatory networks that recruit multiple mechanisms and secreted mediators such as IL-10, IL-35, TGF-β, surface molecules, and regulatory cell types. Immune tolerance may be *natural* or *artificial* achieved for medical purposes (e.g., transplantation).

Pathologic tolerance occurs under conditions that pathologically suppress the immune responses to antigens (e.g., in tumor growth and chronic infection). Chronic inflammation is the antipode of natural tolerance [1] or a sample of pathologic tolerance. Another sample of pathologic tolerance is cancer that is in parallel but significantly different from an allergy [2]. *Allergen tolerance*, a form of immune tolerance, may appear upon natural exposure to environmental allergens due to tolerogenic response, for example, when allergens are at a high dose [3]. However, allergen tolerance is a natural condition for most atopic individuals who have silent sensitization and do not have clinical manifestations [4].

2.2 Tolerance at a Glance

▶ **Definition** Immune tolerance is the unresponsiveness of the immune system to an antigen ("self" and "non-self"). Allergen tolerance, a form of immune tolerance, is the unresponsiveness of the immune system to an allergen ("non-self").

In early experiments, artificial immune tolerance was achieved by the 1960 Nobel Laureate, Sir P.B. Medawar, and other researchers by several methods:

- Previous contact with a particular antigen in fetal life or in the newborn period when the immune system is not yet mature
- Prior contact with the antigen in extremely high or low doses
- Exposure to radiation, the introduction of chemotherapy agents, or other substances damaging the immune system

Later, the other 1960 Nobel Laureate, Sir F. Macfarlane Burnet [5, 6], demonstrated the model of "clonal deletion" as a method by which immune tolerance might be achieved.

Tolerance is commonly accepted as an active process at the central and peripheral levels and with engagements of both tolerogenic T cells and B cells. The tolerance state is not absolute and rarely complete. T cell tolerance may be more often low-dose dependent and long-term, and B cell tolerance is more often high-dose dependent and short-term. The continuous persistence of a tolerogen and its accessibility to the immune system is undoubtedly required to maintain tolerance, which may be subsequently canceled by newly emerging T cells and B cells.

Under natural conditions, the immune system is tolerant to [7]:

1. Self-antigens (or autoantigens of the body)
2. Antigens of own symbiotic and opportunistic microbes in the steady-state
3. Food proteins
4. Allergens of the environment
5. Antigens of spermatozoa (inside women) and the father's antigens of the fetus (in pregnant women)

Many genes and proteins of interest are conserved between humans and other mammals. So, there is a bridge between clinical studies and mechanisms defined in experimental animals to help our understanding of self-tolerance mechanisms and functional defects leading to autoimmune disease [8].

An intriguing subject is tolerance in specific anatomic sites, e.g., the conjunctive and unified airway [3]. More than 30 years ago, non-atopic recipients of bone marrow transplants developed both total and specific IgE antibodies comparable to the atopic donor due to repopulation in the recipient with IgE-specific T cells. After asthmatic lung transplantation to non-asthmatic recipients, they developed asthma, while the asthmatic recipients with healthy lungs no longer had asthma [9]. This subject is open to debate, especially concerning the phenomenon of entopy [10] and allergen-specific immunotherapy (AIT).

There are several physiological processes for the maintenance of natural tolerance [11, 12]:

1. Central mechanisms (T cell and B cell clonal deletion)
2. Peripheral mechanisms [13]
   - Activation-induced apoptosis
   - Clonal anergy
   - Clonal ignorance
   - Peripheral system of immune tolerance maintenance, which includes functioning tolerogenic dendritic cells (tDC) [14–16], peripheral regulatory T (pTreg) cells [17–20], regulatory B (Breg) cells [21], and pro-tolerogenic (immunosuppressive) cytokines, neurotransmitters, neuropeptides, and coinhibitory molecules, and other cells [7, 11, 22–24]
   - Tolerogenic microbiota [25–28]

2.3 Antigen Tolerance Due to Primary Organs in the Fetal Life

▶ **Definition** Central tolerance is the first line of unresponsiveness to a self-antigen when emerged self-reactive T and B cells are being eliminated.

Central tolerance of T cells occurs during thymic development, with the bulk of self-reactive T cells eliminated in the course of negative selection in the thymus termed "*clonal deletion*" (see Fig. 2.1 and the description) [29, 30]. In particular, among different factors, the *gene AIRE* (on 21q22.3) upregulates negative selection via the encoded transcription factor AIRE to prevent autoimmunity in humans [31]. However, the thymic selection is not a perfect process explained by the findings that many "tissue" self-antigens are occasionally expressed in the thymus within thymic medullary epithelial cells and a part of self-reactive T cells may frequently be released into the periphery. Most survived self-reactive T cells are low-affinity. In addition, it is unlikely that all peripheral self-antigens are expressed within the thymus, so high-affinity self-reactive T cells can also enter the bloodstream. The low-affinity and high-affinity cells are potentially dangerous for the body as they can be engaged in an autoimmune response.

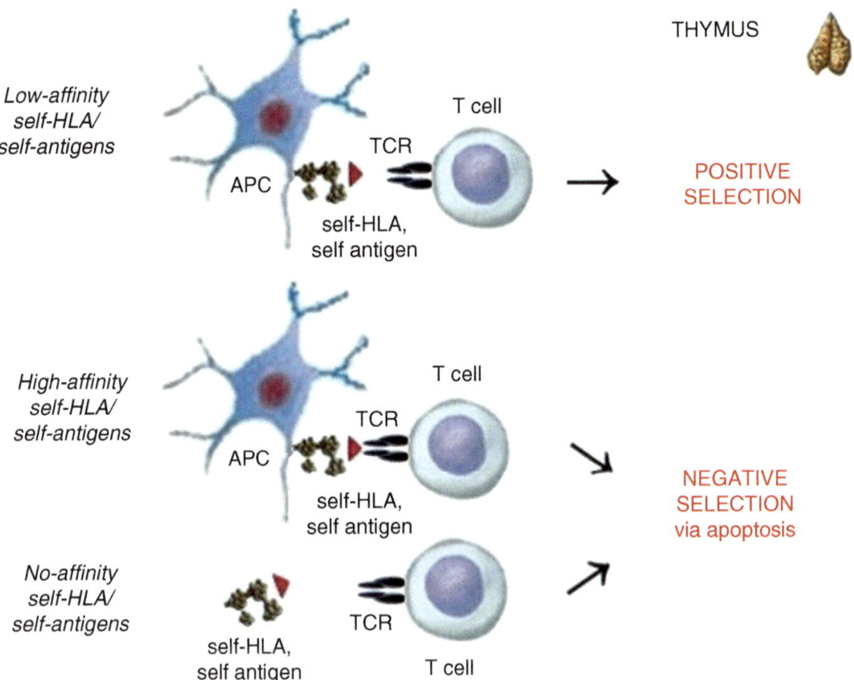

Fig. 2.1 T cell clonal deletion in the thymus. There are two types of thymic selection: positive selection, when TCRs have a low affinity for self-HLA molecules and self-antigens, and negative selection (or *clonal deletion*), which induces apoptosis in thymocytes, which bind self-HLA molecules and self-antigens too well or do not bind them at all. APC antigen-presenting cell, TCR T cell antigen-recognizing receptor, HLA human histocompatibility system

Central B cell tolerance is regulated by clonal deletion of immature B cells in the bone marrow, engaging apoptosis and *receptor editing* (see Fig. 2.2 and description) [32]. However, survived self-reactive low-affinity B cells enter the bloodstream. Some self-reactive B cells in the bone marrow get further chances to express alternative BCRs through a gene rearrangement process known as receptor editing rather than undergo apoptosis [33]. The most recent studies have employed the approach of cloning and expressing antibody genes obtained from single human B cells at different stages of their differentiation [32].

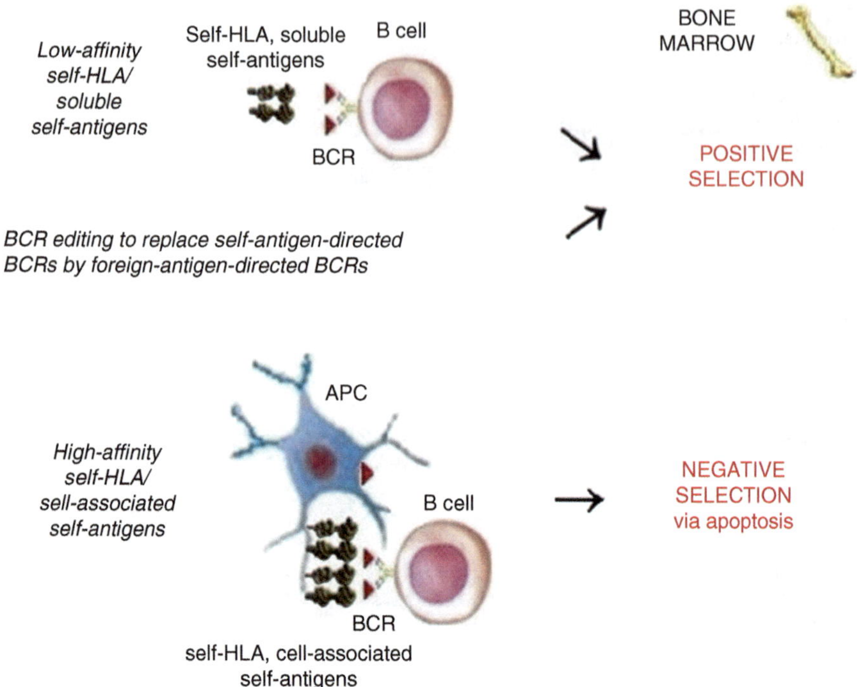

Fig. 2.2 B cell clonal deletion in the bone marrow. There are two types of B cell selection: positive selection, when BCRs have a low affinity for self-HLA molecules and soluble self-antigens or are edited in V gene region to replace self-antigen directed BCRs by non-self-antigen directed BCRs, and negative selection, which induces apoptosis in B cells (*clonal deletion*), which bind self-HLA molecules and cell-associated self-antigens too tightly. APC antigen-presenting cell, BCR B cell antigen-recognizing receptor, HLA human histocompatibility system

2.4 Peripheral Tolerance

▶ **Definition** Peripheral tolerance is the second line of unresponsiveness to a self-antigen when initially escaped self-reactive T and B cells are being eliminated.

Peripheral tolerance expands tolerance initiated centrally in the thymus. For those self-reactive T cells and B cells that escape clonal deletion in the thymus and bone marrow, additional fail-safe mechanisms are operating in the periphery with the deletion option still available. They have been mentioned above.

Activation-induced apoptosis is based on the interaction Fas receptor with FasL in two self-reactive T cells previously activated via their TCRs (see Fig. 2.3 and the description) that lead to promoting the CD95 pathway of apoptosis [34, 35]. The costimulation through a costimulatory molecule like CD28 cancels the process of apoptosis; therefore, this action must be absent. Activation-induced apoptosis is essential for maintaining natural tolerance and preventing autoimmune disorders in target organs.

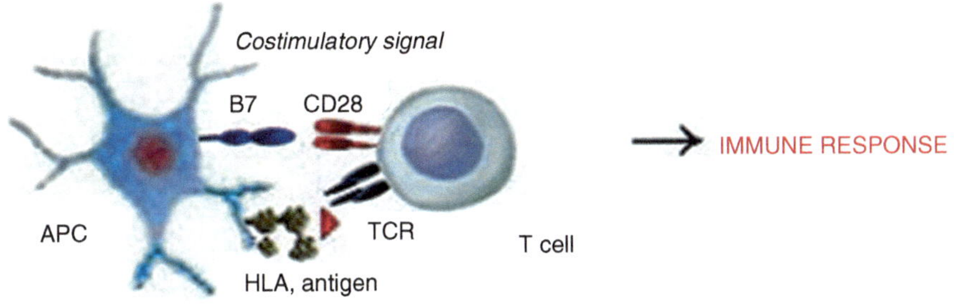

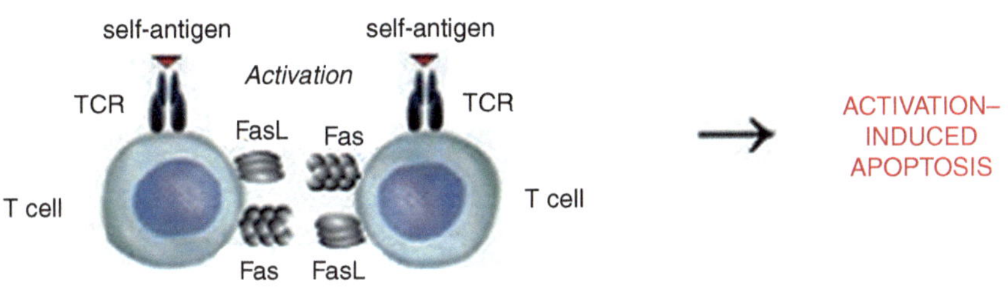

Fig. 2.3 Activation-induced apoptosis. *Activation-induced apoptosis* is the apoptosis in self-reactive T cells previously activated through TCR. TCR ligation upregulates CD95 expression and induces the expression of CD95L (CD178). Apoptosis is mediated by activating the Fas (CD95) pathway, started upon the ligation of cell surface CD95 by CD95L (FasL), and can occur by the interaction of CD95 and CD95L on the second self-reactive T cell. However, costimulation of T cells by the direct ligation of CD28 inhibits activation-induced apoptosis in these cells. So, for activation-induced apoptosis in previously activated self-reactive T cells, maintenance of natural tolerance, and prevention of autoimmune disorders in target organs, the absence of a costimulatory signal is necessary. APC antigen-presenting cell, TCR T cell antigen-recognizing receptor, CD28, B7 costimulatory molecules, Fas, FasL molecules taking part in apoptosis, HLA human histocompatibility system

Clonal anergy [36] (see Figs. 2.4 and 2.5) is a silent state of self-reactive T cells and B cells in the periphery. Some self-reactive T cells with a lower activation profile and B cells at the immature stages whose BCRs were directed to soluble self-antigens at a low concentration can escape from the negative selection in the thymus and bone marrow. These cells become anergic in the periphery.

Typically, T cells participating in immune responses must receive three signals through:

1. TCR
2. Costimulatory molecules, CD28 and ICOS [37–39]
3. Pro-immunogenic cytokines in a set depending on a differentiation route of helper T cells

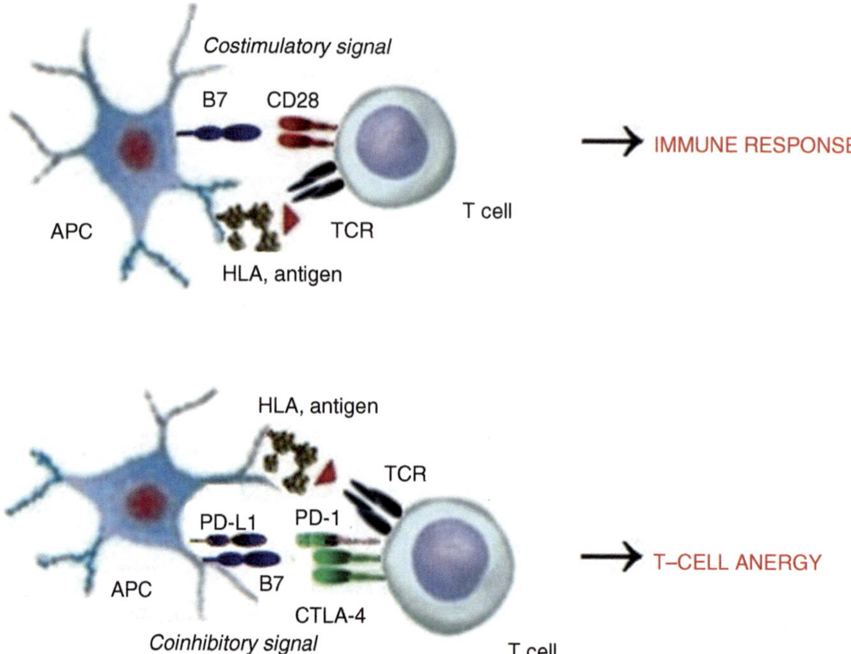

Fig. 2.4 T cell anergy in the periphery. After negative thymic selection, part of the survived self-reactive low-affinity T cells occurs in the periphery. Another part, the high-affinity self-reactive T cells whose TCRs are directed to self-antigens not expressed within the thymus, also occur in the periphery. Peripheral self-reactive T cells become *anergic* due to losing the valuable TCR signaling and getting coinhibitory signals from the expressed coinhibitory molecules like PD-1 and CTLA-4. APC antigen-presenting cell, TCR T cell antigen-recognizing receptor, CD28, B7 costimulatory molecules, CTLA-4, PD-1, PD-L1 coinhibitory molecules, HLA human histocompatibility system

When becoming anergic, T cells lose the valuable TCR signaling and get coinhibitory signals from the expressed coinhibitory molecules instead. These molecules for T cells are CTLA-4, PD-1, BTLA, LAG-3, etc. [24, 40–43].

B cells taking part in advanced immune response must also receive three signals through:

1. BCR
2. Costimulatory molecules, CD40 plus CD30, and OX40L binding ligands on the helper T cells [37]
3. Pro-immunogenic cytokines

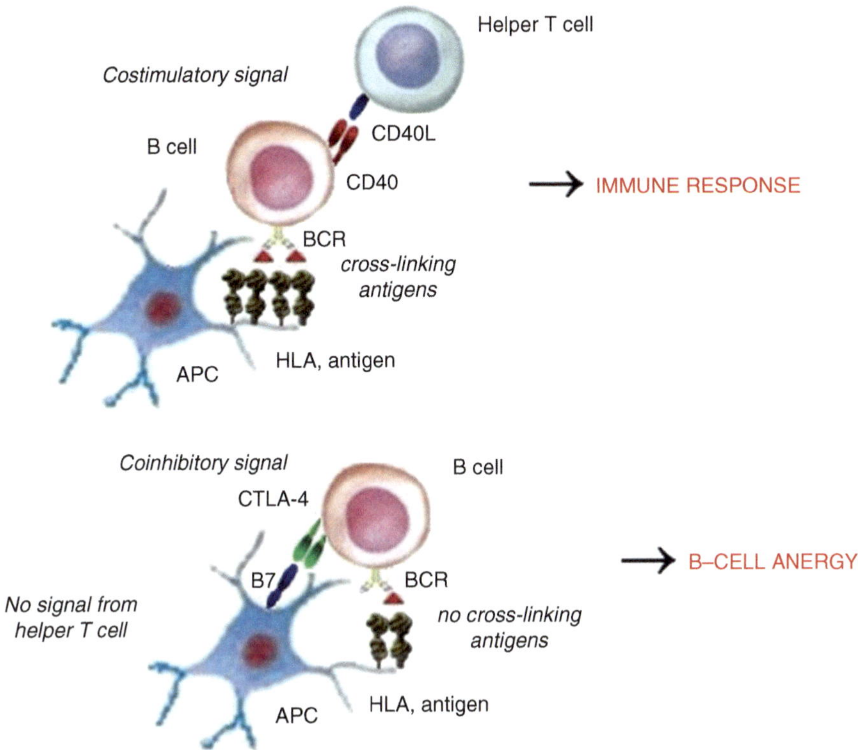

Fig. 2.5 B cell anergy in the periphery. The antigen-recognizing receptors of B cells at the immature stages are directed to soluble self-antigens at a low concentration. These B cells escaped from the negative selection in the bone marrow and appeared in the periphery. When self-reactive B cells become *anergic*, they lose the BCR signaling, get coinhibitory signals from the coinhibitory molecules, and do not receive aid from helper T cells. APC antigen-presenting cell, BCR B cell antigen-recognizing receptor, CD40, CD40L costimulatory molecules, CTLA-4 coinhibitory molecules, HLA human histocompatibility system

If B cells become anergic, they lose the BCR signaling (see Fig. 2.5), and T helpers aid them. Also, they receive coinhibitory signals from the coinhibitory molecules, which are the same as for T cells (CTLA-4, PD-1, BTLA, and LAG-3) plus CD22 and CD72 [44, 45]. In addition, in all cases of anergic processes, pro-tolerogenic (immunosuppressive) cytokines provide cells with negative signals.

Later, passive anergic T cells can convert into FoxP3^{-}Tr1 by antigen stimulus at systemic doses. The conversion into pro-tolerogenic Tr1 cells correlated with the transient intracellular CTLA-4 expression [46].

Regulatory T (Tregs) cells, tolerogenic dendritic (tDCs) cells, and molecules including immunosuppressive cytokines such as IL-10, IL-27, IL-35, and TGF-β, and pro-tolerogenic neurotransmitters by which those mechanisms are operated will be described in Chaps. 3 and 4.

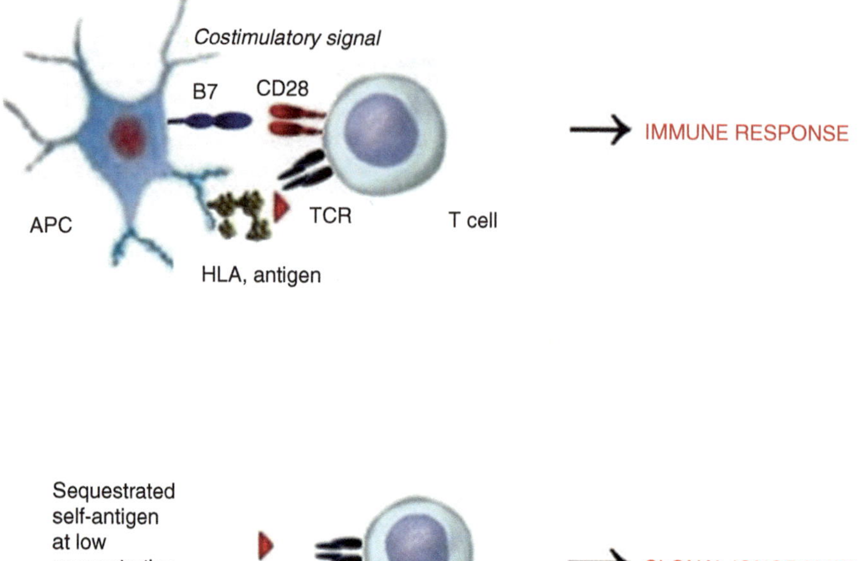

Fig. 2.6 Clonal ignorance in the periphery. *Clonal ignorance* is the unresponsiveness of peripheral T cells to a specific group of self-antigens at a low concentration. These self-antigens are termed "sequestrated" self-antigens, "cryptic determinants" or "hidden self" autoantigens. They originate due to the blood-brain barrier and other physiological barriers. If "sequestrated" self-antigens or other neo-self-antigens enter the bloodstream at a sufficient concentration, they result in immune tolerance breakdown. APC antigen-presenting cell, TCR T cell antigen-recognizing receptor, CD28, B7 costimulatory molecules, HLA human histocompatibility system

Clonal ignorance (see Fig. 2.6) describes the phenomenon when self-reactive T cells ignore self-antigens [47]. These self-antigens are present in the blood in minimal quantities or separated by a physiological barrier (e.g., the blood-brain barrier). The term *immune-privileged organs* [48, 49] containing so-called "sequestrated self-antigens," "cryptic determinants," or "hidden self" autoantigens designate some parts of the brain, the anterior chamber of the eye, the testes, etc., which are isolated from the bloodstream from birth; therefore, these antigens have never been in the thymus. A uniquely immunologically privileged organ is the liver [50]. However, self-ignorant T cells represent one of the most significant threats to the maintenance of tolerance as self-antigens from the immune-privileged organs or other neo-self-antigens can, upon certain conditions (e.g., trauma or viral infection), enter the bloodstream at a sufficient concentration and lead to immune tolerance breakdown and autoimmune process.

According to the expanding problem of autoimmune diseases, research in the field of peripheral immune self-tolerance is at the cutting-edge, and tolerogenic dendritic (tDCs) cells and peripheral regulatory CD4+CD25+FoxP3+ T (pTregs) cells occupy two central places. Tolerogenic dendritic (tDC) cells establish and maintain peripheral immune tolerance contrasted with immunogenic DCs [51]. However, immature immunogenic DCs, if maturation factors are absent, can result in the generation of tolerogenic DCs [52], which induce the proliferation of pTregs and secretion of immunosuppressive cytokines. Tolerogenic DCs are crucial in the regulation of tolerance induction and maintenance that are achieved by the following mechanisms: (1) clonal T cell deletion, (2) inhibition of memory T cells, (3) T cell anergy, (4) promotion of regulatory T (Treg) cells [16], (5) production of immunosuppressive cytokines: IL-10, TGF-β, and IL-35, (6) secretion of enzymes: indoleamine-2,3-dioxygenase (IDO) and HO-1 (heme oxygenase-1), inhibiting T cells [16], and (7) negative feedback [53]. Taking into account the contrasting features of two DCs subsets, immunogenicity and tolerogenicity [51], they are also used as therapeutic tools for prevention and therapy for both cancer and autoimmune disorders [14, 54, 55].

Thymus-derived natural Tregs (nTregs), and peripherally induced antigen-specific regulatory T (pTreg) cells, provide essential suppressive mechanisms of immune tolerance maintenance: (1) competing with proliferating lymphocytes for IL-2 by CD25+ molecule, a part of the IL-2 receptor, (2) inducing immunosuppressive cytokines IL-10, TGF-β, and IL-35, (3) inhibiting helper T cells and ILC2, (4) triggering apoptosis in target and (5) promoting the expression of coinhibitory molecules [18]. These specialized T cell subsets are clonal groupings within a much larger, heterogeneous population of CD4+ T cells, including Th1, Th2, Th9, Th17, and Th22 cells. It has been supposed that Th17 is the most potent detractor of pTregs performing opposite functions. Treg cells and Th17 cells originate from the same precursor cells, and their differentiation involves TGF-β signaling pathway. Moreover, in autoimmune conditions, such as type 1 diabetes mellitus, juvenile arthritis, and multiple sclerosis, a plasticity fraction of pTregs can undergo the pathologic conversion to IL-17+ or IFNγ+ "exFoxP3" T cells that phenotypically do not differ from effector Th17 or Th1 cells [56, 57].

From a clinical viewpoint, researchers are continuing work on different approaches to dendritic cell-based vaccines and tDCs and Treg cell therapy in cancer, autoimmune diseases, allergies, and organs transplantation [50]. Some *dendritic cell-based vaccines* are already in use correlating with favorable prognosis in cancer. Immunogenic dendritic cell-based vaccines are mainly used in immunotherapy for melanoma, prostate cancer, glioblastoma, or renal cell carcinoma [58]. To induce anti-cancer NK cell, CD8+ T cell, and CD4+ T cell immune responses in cancer patients, autologous delivered into cancer patient's dendritic (DCs) cells have to present the relevant tumor antigens. However, concerning DC-based vaccines, there are still some limitations. Conversely, an interesting strategy is to reestablish antigen-specific tolerance using tolerogenic dendritic cell-based vaccines in the treatment option for autoimmune diseases [59, 60].

In addition, *cell therapy using regulatory T (Treg) cells* is currently undergoing clinical trials for the treatment of autoimmune diseases, transplant rejection, and graft-versus-host disease [61]. Besides, genetic engineering is being exploited to express chimeric antigen receptors in Tregs for an increase in their efficacy by conferring antigen-specificity [62]. In an experiment on mice, a regulatory T (Treg) cell-based therapy has been explored for allergic airway inflammation, a model of asthma characterized by the chronic, Th2 cell-dominated immune response to ovalbumin. Tregs with chimeric antigen receptors were more efficient in controlling airway inflammation than non-modified Tregs, confirming the pivotal role of specific Treg cell activation in the lung [63].

Key Points

1. Immune tolerance to an antigen develops at central and peripheral levels and depends on the antigen dose. There are some mechanisms of tolerance such as T cell and B cell clonal deletion and anergy, activation-induced apoptosis, and clonal ignorance.
2. Normally, the immune system is tolerant to self-antigens, antigens of its own symbiotic and opportunistic microbes in the steady-state, food proteins, environmental allergens, and antigens of spermatozoa (inside women), and the father's antigens of the fetus (in pregnant women).
3. Peripheral immune tolerance is maintained by tolerogenic dendritic (tDC) cells, peripheral regulatory T (pTreg) cells, regulatory B (Breg) cells, expression of coinhibitory molecules, and pro-tolerogenic cytokines and neurotransmitters, as well as tolerogenic microbiota.

Take-Home Messages

1. Write a paragraph about two levels of immune tolerance.
2. Write an essay about central tolerance.
3. Write a flyer about immunosuppressive cytokines.
4. Write an essay about activation-induced apoptosis.
5. Write an essay about T cell anergy in the periphery.
6. Write an essay about B cell anergy in the periphery.
7. Write an essay about clonal ignorance in the periphery.
8. Write a paragraph about cells and molecules taking part in peripheral tolerance.
9. Describe central tolerance in fetal life.
10. Name methods by which P.B. Medawar achieved artificial tolerance in experiments.
11. Name primary and secondary organs of the immune system.
12. Write a paragraph about high-dose and low-dose tolerance.

Quiz

Reading a question, please choose only one right answer.

Question 1

Typically, the immune system is tolerant to:

1. Self-antigens.
2. Food allergens.
3. All points.
4. Antigens of own microbiota.

Question 2
Typically, the immune system is intolerant to:

1. Environmental pathogens.
2. Grass allergens.
3. Birch allergens.
4. Spermatozoa.

Question 3
This mechanism is related to peripheral tolerance:

1. Activation-induced apoptosis.
2. Clonal anergy.
3. Clonal ignorance.
4. All points.

Question 4
A coinhibitory molecule for T cells is:

1. CD22.
2. CTLA-4.
3. CD72.
4. CD40.

Question 5
A costimulatory molecule for B cells is:

1. CD40.
2. PD-1.
3. CD28.
4. BTLA.

Question 6
Ligand for CD28 is:

1. PD-L1.
2. B7.
3. CD40L.
4. FasL.

Question 7
Passive anergic T cells can convert into Tr1 cells:

1. Never.
2. No way.
3. It is impossible.
4. It is possible.

Question 8
Tolerogenic dendritic (tDCs) cells are generated from:

1. Regulatory T (Treg) cells.
2. Immature dendritic cells.
3. Regulatory B (Breg) cells.
4. Myeloid-derived suppressor cells.

Question 9
Activation-induced apoptosis occurs if:

1. Two self-reactive T cells interact with each other.
2. B cells undergo phagocytosis and apoptosis.
3. Neurons undergo apoptosis.
4. Macrophages phagocyte T cells.

Question 10
For clonal deletion, negative selection in the thymus includes:

1. Apoptosis of self-reactive B cells.
2. Apoptosis of thymic dendritic cells.
3. Anergy of M1 macrophages.
4. Apoptosis of self-reactive T cells.

Question 11
The receptor editing is:

1. Hypermutations in B cells during B cell response.
2. Apoptosis in B cells.
3. Alternative splicing in the process of synthesis of BCR.
4. A gene rearrangement process in bone marrow's B cells.

Question 12
Immune tolerance breakdown may result in:

1. Cancer.
2. Benign tumors.
3. Severe combined immunodeficiency.
4. Autoimmune diseases.

Question 13
"Cryptic determinants or hidden self" are self-antigens located in:

1. The gut.
2. The immune-privileged organs.
3. The bone marrow.
4. The lymph nodes.

Question 14
Clonal ignorance is related to:

1. Self-antigens at a low concentration.
2. Self-antigens at a medium concentration.
3. Self-antigens at a high concentration.
4. Foreign antigens.

Question 15
Immune tolerance is:

1. Increased responsiveness of the immune system to an antigen.
2. Unresponsiveness of the immune system to an antigen.
3. Allergic immune response.
4. Simple B cell immune response.

Question 16
The group of immunosuppressive cytokines includes:

1. IFN-γ, TNF-β, and IL-2.
2. IL-4, IL-5, and IL-13.
3. TNF-β, IL-1, and GM-CSF.
4. IL-10, IL-27, IL-35, and TGF-β.

References

1. Rogovskii V. Immune tolerance as the physiologic counterpart of chronic inflammation. Front Immunol. 2020;11:2061. https://doi.org/10.3389/fimmu.2020.02061.
2. Jensen-Jarolim E, Baz HJ, Bianchini R, Crescioli S, Daniels-Wells TR, Dombrowicz D, et al. AllergoOncology: opposite outcomes of immune tolerance in allergy and cancer. Allergy. 2018;73:328–40. https://doi.org/10.1111/all.13311.
3. Wisniewski J, Agrawal R, Woodfolk JA. Mechanisms of tolerance induction in allergic disease: integrating current and emerging concepts. Clin Exp Allergy. 2013;43(2):164–76. https://doi.org/10.1111/cea.12016.
4. Calderón MA, Linneberg A, Kleine-Tebbe J, De Bay F, de Rojas DHF, Virchow JC. Respiratory allergy caused by house dust mites: what do we really know? J Allergy Clin Immunol. 2015;136(1):38–47. https://doi.org/10.1016/j.jaci.2014.10.012.
5. Burnet MF. Immunological recognition of self: Nobel lecture. Nobel Foundation; 1960. Archived from the original on 15 Dec 2010.
6. Burnet MF. The clonal selection theory of acquired immunity. Nashville, TN: Vanderbilt University Press; 1959.
7. Klimov VV. Adaptive immune response. In: From basic to clinical immunology. Cham: Springer; 2019. https://doi.org/10.1007/978-3-030-03323-4.
8. Goodnow CC, Sprent J, de St Groth BF, Vinuesa CG. Cellular and genetic mechanisms of self tolerance and autoimmunity. Nature. 2005;435:590–7. https://doi.org/10.1038/nature03724.
9. Pucci S, Incorvaia C. Allergy as an organ and a systemic disease. Clin Exp Immunol. 2008;153(Suppl 1):1–2. https://doi.org/10.1111/j.1365-2249.2008.03712.x.
10. Powe DG, Bonnin AJ, Jones NS. "Entopy": local allergy paradigm. Clin Exp Allergy. 2010;40(7):987–97. https://doi.org/10.1111/j.1365-2222.2010.03536.x.

11. Waldmann H. Immunological tolerance. In: Reference module in biomedical sciences. Oxford: Elsevier; 2014. p. 1–7. https://doi.org/10.1016/B978-0-12-801238-3.00116-1.
12. Waldmann H, Adams E, Cobbold S. Reprogramming the immune system: co-receptor blockade as a paradigm for harnessing tolerance mechanisms. Immunol Rev. 2008;223(1):361–70. https://doi.org/10.1111/j.1600-065X.2008.00632.x.
13. Zouali M. Immunological tolerance: mechanisms. In: eLS. Paris: Wiley; 2007. p. 1–9. https://doi.org/10.1002/9780470015902.a0000950.pub2.
14. Audiger C, Rahman MJ, Yun TJ, Tarbell KV, Lesage S. The importance of dendritic cells in maintaining immune tolerance. J Immunol. 2017;198:2223–31. https://doi.org/10.4049/jimmunol.1601629.
15. Iberg CA, Hawiger D. Natural and induced tolerogenic dendritic cells. J Immunol. 2020;204(4):733–44. https://doi.org/10.4049/jimmunol.1901121.
16. Raker VK, Domogalla MP, Steinbrink K. Tolerogenic dendritic cells for regulatory T cell induction in man. Front Immunol. 2015;6:569. https://doi.org/10.3389/fimmu.2015.00569.
17. Kupriyanov SV, Sinitsky AI, Dolgushin II. Multiple subsets of regulatory T-cells. Bull Sib Med. 2020;19(3):144–55. https://doi.org/10.20538/1682-0363-2020-3-144-155.
18. Shevyrev D, Tereshchenko V. Treg heterogeneity, function, and homeostasis. Front Immunol. 2020;10:3100. https://doi.org/10.3389/fimmu.2019.03100.
19. Lee W, Lee GR. Transcriptional regulation and development of regulatory T cells. Exp Mol Med. 2018;50:e456. https://doi.org/10.1038/emm.2017.313.
20. Ohkura N, Kitagawa Y, Sakaguchi S. Development and maintenance of regulatory T cells. Immunity. 2013;38(3):414–23. https://doi.org/10.1016/j.immuni.2013.03.002.
21. Abebe EC, Dejenie TA, Ayele TM, Baye ND, Teshome AA, Muche ZT. The role of regulatory B cells in health and diseases: a systemic review. J Inflamm Res. 2021;14:75–84. https://doi.org/10.2147/JIR.S286426.
22. Bluestone JA, Bour-Jordan H, Cheng M, Anderson M. T cells in the control of organ-specific autoimmunity. J Clin Invest. 2015;125(6):2250–60. https://doi.org/10.1172/JCI78089.
23. Commins SP, Borish L, Steinke JW. Immunologic messenger molecules: cytokines, interferons, and chemokines. J Allergy Clin Immunol. 2010;125(2):S53–72. https://doi.org/10.1016/j.jaci.2009.07.008.
24. Keir ME, Butte MJ, Freeman GJ, Sharpe AH. PD-1 and its ligands in tolerance and immunity. Annu Rev Immunol. 2008;26:677–704. https://doi.org/10.1146/annurev.immunol.26.021607.090331.
25. Mangalam AK, Ochoa-Reparaz JO. Editorial: the role of the gut microbiota in health and inflammatory diseases. Front Immunol. 2020;11:565305. https://doi.org/10.3389/fimmu.2020.565305.
26. Vitetta L, Vitetta G, Hall S. Immunological tolerance and function: associations between intestinal bacteria, probiotics, prebiotics, and phages. Front Immunol. 2018;9:2240. https://doi.org/10.3389/fimmu.2018.02240.
27. Belkaid Y, Harrison OJ. Homeostatic immunity and the microbiota. Immunity. 2017;46:562–76. https://doi.org/10.1016/j.immuni.2017.04.008.
28. Jiao Y, Wu L, Huntington ND, Zhang X. Crosstalk between gut microbiota and innate immunity and its implication in autoimmune diseases. Front Immunol. 2020;11:282. https://doi.org/10.3389/fimmu.2020.00282.
29. Pobezinsky LA, Angelov GS, Tai X, Jeurling S, Van Laethem F, Feigenbaum L, Park J-H, Singer A. Clonal deletion and the fate of autoreactive thymocytes that survive negative selection. Nat Immunol. 2012;13:569–78. https://doi.org/10.1038/ni.2292.
30. Labrecque N, Baldwin T, Lesage S. Molecular and genetic parameters defining T-cell clonal selection. Immunol Cell Biol. 2011;89(1):16–26. https://doi.org/10.1038/icb.2010.119.
31. Perniola R, Musco G. The biophysical and biochemical properties of the autoimmune regulator (AIRE) protein. Biochem Biophys Acta. 2014;1842(2):326–37. https://doi.org/10.1016/j.bbadis.2013.11.020.

32. Nemazee D. Mechanisms of central tolerance for B cells. Nat Rev Immunol. 2017;17(5):281–94. https://doi.org/10.1038/nri.2017.19.
33. Pillai S, Mattoo H, Cariappa A. B cells and autoimmunity. Curr Opin Immunol. 2011;23(6):721–31. https://doi.org/10.1016/j.coi.2011.10.007.
34. Arakaki R, Yamada A, Kudo Y, Hayashi Y, Eshimaru N. Mechanism of activation-induced cell death of T cells and regulation of FasL expression. Crit Rev Immunol. 2014;34(4):301–14. https://doi.org/10.1615/critrevimmunol.2014009988.
35. Badami E, Cexus ONF, Quaratino S. Activation-induced cell death of self-reactive regulatory T cells drives autoimmunity. PNAS. 2019;116(52):26788–97. https://doi.org/10.1073/pnas.1910281116.
36. Müeller DL. Anergy. In: AccessScience. Columbus, OH: McGraw-Hill Education; 2019. https://doi.org/10.1036/1097-8542.033880.
37. von Knethen A. Costimulatory receptors. In: Parnham MJ, editor. Compendium of inflammatory diseases. Basel: Springer; 2016. https://doi.org/10.1007/978-3-7643-8550-7_101.
38. Watanabe M, Lu Y, Breen M, Hodes RJ. B7-CD28 co-stimulation modulates central tolerance via thymic clonal deletion and Treg generation through distinct mechanisms. Nat Commun. 2020;11:6264. https://doi.org/10.1038/s41467-020-20070-x.
39. Wikenheiser DJ, Stumhofer JS. ICOS co-stimulation: friend or foe? Front Immunol. 2016;7:304. https://doi.org/10.3389/fimmu.2016.00304.
40. Chen L, Flies DB. Molecular mechanisms of T cell co-stimulation and co-inhibition. Nat Rev Immunol. 2013;13(4):227–42. https://doi.org/10.1038/nri3405.
41. Mitsuiki N, Schwab C, Grimbacher B. What did we learn from CTLA-4 insufficiency on the human immune system? Immunol Rev. 2018;287(1):33–49. https://doi.org/10.1111/imr.12721.
42. Jones A, Bourque J, Kuehm L, Opejin A, Teague RM, Gross C, Hawiger D. Immunomodulatory functions of BTLA and HVEM govern induction of extrathymic regulatory T cells and tolerance by dendritic cells. Immunity. 2016;45:1066–77. https://doi.org/10.1016/j.immuni.2016.10.008.
43. Hu S, Xu Liu X, Li T, Li Z, Hu F. LAG3 (CD223) and autoimmunity: emerging evidence. J Autoimmun. 2020;112:102504. https://doi.org/10.1016/j.jaut.2020.102504.
44. Sage PT, Peterson AM, Lovitch SB, Sharpe AH. The coinhibitory receptor CTLA-4 controls B cell responses by modulating T follicular helper, T follicular regulatory, and T regulatory cells. Immunity. 2014;41(6):1026–39. https://doi.org/10.1016/j.immuni.2014.12.005.
45. Tsubata T. Inhibitory B cell co-receptors and autoimmune diseases. Immunol Med. 2019;42(3):108–16. https://doi.org/10.1080/25785826.2019.1660038.
46. Thorman AS, Schneider T, Cyran L, Eckert IN, Kerstan A, Lutz MB. Conversion of anergic T cells into Foxp3- IL-10+ regulatory T cells by a second antigen stimulus in vivo. Front Immunol. 2021;12:704578. https://doi.org/10.3389/fimmu.2021.704578.
47. Parish IA, Heath WR. Too dangerous to ignore: self-tolerance and the control of ignorant autoreactive T cells. Immunol Cell Biol. 2008;86(2):146–52. https://doi.org/10.1038/sj.icb.7100161.
48. Benhar I, London A, Schwartz M. The privileged immunity of immune privileged organs: the case of the eye. Front Immunol. 2012;3:296. https://doi.org/10.3389/fimmu.2012.00296.
49. Wang T, Feng X, Han D. Mechanisms of testicular immune privilege. Front Biol. 2011;6:19–30. https://doi.org/10.1007/s11515-011-1010-4.
50. Ellias SD, Larson EL, Taner T, Nyberg SL. Cell-mediated therapies to facilitate operational tolerance in liver transplantation. Int J Mol Sci. 2021;22:4016. https://doi.org/10.3390/ijms22084016.
51. Nam J-H, Lee J-H, Choi S-Y, Jung N-C, Song J-Y, Seo H-G, et al. Functional ambivalence of dendritic cells: tolerogenicity and immunogenicity. Int J Mol Sci. 2021;22:4430. https://doi.org/10.3390/ijms22094430.

52. Probst HC, Muth S, Schild H. Regulation of the tolerogenic function of steady-state DCs. Eur J Immunol. 2014;44(4):927–33. https://doi.org/10.1002/eji.201343862.
53. Peters M, Peters K, Bufe A. Regulation of lung immunity by dendritic cells: implications for asthma, chronic obstructive pulmonary disease and infectious disease. Innate Immun. 2019;25(6):326–36. https://doi.org/10.1177/1753425918821732.
54. Hasegawa H, Matsumoto T. Mechanisms of tolerance induction by dendritic cells *in vivo*. Front Immunol. 2018;9:350. https://doi.org/10.3389/fimmu.2018.00350.
55. Fucikova J, Palovs-Jelinkova L, Bartunkova J, Spisek R. Induction of tolerance and immunity by dendritic cells: mechanisms and clinical applications. Front Immunol. 2019;10:2393. https://doi.org/10.3389/fimmu.2019.02393.
56. Hua J, Inomata T, Chen Y, Foulsham W, Stevenson W, Shiang T, et al. Pathological conversion of regulatory T cells is associated with loss of allotolerance. Sci Rep. 2018;8:7059. https://doi.org/10.1038/s41598-018-25384-x.
57. Zhu L, Ding W, Ding K, Zhang Y, Xu C. The correlation between the Th17/Treg cell balance and bone health. Immun Ageing. 2020;17:30. https://doi.org/10.1186/s12979-020-00202-z.
58. Wculek S, Cueto FJ, Mujal AM, Melero I, Krummel M, Sancho D. Dendritic cells in cancer immunology and immunotherapy. Nat Rev Immunol. 2020;20(1):7–24. https://doi.org/10.1038/s41577-019-0210-z.
59. Moorman CD, Sohn SJ, Phee H. Emerging therapeutics for immune tolerance: tolerogenic vaccines, T cell therapy, and IL-2 therapy. Front Immunol. 2021;12:657768. https://doi.org/10.3389/fimmu.2021.657768.
60. Cifuentes-Rius A, Desai A, Yuen D, Johnson PR, Voelcker NH. Inducing immune tolerance with dendritic cell-targeting nanomedicines. Nat Nanotechnol. 2021;16:37–46. https://doi.org/10.1038/s41565-020-00810-2.
61. Raffin C, Vo LT, Bluestone JA. Treg cell-based therapies: challenges and perspectives. Nat Rev Immunol. 2020;20:158–72. https://doi.org/10.1038/s41577-019-0232-6.
62. Mohseni YR, Tung SL, Dudreuilh C, Lechler RI, Fruhwirth GO, Lombardi G. The future of regulatory T cell therapy: promises and challenges of implementing CAR technology. Front Immunol. 2020;11:1608. https://doi.org/10.3389/fimmu.2020.01608.
63. Skuljec J, Chmielewski M, Happle C, Habener A, Busse M, Abken H, Hansen G. Chimeric antigen receptor-redirected regulatory T cells suppress experimental allergic airway inflammation, a model of asthma. Front Immunol. 2017;8:1125. eCollection 2017. https://doi.org/10.3389/fimmu.2017.01125.

Immune-Derived Maintenance of Allergen Tolerance

3

Contents

Supplementary Information The online version contains supplementary material available at [https://doi.org/10.1007/978-3-031-04309-3_3].

V. V. Klimov, *Textbook of Allergen Tolerance*,
https://doi.org/10.1007/978-3-031-04309-3_3

Didactics

Knowledge. Upon successful completion of this chapter, students should be able to:

1. Draw the immune-derived system of allergen tolerance maintenance.
2. Distinguish between typical allergen adaptive response and tolerogenic response.
3. Name and describe two cellular lineages occupying central places in the system of allergen tolerance maintenance.
4. List pro-tolerogenic molecules and their functions.
5. Describe tolerogenic dendritic (tDCs) cells.
6. Describe peripheral regulatory T (pTregs) cells.
7. Characterize immunosuppressive cytokines in detail.
8. Characterize coinhibitory molecules and their role in allergen tolerance maintenance.
9. Briefly describe cells in allergic inflammation.
10. Explain the principles of helper T cells suppression.
11. Describe the role of microbiota in allergen tolerance maintenance.

Acquired Skills. Upon successful completion of this chapter, students should demonstrate the following skills, including:

1. Interpret the knowledge related to the system of allergen tolerance maintenance.
2. Critically evaluate the scientific literature about allergen tolerance.
3. Discuss the scientific articles from the current research literature to criticize experimental data and formulate new hypotheses in allergy.
4. Have a clear perception of the presented allergy definitions expressed orally and in written form.
5. Formulate the presented allergy terms.
6. Correctly answer the quiz questions.

Attitude and Professional Behaviors. Students should be able to:

1. Have the readiness to be hard-working.
2. Behave professionally at all times.
3. Recognize the importance of studying and demonstrate a commitment.

3.1 Introduction

▶ **Definition** The tolerogenic response is an immunologic process leading to the establishment of allergen tolerance. Allergen tolerance is the unresponsiveness of the immune system to an allergen. The system of allergen tolerance maintenance enables the body to avoid allergic diseases even if an individual is atopic.

In human populations, allergen tolerance is the consequence of many tolerogenic responses to many environmental allergens. Most people with atopic heredity have

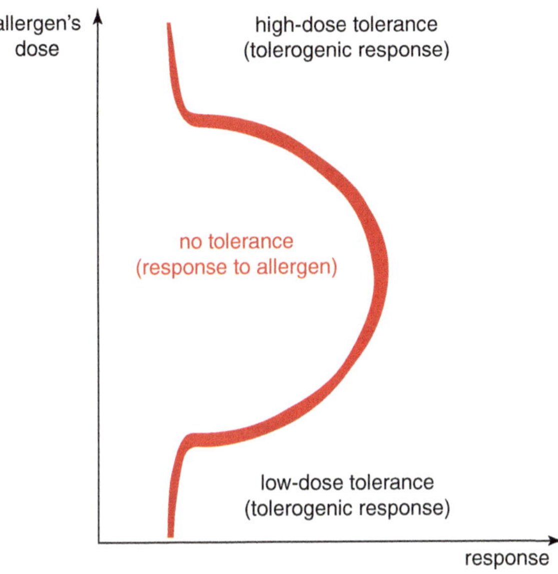

Fig. 3.1 Dose-dependent allergen tolerance. Allergen tolerance depends on the dose of the allergen and may be a low-dose or high-dose tolerance. In a medium-dose zone, there is no tolerance

IgE-sensitization but do not suffer from any atopic disease. Sufferers do not coincide with the number of practically healthy persons with atopic predisposition but without clinical symptoms who are significantly prevalent [1–4].

A tolerogenic response to a causative allergen, in the beginning, resembles the adaptive immune response since a tolerogenic dendritic cell exerts itself as an allergen-presenting cell, whereas a regulatory T cell is similar to an allergen recognizing cell. Further, there is no activation to make an "army" of effector cells and molecules (IgE), leading to a "battle," i.e., allergic inflammation and allergic disease. Such is the course of nature. Instead of a "battle," a series of tolerogenic effects are observed, such as the inactivation of helper T cells, inflammatory cells, and molecules. Some allergens at a high dose (for example, cat's *Fed d 1*) can promote an increase in IgG_4 antibodies in the absence of detectable IgE antibodies and allergic manifestations [1]. In allergen-specific immunotherapy (AIT), allergens are first administered at low concentrations, and allergen tolerance is established [5]. Undoubtedly, a "tolerogenic allergen" causing a tolerogenic response may be associated with either a high dose or low dose corresponding to the classical concept of high-dose/low-dose tolerance (see Fig. 3.1).

However, we should always take into consideration the presence of individual factors. One group of individuals has a different immune system compared to another and recognizes some antigens as allergens. Another group does not sense these antigens as allergens despite the equal level of allergenicity exhibited by these antigens [6].

The discovery of a local respiratory allergy [7] raised one more challenge in the theory of allergen tolerance, implying different levels of tolerance breakdown in the body. There are two such levels: the systemic and local, namely respiratory level. The allergen tolerance breakdown at the regional level leading to a local respiratory allergy is not yet understood (see Chap. 6).

The system of allergen tolerance maintenance consists of two main cell lineages: tolerogenic dendritic (tDCs) cells and allergen-specific peripheral (pTreg) cells. It also includes regulatory B cells, macrophages (M2), myeloid-derived suppressor cells, helper T cells inhibition mechanisms, via immunosuppressive cytokines, coinhibitory molecules, and transcription factors, as well as blocking antibodies, pro-tolerogenic neurotransmitters, and neuropeptides, enzymes, and tolerogenic microbiota.

Neurotransmitters and neuropeptides will be described in Chap. 4.

3.2 Tolerogenic Dendritic (tDCs) Cells

► **Definition** Tolerogenic dendritic cells occupy one of two central places in the system of allergen tolerance maintenance. Cell signaling is the signal transduction from a cellular receptor through signaling pathways to transcription factors for the gene expression to get downstream effects of the cell.

Polymorphisms and functional plasticity are inherent in *tolerogenic dendritic (tDCs) cells* (see Fig. 3.2) [8]. The main designations of DCs are the ability to

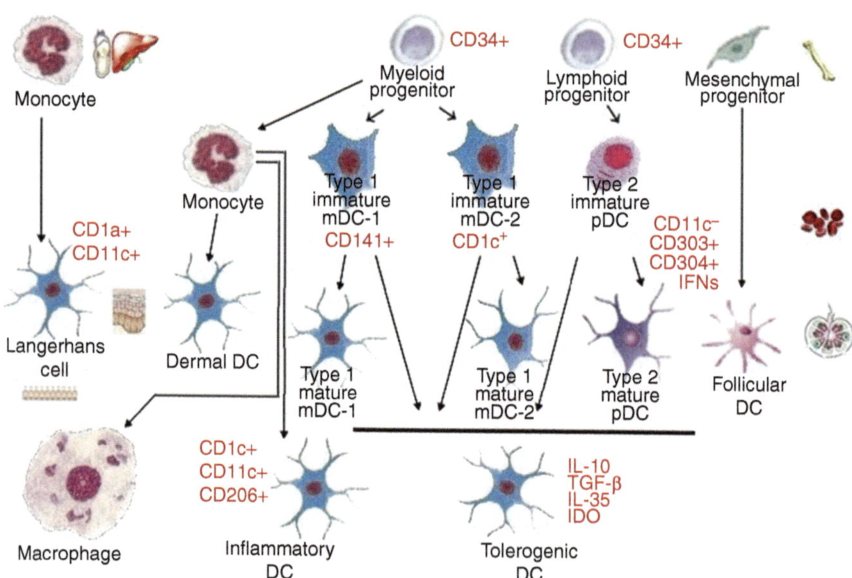

Fig. 3.2 Ontogeny and polymorphism of dendritic cells. Human dendritic cells originated from distinct precursors are differentiated into some subsets and develop maturating from immature to mature cells. Dendritic cells function as antigen-presenting, inflammatory, and tolerogenic cells

perform highly specialized professional antigen presentation, superior migration, and activation of naïve lymphocytes via cytokines and costimulatory molecules [9]. tDCs are not lineage-specific. Due to DCs' extensive functional plasticity and particular extracellular microenvironment, conventional, mainly immature DCs can turn into the tDCs, which are, in fact, "induced tolerogenic DCs" [10]. Unfortunately, the phenotypical division between "immature DCs" and "mature DCs" does not necessarily correspond to "tolerogenic DCs" and "immunogenic DCs," respectively. Besides, tolerogenic properties are constitutively present in some "natural tolerogenic DCs" participating in the promotion of peripheral tolerance [10].

In total, DCs are ambivalent as they possess the features of both tolerogenicity and immunogenicity, and their activation state dictates the ability of DCs to promote either immunity or tolerance [11]. So, the main source of tDCs is immature DCs [12, 13]. tDCs are induced by IL-2, IL-10, TGF-β, vitamin D_3, retinoid acid, numerous immunosuppressive agents, which can represent cytokines such as IL-10, TGF-β, IL-27 [14, 15], endogenous immunosuppressants such as glucocorticoids, vasoactive intestinal peptide (VIP), several synthetic immunosuppressive drugs (e.g., rapamycin, cyclosporine, aspirin), and natural products (e.g., curcumin, resveratrol). Atypical neurotransmitter adenosine upregulates DCs' tolerogenic phenotype. Then tDCs promote in turn pTregs differentiation [16].

Mechanisms of tDCs that provide tolerance include (1) T-clonal deletion, (2) T cell anergy (see Chap. 2), (3) promotion of pTregs proliferation, (4) inhibition of memory cells, (5) production of immunosuppressive cytokines, (6) secretion of enzymes inhibiting T cells, and (7) negative feedback regulation [9, 10, 17, 18]. The promotion of pTregs proliferation is described as a bidirectional coinfluence between tDCs and naïve T cells, leading to the main pTreg subset differentiation (see Fig. 3.3). Next, pTregs suppress helper T cells and associated cytokines, particularly via specific transcription factors. As a result, allergic response and allergic inflammation are stopped before manifestation. Upon the negative feedback regulation, tDCs lose their costimulatory molecules if there is strong adherence of pTregs with tDCs via cell adhesion molecules and activation of an ITIM-containing C-type lectin receptor (e.g., DC-SIGN) on tDCs (see Sect. 3.9.9) [17].

Among tolerogenic DCs subsets [9], there are natural tDCs, induced tDCs, tumor-induced tDCs, pharmacologically induced tDCs, DC-10 (DCs secreting significantly increased value of IL-10), CD103+ tDCs (in the gut and mesenteric lymph nodes) [19], etc. On the one hand, tDCs express an immature or semi-mature phenotype characterized by low-affinity costimulatory molecules and high-affinity coinhibitory molecule pattern, and poor HLA expression [9]. On the other hand, tDCs produce immunosuppressive profile's cytokines such as IL-10, TGF-β, IL-35, atypical neurotransmitter nitric oxide, and enzymes: IDO (indoleamine-2,3-dioxygenase) and HO-1 (heme oxygenase-1), which inhibit T cell proliferation. IDO indirectly drives Treg differentiation by degradation of the essential amino acid tryptophan around effector T cells and concurrent production of toxic metabolites like kynurenines leading to apoptosis in T cells [20].

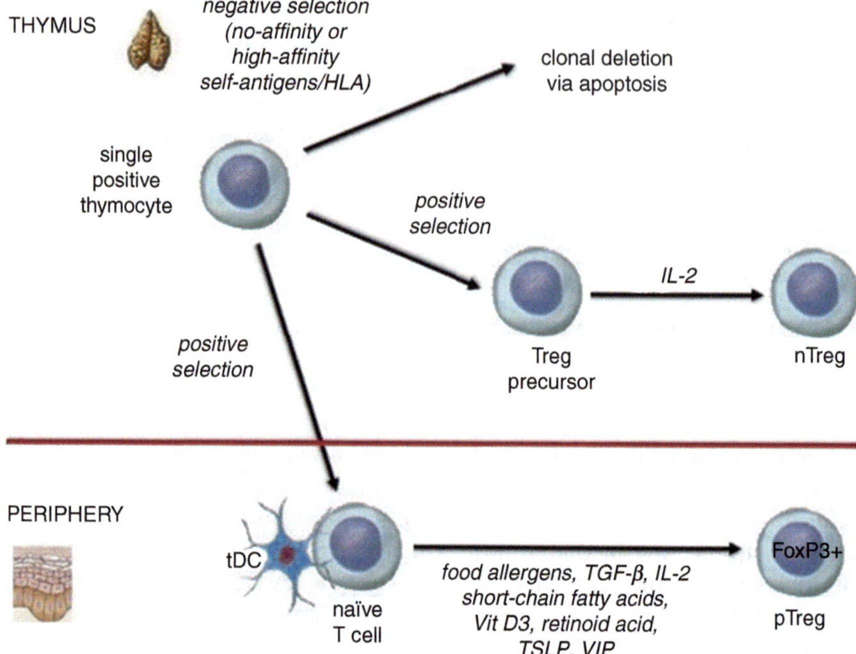

Fig. 3.3 Differentiation of peripheral regulatory T (pTreg) cells. In the periphery, naïve T cells under the influence of environmental factors differentiate into immunosuppressive pTreg cells. Other cells, thymic nTregs and even Th17, may also convert into pTregs

Signal transduction from enormous receptors on cells through signaling pathways provides cells with downstream effects. Before end-effects develop, transcription factors turn on the proper gene expression. A precise set of signaling molecules depends on certain ligands and receptors. Natural or artificial modifications of signaling molecules and transcription factors (e.g., pharmacological) may destruct typical downstream effects of the cells.

From a clinical viewpoint, tDCs are promising candidates for specific cellular therapy in allergic and autoimmune diseases [18].

3.3 Regulatory T (Tregs) Cells

▶ **Definition** Allergen-specific peripheral regulatory T (pTreg) cells occupy one of two central places in the system of allergen tolerance maintenance. A Th17/pTreg balance is considered as the marker of allergen tolerance maintenance or breakdown.

Peripheral naïve T cells, maybe thymic natural regulatory T (nTregs) cells, and sometimes other cells can differentiate into *peripheral T (pTreg) cells* [21], acquiring higher TCR affinity, a transcription factor Forkhead Box P3 (FoxP3), and transcription factor Helios [22]. However, the major source of pTregs is naïve T cells (see Fig. 3.3). Most pTreg cells (the main subset) express CD4+CD25^{hi}FoxP3+, representing approximately 5–10% of the total CD4+ T cell population and exhibiting their pro-tolerogenic potency via cell-to-cell contacts [9]. In the periphery, they mainly exert their pro-tolerogenic properties in five ways: (1) competing with proliferating lymphocytes for IL-2 by CD25+ molecule, a part of the IL-2 receptor, (2) inducing immunosuppressive cytokines such as IL-10, TGF-β, and IL-35 plus galectin-1, (3) inhibiting helper T cells and ILC2, (4) triggering apoptosis in target cells (see Fig. 3.4), and (5) promoting the expression of coinhibitory molecules, CTLA-4, LAG-3 [21, 23]. Treg cells use SMAR1 transcription factor, whereas STAT3 is an inhibitor of FoxP3 in Tregs [24].

From a clinical viewpoint, interestingly, an increase in the pTreg cells in serum is often seen in tumor growth and helminth invasion, whereas a decrease in the cells is found in atopic allergic diseases and autoimmune disorders.

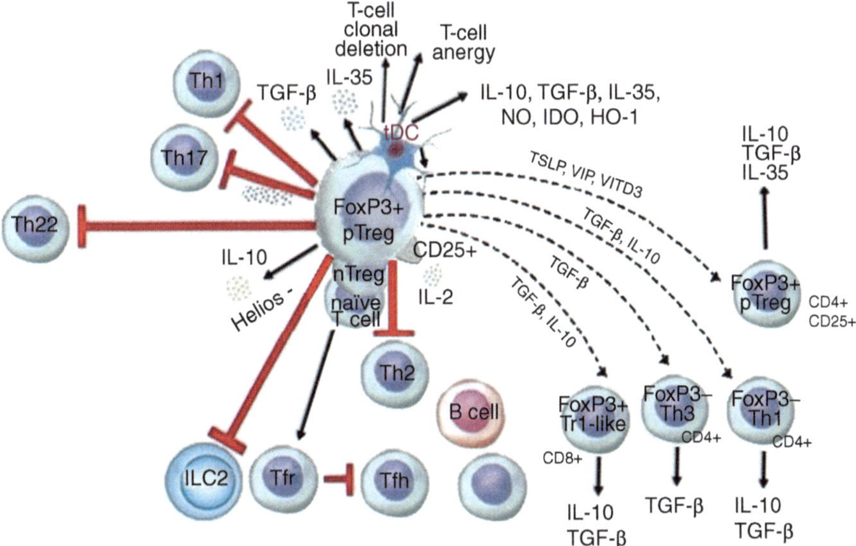

Fig. 3.4 Tolerogenic DCs (tDCs) and regulatory T (Tregs) cells in the system of allergen tolerance maintenance. The principal pro-tolerogenic cells, tDCs and pTregs, function together. Effects of tDCs in part exert through the promotion of pTregs, leading to the proliferation of naïve T cells and nTregs to allergen-specific pTregs. The impacts of pTregs include competing with proliferating lymphocytes for IL-2 by CD25+ molecule (a part of the IL-2 receptor), inducing immunosuppressive cytokines, IL-10, TGF-β, and IL-35, inhibiting helper T cells and ILC2, generating pro-tolerogenic subsets, particularly type 1 regulatory T (Tr1) cells and type 3 helper T (Th3) cells, etc. tDC tolerogenic DC, Tr1 type 1 regulatory T cell, Th3 type 3 helper T cell, TSLP thymic stromal lymphopoietin, IDO indoleamine-2,3-dioxygenase, HO-1 heme oxygenase-1, VIP vasoactive intestinal peptide, Tfh follicular helper T cell, Tfr T follicular regulatory cell

Current extensive research in the field of Tregs resulted in the emergence of many new classifications and understanding heterogeneity of these cells [21, 25]. Many factors acting on the main pTregs subset and these CD4+FoxP3+ T cells cause the establishment of some subpopulations of Tregs: type 1 regulatory T (Tr1) cells, type 3 helper T (Th3) cells, CD8+Treg cells and CD8+Tr1-like Treg cells, helper-specific Tregs, T follicular regulatory (Tfr) cells, FoxP3+RORγt Treg cells, and central memory (cmTreg) and effector memory (emTreg) cells.

1. The Type 1 regulatory T (Tr1) cell, a subset of pTreg cells, induced by TGF-β and IL-10, has a particular phenotype CD4+FoxP3^{-} [9]. Tr1 cells may originate from circulating passive anergic T cells upon short-term restimulation of high and systemic doses of antigen [26]. Tr1 cells must meet the following criteria: (1) secreting a high level of IL-10; (2) promoting extensive tolerogenic properties contrasted to other IL-10-secreting cells; (3) constant expressing coinhibitory molecule LAG-3; and (4) not constitutively expressing FoxP3 [27]. So, this subset is also known as FoxP3^{-} IL-10-secreting Treg. In addition, Tr1 cells cause apoptosis in effector T cells and use other coinhibitory molecules such as PD-1 and CTLA-4 to provide pro-tolerogenic action at mucosal sites independent from the main pTreg subset [27]. Notably, the Tr1 subset exerts its pro-tolerogenic capacity in a cytokine-mediated/cell-to-cell contact manner. However, it has been experimentally shown that Tr1 cells did not contribute to tolerogenic memory [28]. Tr1 cells use IRF4, c-Maf, and AHR transcription factors upon signal transduction [27].
2. The Type 3 helper T (Th3) cell, CD4+Th3 subset of pTreg cells, induced by TGF-β, also has a particular phenotype CD4+CD25^{-}FoxP3^{-}LAP+ [3, 29], and can secrete TGF-β functioning at mucosal sites and preventing allergy and autoimmunity. This subset is also known as FoxP3^{-} TGF-β-secreting Treg.
3. Naïve T cells, which interact with mature DCs in a lymphoid microenvironment rich in TGF-β and IL-2 [30], differentiate into "induced Treg" (iTreg) cells. So far, most researchers employ the term "induced Treg" for all subsets originated from immature T cells contrasted with nTregs. iTreg were described as cells possessing a typical pTregs phenotype CD4+CD25+FoxP3+ and inhibiting effector T cells via immunosuppressive cytokines IL-10 and TGF-β at mucosal sites [25]. Also described were CD8+CD25+CTLA-4+CD28^{-} Tregs exerting pro-tolerogenic properties in tonsils by secreting IL-10, TGF-β in the presence of IFN-γ [3, 25, 29]. CD8+Treg cells and CD8+Tr1-like Treg cells may be the same cells.
4. Some subpopulations of pTregs are functionally directed to certain subsets of helper T cells suppressing particular helper T cell subsets [3, 31]. Also identified were pTregs specific for Th1, Th2, Th17, and Tfh [32]. Those pTregs are characterized by a specific set of cytokines and transcription factors [33]. For example, for Th1 suppression by pTregs and inactivation of Th1 associated cytokines, such as IFN-γ and IL-2, the expression of T-bet is necessary. For the

development of Th2-specific pTregs and inhibition of Th17 by pTregs, expression of GATA3 and RORγt is necessary, respectively [34, 35]. Conversely, for increased IL-10 production, pTregs must not have transcription factor Helios (Helios$^-$ pTregs).
5. Natural regulatory T (nTreg) cells differentiate into T follicular regulatory (Tfr) cells [32, 36] that depend on Bcl6 and other transcription factors. Tfr cells allow the suppression of adaptive responses and re-switching antibodies' isotype in the lymph node germinal center, which Tfh cells activate and maintain. Tfr cells also prevent potential autoimmunity [36].

In summary, in terms of differentiation, there are three developmental categories of all Tregs: (1) naïve, (2) central memory (cmTreg) cells, and (3) effector memory (emTreg)cells[21,37].Innewborns,mostTregsarenaïveCD45RA^{hi}CD45R0$^-$FoxP3$^-$T cells (85.2%), whereas cmTregs account for 5.6% and emTregs make up 4.5%. In healthy adult individuals, up to 30% of Tregs are naïve, and, in aging due to thymic involution, the proportion of naïve Tregs diminishes to 15.2%. Most Tregs are FoxP3^{hi} memory cells, in particular, CD45R0^{hi}CD62L$^+$cmTregs (56.5%) and CD45R0^{hi}CD62L$^-$emTregs (25.2%) [37].

Currently, Th17 is thought to be the main powerful detractor of pTregs [38]. The ratio of Th17/pTreg is considered the marker of processes related to allergen tolerance. Paradoxically, pTregs may sometimes produce pro-inflammatory cytokines that can potentially disrupt the action of tolerogenic mechanisms induced by immunosuppressive pTregs. The pathological conversion of pTreg to Th17+'exFoxP3' T cells has been described [39]. However, Th17 can convert into FoxP3+IL-17$^-$, and then FoxP3+Treg cells in allergen-specific immunotherapy (AIT) [40]. Immunosuppressive FoxP3+RORγt Treg cells are a unique Tregs subset, which differentiated from pro-inflammatory IL-17–producing CD4+ Th17 cells under the influence of IL-2, TGF-β, IL-6, IL-21, IL-23, and retinoid acid [41, 42].

One more pathological conversion of pTregs has been reported. Under certain circumstances of allergic response, pTregs can acquire a Th2 phenotype, express GATA3/IRF4 transcription factors, release IL-4 and IL-13, and lose their potency to immunosuppresion, becoming "pathogenic" [2, 43].

Atopic allergic responses develop in the context of the failure of tolerance toward specific allergens. This event is marked by the production of allergen-specific IgE under the type 2 helper CD4+ T cells control. The proliferation and differentiation of "normal" pTregs can limit progressing allergic response. As mentioned above, in terms of memory, Tregs are subdivided into central memory Tregs (cmTregs) and effector memory Tregs (emTregs) [21].

Some examples illustrate the evolutionary rationale of memory Tregs production. The evolutionary target-antigens of memory Tregs are food allergens, microbiota antigens, fetal antigens, and many environmental allergens. Exposure to a husband's antigens or fetal antigens can recruit antigen-specific memory Tregs to the appropriate tissue like the uterus to have a subsequent successful pregnancy.

Memory Tregs might be a valuable mechanism for avoiding inflammation if previous reactivation of normal microbial microflora at the barrier surfaces was available. The efficacy of AIT persisting over a long time relies on the induction of memory Tregs [44].

3.4 Other Pro-Tolerogenic Cells

3.4.1 Regulatory B (Breg) Cells

The *regulatory B (Bregs) cells* have been identified later than Tregs being isolated from beekeepers who displayed bee venom tolerance in allergic patients before and after AIT [45, 46]. So far, Bregs are phenotypically (CD19+, CD24+, CD38+, PD-L1+) [47] and functionally characterized as IL-10-secreting and anti-inflammatory cells [40, 48]. Bregs can also secrete TGF-β, IL-35, and IL-1-receptor antagonist (IL-1RA), use indoleamine-2,3-dioxygenase (IDO), and interact with myeloid-derived suppressor (MDSC) cells [49].

In allergies, a Breg subset, Br1 cells, CD25+CD71+CD73^{-}, have high IL-10 production, suppress allergen-specific CD4+ T cell proliferation, and upregulates IgG_4 antibodies production as a consequence of AIT [50]. The ratio of Th17/Breg is supposed to be the second biomarker predicting AIT success [40]. Breg cells use Jak/STAT signaling pathway and TLR-related pathways for signal transduction [48].

3.4.2 Macrophages (M2)

Macrophages are prevalent cells in many target organs, making up 70% of all immune cells in the lung. There are two sources of macrophage origin, yolk sac/fetal liver in early embryonic development and recruited due to emergency monopoiesis monocytes in adult life [51–53]. It is poorly understood from which kind of monocytes, classical, intermediate or nonclassical "patrolling" cells, M1 and M2 macrophages generate [52].

Type 2 macrophages (M2), CD163+CD206+, are subdivided into four subsets, M2a, M2b, M2c, and M2d, which differ from each other, considering their properties and numerous phenotypic markers. Particularly, IL-4 and IL-13 promote M2a (alternatively activated) macrophages, which mainly exert pro-tolerogenic properties; in contrast, M2b cells (type II activated macrophages) may be pro-inflammatory; M2c (deactivated) macrophages perform phagocytic clearance of dead cells; M2d or M2-like (tumor-associated) macrophages (TAM) stimulate tumor growth [51, 54].

M2a and M2b macrophages are reported as ambivalent cells possessing pro-inflammatory and anti-inflammatory potential in allergies [55, 56]; among them, M2a macrophages contribute to allergic inflammation suppressing, tissue repair, wound healing, and pattern-associated molecular patterns (PAMP) sensing.

Eventually, all M2 subsets are anti-inflammatory as they produce the potent immunosuppressive cytokine IL-10 and some TGF-β. The gut is a zone of tolerance where M2 macrophages (mucosal, lamina propria's, and muscular) are predominant compared to M1 macrophages [57]. M2 macrophages express many receptors and involve many signaling pathways for signal transduction, but they preferentially engage the Jak/STAT and PI3K/Akt signaling pathways [56] and KLF4 and IRF4 transcription factors in M2 polarization [51].

Upon resolution of allergic inflammation, inflammatory cells die by apoptosis when apoptotic cell fragments are released in the form of apoptotic bodies as well as *extracellular vesicles (microvesicles and exosomes)* recruiting macrophages to engulf them in a process known as *efferocytosis* [53]. The extracellular vesicles contain powerful mediators and enzymes required for the communication between dying cells and macrophages, a phenotypic shift within macrophages toward M2 phenotype, and prevention of tissue damage. Besides, extracellular vesicles have an immunoregulatory action [58].

3.4.3 Myeloid-Derived Suppressor (MDSC) Cells

Myeloid-derived suppressor (MDSC) cells have pro-tolerogenic activity appearing during immunosenescence and making a poor prognosis in cancer. MDSCs are divided into two subpopulations, polymorphonuclear (granulocyte)-MDSCs and monocyte-MDSCs [59]. The function of MDSCs in allergic conditions has not yet been studied sufficiently because most research was carried out in cancer in murine models [60]. Monocytic MDSC isolated from the blood of COVID-19 patients demonstrated immunosuppressive activity via a typical arginase 1-dependent mechanism that led to increased uptake of L-arginine and blockade of the proliferation of T cells. The elevated level of these MDSCs correlated with disease severity [61]. It is known the main MDSC immunosuppressive mechanism is linked to the production of metabolites.

In the experiment, granulocyte-MDSCs canceled T cell activation, upregulated Treg cells, and decreased airway hyperresponsiveness in ovalbumin-sensitized mice with induced allergic asthma [62]. In another experiment, granulocyte-MDSCs inhibited Th2 activity and diminished lung hyperreactivity in allergen-challenged aspirin-treated mice [63]. In the third study, granulocyte-MDSCs suppressed Th2 cells and, compared to monocyte-MDSCs, inhibited ILC2 in humans [64].

MDSCs use Jak/STAT, and SMAD signaling pathways depending on ligands in the myeloid development [65].

3.5 Immunosuppressive Cytokines

▶ **Definition** Cytokines are specialized regulatory molecules, which mainly act on target cells in a short distance manner, either as pro-immunogenic or pro-tolerogenic factors.

The main immunosuppressive cytokines are IL-10, TGF-β, and IL-35, involved in both pTregs and tDCs functioning. IL-27 is also related to immunosuppressive cytokines [13, 15]. IL-10 is the most potent immunosuppressive cytokine. A primary source for IL-10 is pTregs, tDCs, monocytes, and B cells, but its sources are many human cells. It has been known IL-10 inhibits the production of IFN-γ by Th1 cells; IL-4 and IL-5 by Th2 subsets; IL-1β, IL-6, CXCL8, IL-12, and TNF-α by mononuclear phagocytes; and IFN-γ and TNF-α by NK cells [14]. Constitutive expression of IL-10 in the respiratory tract plays a role in the allergen tolerance maintenance of practically healthy atopic subjects. IL-10 binding IL-10R1 and IL-10R2 turns on Jak/STAT signaling pathway [66].

Recently, well-established immunosuppressive cytokine IL-10 has been revised in tDCs induction, called DC-10. It has been shown that DC-10 can express both costimulatory and coinhibitory molecules and specifically induce the generation of Tr1 cells. IL-10-treatment of monocyte-derived DC-10 resulted in two subtypes of DCs, $CD83^{high}CCR7+$ with high immunosuppressive potential and $CD83^{low}CCR7^{-}$ with low suppressive activity [16].

In some cases, e.g., in COVID-19, an elevated level of IL-10 was found corresponding to the nonclassical pro-inflammatory effect of this cytokine in the face of systemic inflammation [67].

TGF-β existing in three isoforms, TGF-β_1, TGF-β_2, and TGF-β_3, is the most pleiotropic among immunosuppressive cytokines [68]. In immunity, it is mainly inhibitory for B cells, CD8+ T cells, mononuclear phagocytes, and NK cells. TGF-β production by mucosal Th3 cells, a Treg's subset, supports the isotype switch, including secretory IgA by B cells, and is critical for maintaining immune unresponsiveness to food allergens [14]. TGF-β activates downstream signaling pathway, SMAD, leading to the pro-tolerogenic polarization of target cells functioning [68].

IL-35 activates Jak/STAT signaling pathway to get the following pro-tolerogenic downstream effects: (1) suppression of T cell proliferation; (2) stimulation of naïve T cells into IL-35+Treg cells conversion; (3) inhibition of Th17 cells; and (4) promotion of Breg cells into a Breg subset producing IL-35 and IL-10 [69]. In the clinical study, it has been shown that IL-35 can suppress Th17 activity in allergic rhinitis in children [70].

In the past, IL-27 was recognized as a pro-inflammatory cytokine stimulating the IFN-γ production and development of Th1 cells. But the past decade has seen a more nuanced appreciation of its functional activities, namely, that IL-27 is a potent antagonist of distinct classes of inflammation and inductor of IL-10 synthesis, pTreg and Tr1 differentiation [15]. Besides, IL-27 downregulates receptors of IL-1 and TNF, allergen-presenting by DCs, and upregulates coinhibitory molecules expression. For signal transduction, IL-27 uses Jak/STAT and MAPK signaling pathways [15].

See allergen tolerance in the nose in Fig. 3.5.

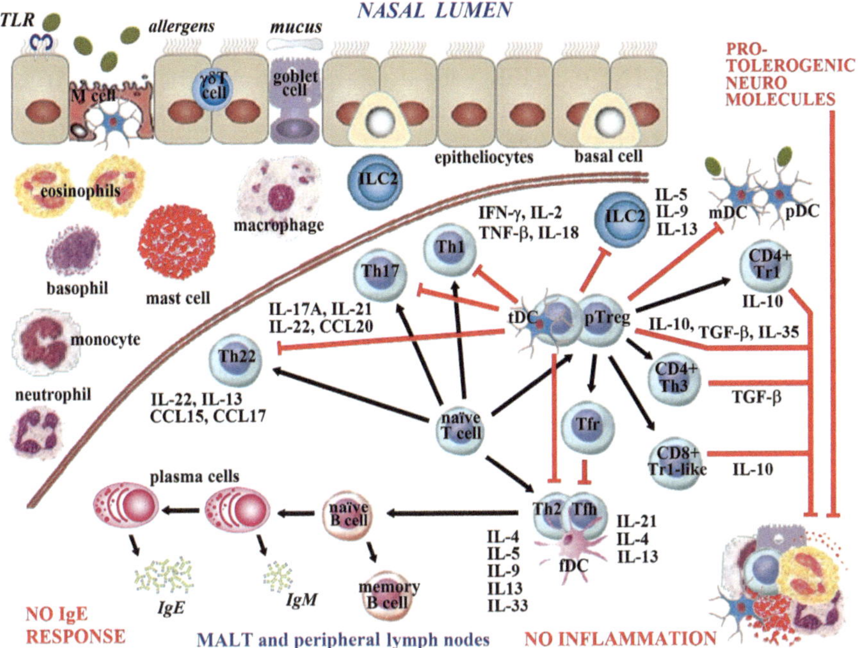

Fig. 3.5 Allergen tolerance in the nose. The principal pro-tolerogenic cells, tDCs, pTregs, and Tregs' subsets through immunosuppressive cytokines and coinhibitory molecules suppress helper T cells, including Th2 cells plus ILC2. So, allergic inflammation cannot continue without the help of Th2 cells and ILC2, and recent portions of IgE and activated eosinophils, neutrophils, and monocytes. Pro-tolerogenic neurotransmitters in the nose also take part in the process. *NB.* Th1 cells are suppressed in part of adaptive T cell responses, not of control for IgG production. ILC2 group 2 innate lymphoid cell, TSLP thymic stromal lymphopoietin, tDC tolerogenic dendritic cell, pTreg peripheral regulatory T cell, mDC myeloid DC, pDC plasmacytoid DC, Tfh follicular helper T cell, Tfr T follicular regulatory cell, fDC follicular DC, Tr1 type 1 regulatory T cell, Th3 type 3 helper T cell

3.6 Coinhibitory Molecules

▶ **Definition** Coinhibitory molecules are the antipode of costimulatory molecules. The coinhibitory molecules suppress the course of the adaptive immune response.

Coinhibitory molecules are essential in maintaining the balance between the capacity to generate effector T cells, allergic inflammation, and preservation of tolerance. In adaptive responses, key coinhibitory molecules control the fate of effector and memory T cells. An important role in immunosuppression is played by such coinhibitory molecules as PD-1, CTLA-4, BTLA, and LAG-3 expressed on T cells and DCs. Importantly, T cells and B cells differ in terms of their set of costimulatory molecules, but the recruitment of coinhibitory molecules is the same.

It has been shown that a blockade of PD-1 strongly enhances proliferation of allergen-specific CD4+ T cells in response to allergens and Th1 and Th2 cytokines profiles (IFN-γ and TNF-α, and IL-5 and IL-13, respectively). Blocking of BTLA resulted in an influence on the allergen-specific T cell growth but not cytokine secretion, whereas CTLA-4 competed with LAG-3 [71].

From a clinical viewpoint, only some coinhibitory molecules have been investigated in clinical trials, that is, PD-1 and CTLA-4. The 2018 Nobel Laureates J Allison (USA) and T. Honjo (Japan) have shown the reliable efficacy of combination anti-CTLA-4 (ipilimumab) and anti-PD-1 (nivolumab), respectively, in therapy for metastatic melanoma patients.

However, tolerance may be reversed by blocking the interactions between coinhibitory molecules and their ligands [72]. For signaling, coinhibitory molecules specifically use different signaling pathways depending on the ligand-receptor interactions.

3.7 Blocking or Competing Antibodies

Over some years, AIT allowed the accumulation of many facts about the pro-tolerogenic mechanism showing an increase in IgG and IgA during therapy. AIT is a tolerance-inducing approach, which causes allergen tolerance re-switching the IgE synthesis on IgG_4 and IgA_2 production. It has been found for the first time that allergen-specific IgG_1 antibodies could be the prevalent protective blocking subisotype in the early phase of sublingual AIT with *Mad d 1*. However, IgG_1 to *Bet v 1* competed with IgE better than IgG_1 binding to *Mal d 1* [73].

It has been shown that the antibody subisotype titer did not correlate with clinical AIT efficacy. During AIT with *Bet v 1*, different antibody subisotypes had heterogeneous patterns of avidity for *Bet v 1*. Inhibition significantly increased during AIT, revealing that induced IgG achieved the ability to block IgE-specific epitopes, i.e., competed with them [74].

Oral AIT with *Ara h 1* and *Ara h 2* resulted in changing the amount and specificity of blood B cells. First, B cells in baseline blood were enhanced approximately three-fold higher. Second, AIT stimulated somatic hypermutations of allergen-specific B cells, and blocking IgG_4 took place [75].

A Breg subset, Br1 cells, CD25+CD71+$CD73^-$, and Treg subsets are responsible for the promotion of blocking antibodies production in constituting allergen tolerance.

3.8 Tolerogenic Microbiota

The microbiota plays a significant role in the human body since it is sometimes referred to as our "forgotten organ" containing at least 100 trillion (10^{14}) microbial cells [76]. Starting at birth, then during life, microbiota settles the skin and all mucosal barrier organs with prevalence in the gut. The role of the host immune system concerning microbiota is paradoxical: first, it has to tolerize "non-self" commensals-symbionts; second, it must protect the host against possible microbial pathogens [77]; third, the immune system has to tolerize contacted, ingested, inhaled, and injected environmental noninfectious proteins and not sense them as allergens ("non-self"). Fortunately, a particular part of microbiota can help the host perform this tolerizing function due to their metabolites, promoting the allergen tolerance maintenance system [78].

Upon dietary fiber fermentation, the gut microbiota produces eight short-chain fatty acids: butyrate, propionate, acetate, formate, isobutyrate, valerate, isovalerate, and 2-methyl butanoate. Part of them possesses tolerogenic activity promoting pTreg cells maturation [79] and downregulating IL-17 in the lamina propria, inhibiting Th2 cells and Th2-linked cytokines, and activating IgA-secreting B cells in the Peyer's patches [78, 80]. Pro-tolerogenic neurotransmitters and neuropeptides (see Chap. 4) in which the gut is rich also contribute to this process. In addition, the excess of gut microbiota metabolites if dysbiosis absent allows the upregulation of tolerogenic systems in the unified airway, skin, and genitourinary organs [78]. Notably, multidirectional interrelations exist between the microbiota of these barrier organs.

Tolerogenic microbiota must meet the following main criteria:

1. producing metabolites that promote allergen tolerance maintenance systems in the whole body at all times,
2. competing with other microbes, which may cause inflammation, and
3. dynamic, positive changes in dependency on the flux microenvironment.

Without taking into account their high level of variability and taxonomic diversity, the influence of the season, topographical and interpersonal aspects, etc., the most critical part of tolerogenic human gut microbiota consists of *Bifidobacterium spp, Clostridia spp, Bacteroides spp,* and *Lactobacillus spp*, particularly *Lactobacillus rhamnosus* [81–83]. In healthy human lungs, normal microbiota, in part tolerogenic, consist of commensals, *Prevotella spp, Veilonella spp, Streptococcus spp,* and *Fusobacterium spp* [84, 85]. Commensals (in part tolerogenic), *Staphylococcus epidermidis, Corynebacterium spp*, and *Malassezia spp*, predominantly colonize the skin sites [83, 86, 87]. Among tolerogenic vaginal microbiota of healthy nonpregnant females, lactate-producing *Lactobacillus spp,* including *Lactobacillus acidophilus* (Döderlein's microflora), is prevalent [88, 89]. In uncircumcised and circumcised men, the composition of normal urethral microbiota differs in terms of a decrease in anaerobic bacteria (*Prevotella spp, Porphyromonas spp*, and *Anaerococcus spp*) except for *Gardnerella spp* and the presence of *Corynebacterium spp* and *Staphylococcus spp* in circumcised males [90, 91].

Quiz A

Reading a question, please choose only one right answer.

Question 1

Depending on allergen's dose, there is no tolerance in a zone:

1. In a high-dose zone.
2. In a medium-dose zone.
3. In a low-dose zone.
4. Outside dose-defined zone.

Question 2
"Tolerogenic allergen" causing tolerogenic response may be associated with:

1. Only a low dose.
2. Only a medium dose.
3. Either a high dose or a low dose.
4. Only a high dose.

Question 3
The source of tolerogenic dendritic (tDC) cells is:

1. Immature dendritic cells.
2. Lymphocytes.
3. Mature dendritic cells.
4. ILC2 cells.

Question 4
Peripheral allergen-specific regulatory T (pTreg) cells originate from:

1. Type 3 helper T cells.
2. Immature dendritic cells.
3. Macrophages.
4. Naïve T cells.

Question 5
Tolerogenic dendritic (tDC) cell and peripheral regulatory T (pTreg) cell:

1. Operate in the ensemble.
2. Counteract each other.
3. Operate on separation.
4. Do not interact with each other.

Question 6
Peripheral regulatory T (pTreg) cells generate the following subsets:

1. DC-10.
2. Th1 and Th17 cells.
3. Tr1 and Th3 cells.
4. Tfr cells.

Question 7
Immunosuppressive cytokines are:

1. IL-10, IL-27, IL-35, and TGF-β.
2. IFN-γ, TNF-β, and IL-2.
3. TNF-β, IL-1, and IL-6.
4. IL-4, IL-5, and IL-13.

Question 8
A pro-tolerogenic effect of pTregs is:

1. Promoting the expression of coinhibitory molecules.
2. Promoting immune responses.
3. Promoting the expression of costimulatory molecules.
4. Promoting the proliferation of ILC2.

Question 9
Coinhibitory molecules for T cells and B cells are:

1. PD-1 and CTLA-4.
2. CD28 and ICOS.
3. Fas and FasL.
4. CD40.

Question 10
Costimulatory molecules for T cells are:

1. PD-1 and CTLA-4.
2. BTLA and LAG-3.
3. CD28 and ICOS.
4. CD40.

Question 11
Costimulatory molecules for B cells are:

1. PD-1 and CTLA-4.
2. BTLA and LAG-3.
3. CD40.
4. CD28 and ICOS.

Question 12
The most potent immunosuppressive cytokine is:

1. IL-27.
2. TGF-β.
3. IL-10.
4. IL-35.

Question 13
Allergen tolerance is:

1. Responsiveness of the immune system to an allergen.
2. Unresponsiveness of the immune system to an allergen.
3. Passive state of the immune system.
4. A form of the immune response.

Question 14
The following effects are not related to pTreg cells:

1. Downregulating helper T cells.
2. Upregulating the immunosuppressive cytokine production.
3. Promoting immune responses.
4. Generating Tr1 and Th3 cells.

Question 15
Tolerogenic microbiota meets this criterium:

1. Producing metabolites that promote allergen tolerance maintenance systems in the whole body at all times.
2. Producing toxins.
3. Causing inflammation in the target organ.
4. Stimulating production of pro-inflammatory cytokines and chemokines.

Question 16
Myeloid-derived suppressor (MDSC) cells have:

1. Pro-inflammatory action.
2. Pro-immunogenic action.
3. Pro-tolerogenic effect.
4. Antiproliferative effect.

3.9 Pro-Inflammatory Factors

Definition Pro-inflammatory cells like mast cells and eosinophils, pro-inflammatory cytokines, chemokines, and neurotransmitters counteract the system of allergen tolerance maintenance.

Allergic inflammation is a well-organized anti-immunosuppressive system containing mast cells, basophils, eosinophils, ILC2, neutrophils, monocytes, macrophages, and inflammatory biomolecules [1], which counteract systemic and local balance in the body even in practically healthy atopic individuals (see Fig. 3.6). Essentially, mast cells, eosinophils, and neutrophils occupy a central place in allergic inflammation.

3.9.1 Mast Cells and Basophils

Mast cell progenitors enter the circulation and complete their tissue maturation, and mature mast cells do not circulate in the bloodstream [92]. They are highly heterogeneous and divided into mast cells expressing tryptase and chymase (MC_{TC}), mast cells

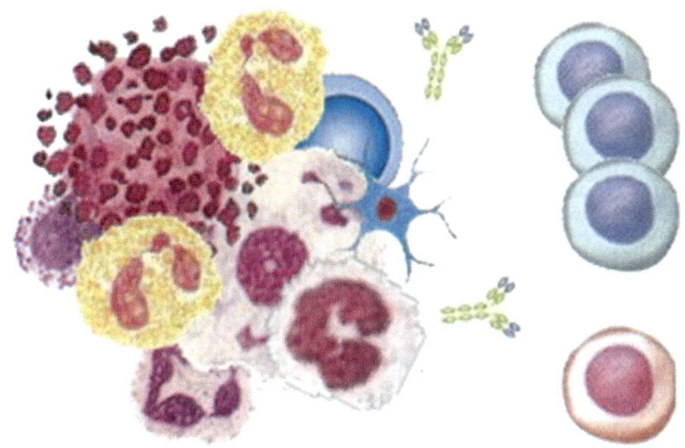

Fig. 3.6 Cells and IgE of allergic inflammation. Activated mast cells, basophils, eosinophils, neutrophils, ILC2, monocytes, and M1 macrophages are related to allergic inflammation cells

expressing only tryptase (MC_T), and the rare mast cells expressing only chymase (MC_C) [93]. MC_{TC}s are mainly located at nonmucosal areas ("connective-tissue mast cells"), but MC_Ts are primarily found at mucosal surfaces ("atypical, or mucosal mast cells"). Human mast cells express the high-affinity receptors for IgE (FcεRI), pro-inflammatory and anti-inflammatory cytokines, chemokines, histamine, prostaglandins, cysteinyl leukotrienes, costimulatory molecules, neuro molecules, and many others [94].

A mast cell contains 50–200 large granules that store inflammatory mediators, which are rich in the following: (1) *preformed mediators*, including histamine, serotonin, dopamine, tryptase, chymase, heparin, chondroitin sulfate, TNF-α, IL-4, IL-15, TGF-β, CCL2 (MCP-1), CCL5 (RANTES), CCL7 (MCP-3), and chemotactic peptides for eosinophils and neutrophils; (2) *neoformed mediators* such as cysteinyl leukotrienes (LTC_4, LTD_4, and LTE_4), leukotriene B_4 (LTB_4), prostaglandin D_2 (PGD_2), prostaglandin E_2 (PGE_2), and platelet-activating factor (PAF); (3) *neosynthesized mediators*: a variety of cytokines and chemokines, growth factors, nitric oxide, and components of complement (C3 and C5) [95, 96]. Preformed mediators are released during the degranulation of mast cells, whereas neoformed mediators are secreted rapidly after preformed, and neosynthesized molecules require little time for production and release. Tryptase is the most excessive mast cells' secretary granule-derived proteinase, which has been considered as the main marker in our understanding of the pathophysiology of this type of cell and clinical laboratory marker. The measurement of serum total mast cell tryptase is the "gold standard," which may help differentiate anaphylaxis from its mimics [97].

For a long time, mast cells were viewed canonically as effector cells in allergic disorders. There is now evidence that they and their different products (soluble mediators, extracellular vesicles, and extracellular DNA traps) communicate with nearly all immune cells and neurons and contribute to the homeostasis of the immune and nervous systems, and take part in the host defense against pathogens, pathogenesis of cancer, and other pathologic processes [94]. Upon exposure to an allergen in the unified airway, mast cells' degranulation leads to vascular permeability, local edema, bronchial and nasal obstruction, and a cough. During exposure to an allergen in the gastrointestinal tract, the allergen permeates through the epithelial layer of the gut's mucosa and binds to IgE on mucosal mast cells. Mast cells respond, increasing fluid secretion, smooth muscle contraction, skin itch, peristalsis, vomiting, and diarrhea.

While basophils and mast cells share the ability to degranulate rapidly and release histamine following high-affinity IgE receptor cross-linking, they differ in their precursors, the capacity of generating inflammatory eicosanoids, and releasing immunomodulating cytokines and chemokines [98]. Besides, basophils leave the bone marrow mature, whereas the mast cells circulate throughout the body in an immature form, maturing once in a tissue site.

Mast cells are upregulated by type 9 helper T cells (IL-9, IL-10), type 2 helper T cells (IL-4, IL-9, IL-13, and particularly IL-33 [99]), and some chemokines, including CCL11 (Eotaxin-1), CCL24 (Eotaxin-2), and CCL26 (Eotaxin-3) [100]. On the other hand, mast cells play a role in the differentiation of type 2 helper T cells and follicular helper T cells.

Activation and degranulation of mast cells occur when allergen/IgE molecules are bound to FcεRI on the cell's surface, and the process proceeds in a phasic manner. Upon binding to allergen/IgE through FcεRI, mast cells use many molecules for signaling, including tyrosine kinase cascade, adapter proteins, Akt/PI3-K and MAPK pathways, and transcription factors (NFAT, AP-1, and NF-κB) to provide the main downstream effect, namely mast cells' degranulation [101].

Meanwhile, many endogenous and exogenous factors can stimulate mast cells to release mediators immediately, causing nonlinked with the immune system *pseudo allergic reactions* (the old term). In the experiment, the mast-cell-specific Mas-related G-protein-coupled receptor (mrgprb2), a murine homolog of human mas-related G-protein-coupled receptor X2 (MRGPRX2), responsible for hyperalgesia possibly due to "neurogenic inflammation" and recruitment of inflammatory cells at the site of injury was identified [102]. Pro-immunogenic neuropeptide substance P, an agonist of MRGPRB2, promoted cells migration via MRGPRB2. In humans, substance P activation of mast cells led to the release of pro-inflammatory cytokines and chemokines via MRGPRX2. As is known, MRGPRX2 meditates mast cell-derived severe IgE-independent allergic manifestation like pseudo allergic reaction [103]. So, mast cells participate in the establishment of "neurogenic inflammation" and may cause IgE-independent allergies.

Recently, the roles of the nervous system in neuronal regulating mast cell actions have been investigated extensively, but much of the current understanding of mechanisms responsible for the neuro molecules' impact on mast cells have been derived from animal models [104].

From a clinical viewpoint, mast cells take part except for allergy in nervous system disorders, angiogenesis, venom detoxification, gastrointestinal and cardiovascular diseases, and some types of cancer; mast cells-derived tryptase is the "gold standard" in diagnosing anaphylaxis.

3.9.2 Eosinophils

For participation in allergic inflammation, eosinophils involve various biomolecules; among them, IL-5 and IL-33 are the main factors required, particularly at the early phase of eosinophil development, for survival, maintenance, and activation of circulating and tissue eosinophils, preventing their apoptosis [105, 106]. IL-5 is produced by Th2 cells, NK cells, mast cells, and eosinophils. IL-5, CCL11 (Eotaxin-1), CCL24 (Eotaxin-2), and CCL26 (Eotaxin-3) [100, 107] serve as essential chemokines for eosinophils. Eosinophils have two types of granules, primary and specific/crystalloid, which contain galectin 10, major basic protein, eosinophilic cationic protein, eosinophilic peroxidase, enzymes, cysteinyl leukotrienes, histaminase, etc. Most of these factors released during degranulation, affect parasites in a toxic manner, and participate in inflammatory processes. Eosinophils degranulate, exhibiting recently described different patterns such as piecemeal degranulation, exocytosis, and cytolysis [108]. Charcot-Leyden (CLC) crystals are found in many biologic fluids, including asthmatic patients' sputum, and consist of a chitinase-like protein, renamed galectin-10 (CLC protein). CLC protein (galectin-10) is overexpressed in eosinophils and identified in basophils, lymphocytes, and macrophages. So, stimulating signals can trigger massive eosinophil release of galectin-10 and even induce eosinophil apoptosis or necrosis. The formation of CLCs may be used as a potential biomarker for eosinophilic inflammation [109]. Analogous to mast cells, eosinophils are capable of phagocytosis and extracellular DNA trapping (NETosis).

It has been shown in many atopic diseases that eosinophils, a main lineage among inflammatory cells, contribute to tissue damage in allergic inflammation. In addition, eosinophil pulmonary tissue infiltration can correlate with the severity of asthma, and the Th2-high/eosinophilic endotype is sometimes a source of uncontrolled asthma [110]. In allergic rhinitis, tissue infiltration by eosinophils occurs during the *late-phase* response, which develops over 4–6 h after exposure to an allergen and lasts for 18–24 h. The duration of eosinophil infiltration may be linked with a nasal epithelial cells injury. In eosinophilic esophagitis, this circumstance can complicate the diagnosis of allergic rhinitis in particular [111]. Esophageal eosinophilic infiltration in gastroesophageal reflux disease also occurs often resulting in damage of the esophageal epithelium. Eosinophil infiltration of the skin in atopic dermatitis and blood eosinophilia correlates with disease severity [107]. Eosinophils binding IL-5 engage two signaling pathways, Jak/STAT and Akt/PI3-K. The transcription factor PU.1 is involved in the transcription of specific genes in eosinophils responsible for granulogenesis and maturation [112], whereas GATA1 is necessary for eosinophil lineage commitment [105].

From a clinical viewpoint, *eosinophilia*, i.e., elevated eosinophil count in the blood, may be caused by parasitic invasions, atopic allergic conditions, drug allergy, some forms of primary immunodeficiencies, an eosinophilic leukemoid reaction, eosinophilic esophagitis, and other nonallergic disorders of tissues.

3.9.3 ILC2

ILC2 shares many functional similarities with Th2 cells [113]. ILC2 is mainly located in the allergen target organs such as the skin, unified airway, and intestinal mucosa and can respond to so-called alarmins, IL-25, IL-33, and thymic stromal lymphopoietin (TSLP), which are produced by the epithelium (particularly, tuft cells) in exposure to allergens. C3a is an additional factor of the ILC2 activation. This process is driven by the pro-inflammatory neurotransmitter neuromedin U [113–115] and, conversely, can ensure an IgE-independent pathway of allergic inflammation [115, 116]. ILC2 secrete the Th2-resemble set of cytokines: IL-4, IL-5, IL-9, IL-13, and IL-17. It has also been shown that ILC2 independently from T cells are present in a higher number in the allergic area, such as in the lungs, nasal polyps, and skin in patients with atopic diseases. Two alarmins, IL-33 and TSLP, are the main cytokines responsible for the skin itch [117]. Upon signal transduction, ILC2 cells use GATA3, RORα and other transcription factors [113].

3.9.4 Neutrophils

Neutrophils are related not only to innate immunity but also to allergies, dividing into two pools, a *circulating pool* and *a marginal pool*, and some subsets, which differ depending on health or pathology [118]. They migrate very fast toward the site of infection, fight the pathogens through phagocytosis and extracellular DNA trapping (NETosis) and take part in allergic inflammation. Circulating neutrophils are a prevalent cell type among leukocytes, making up 45–75%, but in healthy children from 4–5-days-old to 4–5 years of age, lymphocytes predominate over neutrophils in the bloodstream. The cytoplasm of the cells comprises 200 granules of three types: larger azurophilic containing myeloperoxidase, α defensins, neutrophil elastase, and bactericidal/permeability-increasing protein; smaller specific granules possessing NADPH oxidase (responsible for reactive oxygen species—ROS), lysozyme, lactoferrin, cathelicidins, and histaminase; and tertiary granules, which contain metalloproteinases (collagenase, gelatinase).

In the last decade, some new neutrophil phenotypes in homeostasis and diseases have been described, including tumors (e.g., N1 and N2), but the origin of at least part of the additional blood neutrophil phenotypes remains unestablished [118, 119]. A wide range of cytokines and chemokines regulate the neutrophil activity, including IL-17, IL-8 (CXCL8) and chemokines predominantly of the CXCL subfamily: CXCL1 (GROα), CXCL2 (MIP-2α), CXCL3 (MIP-2β), etc., and use chemokine receptors belonging to G-protein coupled receptors family [100, 120]. Neutrophils express many cell surface receptors for recognizing the inflammatory environment. IL-8 binds to IL-8R, then involves MAPK and Akt/PI3-K signaling pathways, phospholipase C and protein kinase C enzymes, and transcription factors NF-κB, AP-1, and others to the gene expression [121, 122]. The various cell surface receptors trigger diverse intracellular signaling [123].

Some years ago, a new role of neutrophils in allergy was revised. Neutrophils and allergen-specific T cells accumulate in patients with allergic late-phase reactions, making allergic inflammation more severe, e.g., Th2-low/Th17/neutrophilic endotype in asthma. In the local cytokine environment, neutrophils are converted into functional antigen-presenting cells [124] and activate allergen-specific effector CD4+ T cells. The upregulation of HLA class II molecules on human neutrophils by GM-CSF, IFN-γ, and IL-3 in vitro and in vivo has been described [125].

3.9.5 Monocytes and Macrophages (M1)

Despite their different morphology, monocytes and M1 macrophages share some functional similarities: phagocytic capacity, producing pro-inflammatory cytokines, and promoting inflammation. At the early phase, activation of monocytes, precursors of macrophages, proceed with supporting the EGR1 transcription factor [126]. Differentiated classical monocytes are short-lived cells that possess some ability to infiltrate inflammatory sites, secrete pro-inflammatory cytokines, and commence the program of differentiation to M1 macrophages, which lasts for 5–7 days [52]. PU.1 acts as a priming transcription factor that allows the process to start. It should be noted that later, EGR1 as the versatile transcriptor factor may exert unexpected repressive activity in tissue-resident macrophages, converting them into anti-inflammatory M2 phenotype [126].

The pro-inflammatory phenotype of macrophages, *type 1 macrophages (M1)* [55], CD64+, originate from yolk/fetal liver and monocytes and operate as participants of any allergic inflammation and antigen presentation for CD4+ T cell-mediated immune response [127], including type IV hypersensitivity. M1 macrophages are a source of a series of pro-inflammatory molecules: IL-1β, TNF-α, IL-6 and other cytokines, chemokines, enzymes including metalloproteinases (e.g., collagenase), complement proteins, reactive oxygen species (ROS) such as nitric oxide and arachidonic acid's metabolites (prostaglandins and leukotrienes) that contribute to atopic allergic inflammation. These molecules can be potentially damaging. Essential chemokines for macrophages are CXCL14 (BRAK), CCL3 (MIP-1α), CCL4 (MIP-1β), and CCL5 (RANTES) [100]. Macrophage's capacity for uncomplete phagocytosis can introduce an imperceptible infectious hazard into inflammation. The excitement of macrophages depends on many factors, among which IFN-γ is a crucial activator for M1 polarization, and binding to IFN-γ, macrophages recruit Jak/STAT signaling pathway [128]. In each case, the precise set of signal transduction is defined by the ligand-receptor interactions.

3.9.6 Inflammatory Dendritic Cells

Monocytes recruited to the sites of allergic inflammation can differentiate into

1. Monocyte-derived "inflammatory" DCs (using transcription factors: BLIMP1, IRF4, and AHR) or
2. Tissue-resident macrophages (using transcription factor MAFB) [129]

The particular DC subset, monocyte-derived inflammatory DCs, meet the following criteria:

1. *Phenotype.* Inflammatory DCs are HLA-DR+CD1c+CD11c+CD206+ cells.
2. *Function.* Inflammatory DCs possess typical DC functions, such as the ability to efficiently stimulate naïve T cells and the capacity to express CCR7, which

allows their migration to lymph nodes. They secrete IL-1β, TNF-α, IL-12, and IL-23 [8].

3. *Morphology.* This DCs subset exhibits a typical DC morphology: the presence of small size and dendrites and lack of large cytoplasmic vacuoles (as opposed to macrophages).
4. *Ontogeny.* Inflammatory DCs derive from monocytes, which can be assessed by analyzing gene signatures or the expression of CCR2. These DCs can be distinguished from monocyte-derived tissue-resident macrophages by the expression of specific transcription factors such as IRF4 and AHR and the absence of MAFB expression [129]. However, the data on the transcription factors are controversial compared with [8].

3.9.7 Helper T Cells

About 30 years ago, Mossmann and Coffman [130] first divided all helper T cells into two helper subsets, Th1 and Th2 cells. This concept was called *Th1/Th2 paradigm.* At the basic level, *type 1 helper T (Th1) cells* trigger the T cell-mediated immune responses becoming effector CD4+ T cells and upregulators for cytotoxic CD8+ T cells. Th1 cells also take part in antibody switching as upregulators. On the contrary, *type 2 helper T (Th2) cells* upregulate only the advanced B cell-mediated immune response. Both helper subsets can inhibit each other and cancel opposite effects to reorder the immune response pathway.

Under an immunopathologic Th1 polarization condition, Th1 cells are overactivated in intracellular infections, Th1-type autoimmune diseases, repeated spontaneous abortion, etc. The Th2 polarization condition is present in atopic diseases, Th2-type autoimmune diseases, survival of HLA-restricted fetal allograft, etc. However, the Th1/Th2 paradigm taken in its simplistic form is prone to several paradoxes and exceptions. This model may not be related to processes at the mucosal level during the defense against some intracellular microbes.

Some "novel" immunoregulatory cells, including helper T cells and ILC have been discovered [131] (see Tables 3.1 and 3.2).

3.9.8 Inflammatory Chemokines

Chemokines are divided into two functional groups, homeostatic and inflammatory, and four structural subfamilies, C, CC, CXC, and CX3C, depending on the location of cysteine (C) between other amino acids (X) in the chemokine's protein molecule sequence [100]. Most chemokines throughout the body are associated with allergic reactions. For example, CCL11 (Eotaxin-1), CCL17 (TARC), and CCL22 (MDC) upregulate allergic inflammation in all target organs. Chemokine CCL11 binds to CCR3, which is responsible for eosinophil and basophil trafficking. Chemokines CCL17 and CCL22 bind to CCR4, which is expressed mainly on Th2 cells [132]. Chemokine receptors are differentially expressed on all immune cells and divided

Table 3.1 Type 1 and type 2 helper T cells

Subset	*Th1*	*Th2*
Name	Type 1 helper T cell	Type 2 helper T cell
Phenotype	CD4+	CD4+
Chemokine receptors	CCR5 CXCR3	CCR3 CCR4
Cytokines which promote generation	*IL-12*, IFN-γ	*IL-4*
Signaling	T-bet	GATA3
Cytokine profile (key cytokines)	*IFN-γ*, IL-2, TNF-β, and IL-18	*IL-4*, IL-5, IL-6, IL-9, IL-10, IL-13, and IL-33
Target cells	T cells, B cells, macrophages, dendritic cells	B cells, eosinophils, mast cells
Functional activity	T cell-mediated and B cell-mediated responses (antibody switching), defense against intracellular pathogens, activation of macrophages	B cell-mediated response, defense against parasites
Pathological conditions	Type IV hypersensitivity and autoimmune diseases	Type I hypersensitivity (IgE-dependent diseases)
Cooperation	Th17, ILC1, and ILC17	Tfh, Th22, Th9, ILC2, and ILC22

Table 3.2 "Novel" type helper T cells

Subset	*Th9*	*Th17*	*Th22*	*Tfh*
Name	Type 9 helper T cell	Type 17 helper T cell	Type 22 helper T cell	Follicular helper T cell
Phenotype	CD4+	CD4+	CD4+	CD4+
Chemokine receptors	CCR6	CCR6	CCR10	CXCR5
Cytokines which promote generation	*IL-4*, TGF-β, IL-2, and IL-25	*IL-23*, IL-21, IL-6, TGF-β	IL-6, TNF-α, PDGF	IL-6, IL-21
Signaling	PU.1, IRF4	RORγt	AHR	Bcl6
Cytokine profile (key cytokines)	*IL-9*, IL-10, and IL-21	*IL-17A*, IL-21, IL-22, and CCL20	*IL-22*, IL-13, FGF, TNF-β, CCL15, and CCL17	*IL-21*, IL-4, and IL-13
Target cells	Mast cells, neutrophils	T cells, B cells, neutrophils, epitheliocytes	T cells, B cells, epitheliocytes, fibroblasts, hepatocytes, neurons	B cells, plasma cells
Functional activity	Defense from helminth and tumor suppression	Pro-inflammatory effects on mucosae and skin, defense against opportunistic infections	Preferentially anti-inflammatory effects on mucosae and skin, epithelium integrity, tissue regeneration	B cell survival and lifelong memory differentiation
Pathological conditions	Type I hypersensitivity (IgE-dependent diseases) and autoimmunity participation	Type IV hypersensitivity and autoimmune diseases	Type I hypersensitivity (IgE-dependent diseases)	Type I hypersensitivity (IgE-dependent diseases)
Cooperation	Th2 and Th17	Th1, ILC1, and ILC17	Tfh, Th9, and ILC22	Th2, Th22, ILC2, and ILC22

into G protein-coupled signaling receptors and atypical nonsignaling receptors [100]. Chemokines binding to these receptors involve many molecules required for signal transduction. In particular, there are Akt/PI3-K and Ras/MAPK signaling pathways, inositol-triphosphate/diacylglycerol metabolic pathway, and phospholipase Cβ and protein kinase C enzymes.

From a clinical viewpoint, the modern chemokines' knowledge must step by step convert into new anti-allergy therapies. Unfortunately, the blockade of one chemokine receptor is not sufficient for successful treatment. Therefore, it could be essential to specific target cells with a mixture of receptor blockers administered in the unified airway, gastrointestinal tract, and skin to overcome this problem.

3.9.9 Molecular Patterns Promote Allergic Inflammation

It is well-known that any infectious process can both downregulate and upregulate allergen tolerance breakdown. There are molecules, pattern recognition receptors (PRRs), expressed on cells of the innate immunity, which are capable of sensing patterns, triggering the reactions of innate immunity such as inflammation and taking part in adaptive immune responses, for example, IgE-dependent responses to allergens. PRRs (for example, toll-like receptors—TLRs) can bind to allergens, and after signaling, promote the release of epithelium-derived alarmins, which activate ILC2, DCs, and Th2 cells. Allergen-associated molecular patterns (AAMP) are specialized to facilitate atopic responses [133]. Typically, PRRs contain one or several C-terminal recognizing or regulatory domains that sense patterns, N-terminal effector domains associated with signaling molecules, and a central domain. To date, some families of PRRs have been described as follows, and most of them concern allergen tolerance:

1. Toll-like receptors (TLRs);
2. C-type lectin receptors (CLRs);
3. NOD-like receptors (NLRs);
4. RIG-1-like receptors (RLRs);
5. AIM-2-like receptors (ALRs).

Viral and bacterial infections mainly enter the body along with TLRs, whereas mycobacterial and fungal infections transmit body using CLRs (see Fig. 3.7). In addition, AAMP and allergens are sensed by PRRs, FcεRI, and IgE.

The concept of allergen-associated molecular patterns (AAMPs) was proposed based on the specific features of immunoglobulin E (IgE), which requires the recognizing of either "continuous epitopes" consisting of a row of consecutive amino acids or "discontinuous epitopes," composed of amino acids from different portions placed close together due to folding the allergen molecule. It makes allergens achievable for recognition by natural or artificial oligomerization [133]. The spacing of IgE epitopes is essential in triggering the IgE-dependent atopic response as it facilitates allergen processing and presentation. An optimal distance of 92–102 Å

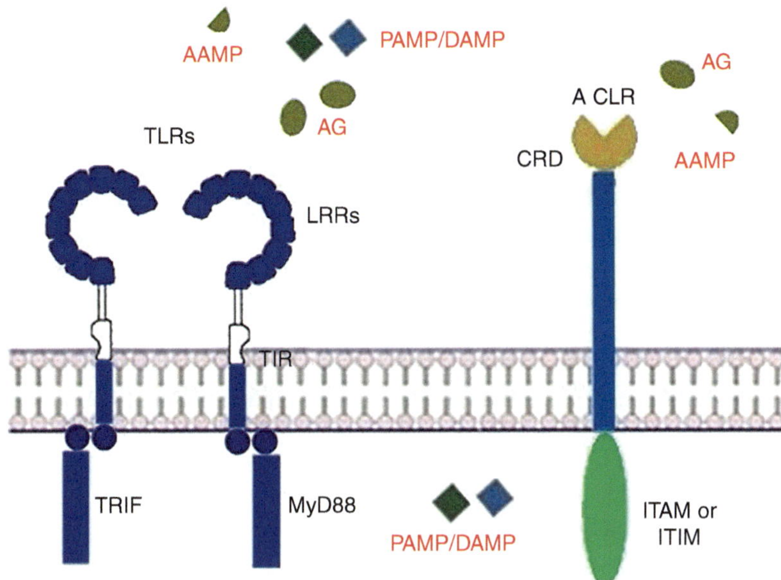

Fig. 3.7 Pattern recognition receptors. Toll-like receptors (TLRs) and C-type lectin receptors (CLRs) are related to pattern-recognizing receptors (PRRs), and ligands for PRRs are molecular patterns (PAMP, DAMP, and AAMP) and allergens. After signaling, the promotion of immune responses appears. AG allergens, TLRs toll-like receptors, TIR toll/IL-1 receptor domain, CLR C-type lectin receptor, PAMP pathogen-associated molecular pattern, DAMP damage-associated molecular pattern, AAMP allergen-associated molecular pattern, LRRs leucine-rich repeat domains, CRD carbohydrate recognition domain, TRIF and MyD88 signaling molecules, ITAM immunoreceptor tyrosine-based activation motif, ITIM immunoreceptor tyrosine-based inhibition motif

between two IgE sites or molecules for cross-linking is created by AAMPs. So, AAMPs upregulate IgE-response and allergic inflammation.

It has long been acknowledged that 10 TLRs respond to a variety of pathogen-associated molecular patterns (PAMPs), including lipopolysaccharide (TLR4), lipopeptides (TLR2 associated with TLR1 or TLR6), bacterial flagellin (TLR5), viral dsRNA (TLR3), viral or bacterial ssRNA (TLR7 and TLR8), and CpG-rich unmethylated DNA (TLR9), among others [134]. TLRs are expressed on the (1) membranes of macrophages, neutrophils, eosinophils, dendritic cells, lymphocytes, epitheliocytes, etc., and present in the (2) cell endosomes. The term "toll" comes from drosophila, in which TLRs were first identified. TLRs contain leucine-rich repeat (LRR) domains and a Toll/IL-1 receptor (TIR) domain, linked to signaling molecules including MyD88, TRIF, etc. After binding to ligands, most TLRs transduce signals in MyD88-dependent and TRIF-dependent pathways and eventually lead to the activation of inflammatory reactions, including allergies. TLRs can recognize PAMPs, AAMPs, and DAMPs and provide a link between innate and adaptive immunity as they can interact with allergens too. A pathogen bound to TLRs may be engulfed, digested, and presented to lymphocytes in immunogenic form.

Table 3.3 C-type lectin receptors

CLR		PRR/ligand	Effects
Dectin 1		PRR binding to β-glucans	Inhibits Th2 response
Dectin 2		PRR binding to rich mannose structure, and AAMP [136]	Induces Th2 response
DC-SIGN		PRR binding to fucose	Induces DC-10
SIGLEC[a]		Receptors binding to sialylated antigens	Downregulates eosinophil and mast cell inflammation
Galactins		Soluble glycoreceptors recognizing galactose	Inhibits eosinophil, mast cell inflammation, and induces pTregs

[a]SIGLEC8 is a target for biologic lirentelimab, which is currently on a clinical trial [137]

A lot of C-type lectin receptors (CLR) have been identified so far [135]. Expressed on myeloid cells, they play a central role in innate immunity. The CLRs are recognized between those that have an "immunoreceptor tyrosine-based activation motif" (ITAM) and those with an "immunoreceptor tyrosine-based inhibition motif" (ITIM). Thus, they can mediate either activating or inhibiting signals to the immune system depending on the ligand (see Table 3.3)

Key Points

1. Allergen tolerance is the unresponsiveness of the immune system to an allergen when the clinical symptoms, despite allergen sensitization in atopic individuals, are absent.
2. The framework of allergen tolerance maintenance consists of two main cell lineages: tolerogenic dendritic (tDCs) cells and allergen-specific peripheral regulatory T (pTreg) cells. It also includes regulatory B cells, macrophages (M2), myeloid-derived suppressor cells, helper T cells inhibition mechanisms, via immunosuppressive cytokines, coinhibitory molecules, and transcription factors, as well as blocking antibodies, pro-tolerogenic neurotransmitters, and neuropeptides, enzymes, and tolerogenic microbiota. IL-10 is the most robust immunosuppressive cytokine.
3. A tolerogenic response to a causative allergen, in the beginning, resembles the adaptive immune response since a tolerogenic dendritic cell exerts itself as an allergen-presenting cell, whereas a regulatory T cell is similar to an allergen-recognizing cell. However, there is neither subsequent activation nor clonal expansion like in the adaptive immune response.
4. On the other hand, there are many anti-tolerogenic mechanisms: inflammatory cells like mast cells and eosinophils, inflammatory chemokines, molecular patterns, including allergen-associated molecular patterns (AAMPs).

Take-Home Messages

1. Write an essay about tolerogenic dendritic cells.
2. Write an essay about peripheral regulatory T cells.
3. Write an essay about immunosuppressive cytokines.

4. Write an essay about coinhibitory molecules.
5. Make a crossword from tolerance's terms (words).
6. Write an essay about mast cells and basophils in the context of allergen inflammation.
7. Write an essay about eosinophils and neutrophils in the context of allergen inflammation.
8. Write a paragraph about ILC2 in the context of allergen inflammation.
9. Write an essay about microbiota in the context of allergen inflammation.
10. Write an essay about macrophages in the context of allergen inflammation.
11. Write an essay about the inactivation of one type helper T cell.
12. Write an essay about inflammatory chemokines.

Quiz B

Reading a question, please choose only one right answer.

Question 1

The source of tolerogenic dendritic (tDC) cells is:

1. Mature dendritic cells.
2. Macrophages.
3. Immature dendritic cells.
4. Lymphocytes.

Question 2

Myeloid-derived suppressor (MDSC) cells have:

1. Pro-tolerogenic action.
2. Pro-immunogenic action.
3. Pro-inflammatory effect.
4. Immune responses-promoting effect.

Question 3

M1 macrophages have:

1. Pro-immunogenic action.
2. Pro-tolerogenic action.
3. Anti-inflammatory effect.
4. Immune responses-suppressing effect.

Question 4

M2 macrophages have:

1. Pro-inflammatory action.
2. Pro-immunogenic action.
3. Pro-tolerogenic effect.
4. Immune responses-promoting effect.

Question 5
Immunosuppressive cytokines are:

1. IFN-γ, TNF-β, and IL-2.
2. IL-10, IL-27, IL-35, and TGF-β.
3. TNF-β, IL-1, and GM-CSF.
4. IL-4, IL-5, and IL-13.

Question 6
Peripheral regulatory T (pTreg) cells originate from:

1. Type 1 regulatory T cells.
2. Naïve T cells.
3. Macrophages.
4. Myeloid-derived suppressor cells.

Question 7
Peripheral regulatory T (pTreg) cells generate the following subsets:

1. Th1 and Th17 cells.
2. DC-10 cells.
3. Tfr cells.
4. Tr1 and Th3 cells.

Question 8
The following effects are not related to pTreg cells:

1. Promoting immune responses.
2. Upregulating the immunosuppressive cytokine production.
3. Downregulating helper T cells.
4. Generating Tr1 and Th3 cells.

Question 9
Peripheral regulatory T (pTreg) cells function together with:

1. M1 macrophages.
2. Eosinophils.
3. Tolerogenic DCs.
4. Th2 cells.

Question 10
Typically, a pro-tolerogenic effect of pTregs is:

1. Triggering apoptosis in target cells.
2. Phagocyting target cells.
3. Upregulating Th1 cells.
4. Downregulating tDCs.

Question 11
Typically, a pro-tolerogenic effect of pTregs is:

1. Promoting the expression of costimulatory molecules.
2. Promoting immune responses.
3. Promoting the expression of coinhibitory molecules.
4. Promoting the proliferation of ILC2.

Question 12
Allergic inflammation cells group does not include:

1. M2 macrophages.
2. Eosinophils.
3. ILC2.
4. Mast cells.

Question 13
T follicular regulatory (Tfr) cells exert an effect:

1. Upregulating re-switching antibodies isotype.
2. Inhibiting follicular helper T (Tfh) cells.
3. Upregulating self-reactive T cells.
4. Promoting B cell immune responses.

Question 14
Regulatory B (Breg) cells exert an effect:

1. Suppressing CD4+ T cell proliferation.
2. Downregulating TGF-β production.
3. Downregulating IL-35 production.
4. Upregulating IgG_4 antibodies production.

Question 15
The most potent immunosuppressive cytokine is:

1. IL-10.
2. TNF-β.
3. IL-4.
4. IL-35.

Question 16
Coinhibitory molecules are:

1. CD40.
2. CD28 and ICOS.
3. Fas and FasL.
4. PD-1 and CTLA-4.

References

1. Wisniewski J, Agrawal R, Woodfolk JA. Mechanisms of tolerance induction in allergic disease: integrating current and emerging concepts. Clin Exp Allergy. 2013;43(2):164–76. https://doi.org/10.1111/cea.12016.
2. Abdel-Gadir A, Massoud AH, Chatila TA. Antigen-specific Treg cells in immunological tolerance: implications for allergic diseases. F1000Res. 2018;7:1–13. https://doi.org/10.12688/f1000research.12650.
3. Calzada D, Baos S, Cremades-Jimeno L, Cárdaba B. Immunological mechanisms in allergic diseases and allergen tolerance: the role of Treg cells. J Immunol Res. 2018;2018:6012053. https://doi.org/10.1155/2018/6012053.
4. Calderón MA, Linneberg A, Kleine-Tebbe J, De Bay F, de Rojas DHF, Virchow JC. Respiratory allergy caused by house dust mites: what do we really know? J Allergy Clin Immunol. 2015;136(1):38–47. https://doi.org/10.1016/j.jaci.2014.10.012.
5. Matsuoka T, Shaji MH, Durham SR. Allergen immunotherapy and tolerance. Allergol Int. 2013;62:403–13. https://doi.org/10.2332allergolint.13-RAI-0650.
6. Zhang J, Tao A. Antigenicity, immunogenicity, allergenicity. In: Tao A, Raz E, editors, Allergy bioinformatics, Chapter 11. Cham: Springer; 2015. https://doi.org/10.1007/978-94-017-7444-4_11.
7. Testera-Montes A, Salas M, Palomares F, Ariza A, Torres MJ, Rondón C, Eguiluz-Gracia I. Local respiratory allergy: from rhinitis phenotype to disease spectrum. Front Immunol. 2021;12:691964. https://doi.org/10.3389/fimmu.2021.691964.
8. Collin M, Bigley V. Human dendritic cell subsets: an update. Immunology. 2018;154:3–20. https://doi.org/10.1111/imm.12888.
9. Raker VK, Domogalla MP, Steinbrink K. Tolerogenic dendritic cells for regulatory T cell induction in man. Front Immunol. 2015;6:569. https://doi.org/10.3389/fimmu.2015.00569.
10. Iberg CA, Hawiger D. Natural and induced tolerogenic dendritic cells. J Immunol. 2020;204(4):733–44. https://doi.org/10.4049/jimmunol.1901121.
11. Nam J-H, Lee J-H, Choi S-Y, Jung N-C, Song J-Y, Seo H-G, et al. Functional ambivalence of dendritic cells: tolerogenicity and immunogenicity. Int J Mol Sci. 2021;22:4430. https://doi.org/10.3390/ijms22094430.
12. Fucikova J, Palovs-Jelinkova L, Bartunkova J, Spisek R. Induction of tolerance and immunity by dendritic cells: mechanisms and clinical applications. Front Immunol. 2019;10:2393. https://doi.org/10.3389/fimmu.2019.02393.
13. Hasegawa H, Matsumoto T. Mechanisms of tolerance induction by dendritic cells in vivo. Front Immunol. 2018;9:350. https://doi.org/10.3389/fimmu.2018.00350.
14. Commins SP, Borish L, Steinke JW. Immunologic messenger molecules: cytokines, interferons, and chemokines. J Allergy Clin Immunol. 2010;125(2):S53–72. https://doi.org/10.1016/j.jaci.2009.07.008.
15. Yoshida H, Hunter CA. The immunobiology of interleukin-27. Annu Rev Immunol. 2015;33:417–43. https://doi.org/10.1146/annurev-immunol-032414-112134.
16. Švajger U, Rožman P. Induction of tolerogenic dendritic cells by endogenous biomolecules: an update. Front Immunol. 2018;9:2482. https://doi.org/10.3389/fimmu.2018.02482.
17. Peters M, Peters K, Bufe A. Regulation of lung immunity by dendritic cells: implications for asthma, chronic obstructive pulmonary disease and infectious disease. Innate Immun. 2019;25(6):326–36. https://doi.org/10.1177/1753425918821732.
18. Domogalla MP, Rostan PV, Raker VK, Steinbrink K. Tolerance through education: how tolerogenic dendritic cells shape immunity. Front Immunol. 2017;8:1764. https://doi.org/10.3389/fimmu.2017.01764.
19. Hansen IS, Krabbendam L, Bernink JH, Loayza-Puch F, Hoepel W, van Burgsteden JA, et al. FcaRI co-stimulation converts human intestinal CD103+ dendritic cells into pro-inflammatory cells through glycolytic reprogramming. Nat Commun. 2018;9(1):863. https://doi.org/10.1038/s41467-018-03318-5.

20. Chen L, Flies DB. Molecular mechanisms of T cell co-stimulation and co-inhibition. Nat Rev Immunol. 2013;13(4):227–42. https://doi.org/10.1038/nri3405.
21. Shevyrev D, Tereshchenko V. Treg heterogeneity, function, and homeostasis. Front Immunol. 2020;10:3100. https://doi.org/10.3389/fimmu.2019.03100.
22. Thornton AM, Korty PE, Tran DQ, Wohlfert EA, Murray PE, Belkaid Y, Shevach EM. Expression of Helios, an Ikaros transcription factor family member, differentiates thymic-derived from peripherally induced Foxp3+ T regulatory cells. J Immunol. 2010;184(7):3433–41. https://doi.org/10.4049/jimmunol.0904028.
23. Liu G, Liu M, Wang J, Mou Y, Che H. The role of regulatory T cells in epicutaneous immunotherapy for food allergy. Front Immunol. 2021;12:660974. https://doi.org/10.3389/fimmu.2021.660974.
24. Zhou L. How smart can it be: transcriptional regulation of T helper cells by SMAR1. Mucosal Immunol. 2015;8(6):1181–3. https://doi.org/10.1038/mi.2015.71.
25. Zhang H, Kong H, Zeng X, Guo L, Sun X, He S. Subsets of regulatory T cells and their roles in allergy. J Transl Med. 2014;12:125. https://doi.org/10.1186/1479-5876-12-125.
26. Thorman AS, Schneider T, Cyran L, Eckert IN, Kerstan A, Lutz MB. Conversion of anergic T cells into Foxp3- IL-10+ regulatory T cells by a second antigen stimulus in vivo. Front Immunol. 2021;12:704578. https://doi.org/10.3389/fimmu.2021.704578.
27. Roncarolo MG, Gregpri S, Bacchetta R, Battaglia M, Gagliani N. The biology of T regulatory type 1 cells and their therapeutic application in immune-mediated diseases. Immunity. 2018;49(6):1004–19. https://doi.org/10.1016/j.immuni.2018.12.001.
28. Yadava K, Medina CO, Ihsak H, Gurevich I, Kuipers H, Shamskhou EA, et al. Natural Tr1-like cells do not confer long-term tolerogenic memory. eLife. 2019;8:e44821. https://doi.org/10.7554/eLife.44821.
29. Martín-Orozco E, Norte-Muñoz M, Martínez-García J. Regulatory T cells in allergy and asthma. Front Pediatr. 2017;5:117. https://doi.org/10.3389/fped.2017.00117.
30. Schmitt EG, Williams CB. Generation and function of induced regulatory T cells. Front Immunol. 2013;4:152. https://doi.org/10.3389/fimmu.2013.00152.
31. Kupriyanov SV, Sinitsky AI, Dolgushin II. Multiple subsets of regulatory T-cells. Bull Sib Med. 2020;19(3):144–55. https://doi.org/10.20538/1682-0363-2020-3-144-155.
32. Sage PT, Sharpe AH. T follicular regulatory cells. Immunol Rev. 2016;271(1):46–259. https://doi.org/10.1111/imr.12411.
33. Hoefig KP, Heissmeyer V. Posttranscriptional regulation of T helper cell fate decisions. J Cell Biol. 2018;217(8):2615–31. https://doi.org/10.1083/jcb.201708075.
34. Valmori D, Raffin C, Raimbaud I, Ayyoub M. Human RORgammat+ TH17 cells preferentially differentiate from naive FOXP3+Treg in the presence of lineage-specific polarizing factors. Proc Natl Acad Sci U S A. 2010;107(45):19402–7. https://doi.org/10.1073/pnas.1008247107.
35. Olivera A, Laky K, Hogan SP, Frischmeyer-Guerreiro P. Editorial: innate cells in the pathogenesis of food allergy. Front Immunol. 2021;2:709991. https://doi.org/10.3389/fimmu.2021.709991.
36. Lu Y, Craft J. T follicular regulatory cells: choreographers of productive germinal center responses. Front Immunol. 2021;12:679909. https://doi.org/10.3389/fimmu.2021.679909.
37. Motos TR, Hirakawa M, Alho AC, Neleman L, Graca L, Ritz J. Maturation and phenotypic heterogeneity of human CD4+ regulatory T cells from birth to adulthood and after allogeneic stem cell transplantation. Front Immunol. 2021;11:570550. https://doi.org/10.3389/fimmu.2020.570550.
38. Zou XL, Chen ZG, Zhang TT, Feng DY, Li HT, Yang HL. Th17/Treg homeostasis, but not Th1/Th2 homeostasis, is implicated in exacerbation of human bronchial asthma. Ther Clin Risk Manag. 2018;14:1627–36. https://doi.org/10.2147/TCRM.S172262.
39. Hua J, Inomata T, Chen Y, Foulsham W, Stevenson W, Shiang T, et al. Pathological conversion of regulatory T cells is associated with loss of allotolerance. Sci Rep. 2018;8:7059. https://doi.org/10.1038/s41598-018-25384-x.

40. Zissler UM, Schmidt-Weber CB. Predicting success of allergen-specific immunotherapy. Front Immunol. 2020;11:1826. https://doi.org/10.3389/fimmu.2020.01826.
41. Voo KS, Wang YH, Santori FR, Boggiano C, Wang YH, Arima K, et al. Identification of IL-17-producing FOXP3+ regulatory T cells in humans. Proc Natl Acad Sci U S A. 2009;106(12):4793–8. https://doi.org/10.1073/pnas.0900408106.
42. Martínez-Blanco M, Lozano-Ojalvo D, Pérez-Rodríguez L, Benedé S, Molina E, López-Fandiño R. Retinoic acid induces functionally suppressive Foxp3+RORγt+ T cells in vitro. Front Immunol. 2021;12:675733. https://doi.org/10.3389/fimmu.2021.675733.
43. Rivas MN, Burton OT, Rachd R, Chatila TF. Regulatory T cell reprogramming toward a Th2-cell-like lineage impairs oral tolerance and promotes food allergy. Immunity. 2015;42(3):512–23. https://doi.org/10.1016/j.immuni.2015.02.004.
44. Gratz IK, Campbell DJ. Organ-specific and memory Treg cells: specificity, development, function, and maintenance. Front Immunol. 2014;5:333. https://doi.org/10.3389/fimmu.2014.00333.
45. Akdis M, Akdis CA. Mechanisms of allergen-specific immunotherapy: multiple suppressor factors at work in immune tolerance to allergens. J Allergy Clin Immunol. 2014;133:621–31. https://doi.org/10.1016/j.jaci.2013.12.1088.
46. Kucuksezer UC, Ozdemir C, Cevhertas L, Ogulur I, Akdis M, Akdis CA. Mechanisms of allergen-specific immunotherapy and allergen tolerance. Allergol Int. 2020;69(4):549–60. https://doi.org/10.1016/j.alit.2020.08.002.
47. Ran Z, Yue-Bei L, Qui-Ming Z, Huan Y. Regulatory B cells and its role in central nervous system inflammatory demyelinating diseases. Front Immunol. 2020;11:1884. https://doi.org/10.3389/fimmu.2020.01884.
48. Peng B, Ming Y, Yang C. Regulatory B cells: the cutting edge of immune tolerance in kidney transplantation. Cell Death Dis. 2018;9:109. https://doi.org/10.1038/s41419-017-0152-y.
49. Abebe EC, Dejenie TA, Ayele TM, Baye ND, Teshome AA, Muche ZT. The role of regulatory B cells in health and diseases: a systemic review. J Inflamm Res. 2021;14:75–84. https://doi.org/10.2147/JIR.S286426.
50. van den Veen W, Stanic B, Yaman G, Wawrzyniak M, Sollner S, Akdis DG, et al. IgG4 production is confined to human IL-10-producing regulatory B cells that suppress antigen-specific immune responses. J Allergy Clin Immunol. 2013;131:1204–12. https://doi.org/10.1016/j.jaci.2013.01.014.
51. Abdelaziz MH, Abdelwahab SF, Wan J, Cai W, Huixuan W, Jianjun C, et al. Alternatively activated macrophages; a double-edged sword in allergic asthma. J Transl Med. 2020;18:58. https://doi.org/10.1186/s12967-020-02251-w.
52. Guilliams M, Mildner A, Yona S. Developmental and functional heterogeneity of monocytes. Immunity. 2018;49:595–613. https://doi.org/10.1016/j.immuni.2018.10.005.
53. Ross EA, Devitt A, Johnson JR. Macrophages: the good, the bad, and the gluttony. Front Immunol. 2021;12:708186. https://doi.org/10.3389/fimmu.2021.708186.
54. Shrivastava R, Shukla N. Attributes of alternatively activated (M2) macrophages. Life Sci. 2019;224:222–31. https://doi.org/10.1016/j.lfs.2019.03.062.
55. Lee J-W, Chun W, Lee HJ, Min J-H, Kim S-M, Seo J-Y, et al. The role of macrophages in the development of acute and chronic inflammatory lung diseases. Cell. 2021;10:897. https://doi.org/10.3390/cells10040897.
56. Wang LX, Zhang SX, Wu HJ, Rong XL, Guo J. M2b macrophage polarization and its roles in diseases. J Leukoc Biol. 2019;106:345–58. https://doi.org/10.1002/JLB.3RU1018-378RR.
57. Chiaranunt P, Tai SL, Ngai L, Mortha A. Beyond immunity: underappreciated functions of intestinal macrophages. Front Immunol. 2021;12:749708. https://doi.org/10.3389/fimmu.2021.749708.
58. Caruso S, Poon IKH. Apoptotic cell-derived extracellular vesicles: more than just debris. Front Immunol. 2018;9:1486. https://doi.org/10.3389/fimmu.2018.01486.
59. Gabrilovich DI, Nagaraj S. Myeloid-derived suppressor cells as regulators of the immune system. Nat Rev Immunol. 2009;9:162–74. https://doi.org/10.1038/nri2506.

60. Bruger AM, Dorhoi A, Esendagli G, Barczyk-Kahlert K, van der Bruggen P, Lipoldova M, et al. How to measure the immunosuppressive activity of MDSC: assays, problems and potential solutions. Cancer Immunol Immunother. 2018;68(4):631–44. https://doi.org/10.1007/s00262-018-2170-8.
61. Falck-Jones S, Vangeti S, Yu M, Falck-Jones R, Cagigi A, Badolati I, et al. Functional monocytic myeloid-derived suppressor cells increase in blood but not airways and predict COVID-19 severity. J Clin Invest. 2021;131(6):e144734. https://doi.org/10.1172/JCI144734.
62. Deshane J, Zmijewski JW, Luther R, Gaggar A, Deshane R, Lai J-F, et al. Free radical-producing myeloid-derived regulatory cells: potent activators and suppressors of lung inflammation and airway hyperresponsiveness. Mucosal Immunol. 2011;4:503–18. https://doi.org/10.1038/mi.2011.16.
63. Shi M, Shi G, Tang J, Kong D, Bao Y, Xiao B, et al. Myeloid-derived suppressor cell function is diminished in aspirin-triggered allergic airway hyperresponsiveness in mice. J Allergy Clin Immunol. 2014;134(5):1163–674.e16. https://doi.org/10.1016/j.jaci.2014.04.035.
64. Cao Y, He Y, Wang X, Liu Y, Shi K, Zheng Z, et al. Polymorphonuclear myeloid-derived suppressor cells attenuate allergic airway inflammation by negatively regulating group 2 innate lymphoid cells. Immunology. 2018;156:402–12. https://doi.org/10.1111/imm.13040.
65. Trikha P, Carson WE. Signaling pathways involved in MDSC regulation. Biochim Biophys Acta. 2014;1846(1):55–65. https://doi.org/10.1016/j.bbcan.2014.04.003.
66. Wei H-X, Wang B, Li B. IL10 and IL22 in mucosal immunity: driving protection and pathology. Front Immunol. 2020;11:1315. https://doi.org/10.3389/fimmu.2020.01315.
67. Islam H, Chamberlain TC, Mui AL, Little JP. Elevated interleukin-10 levels in COVID-19: potentiation of pro-inflammatory responses or impaired anti-inflammatory action? Front Immunol. 2021;12:677008. https://doi.org/10.3389/fimmu.2021.677008.
68. Tirado-Rodriguez B, Ortega E, Segura-Medina P, Huerta-Yepez S. TGF-β: an important mediator of allergic disease and a molecule with dual activity in cancer development. J Immunol Res. 2014;2014:318481. https://doi.org/10.1155/2014/318481.
69. Zhu J-J, Shan N-N. Immunomodulatory cytokine interleukin-35 and immune thrombocytopaenia. J Int Med Res. 2020;48(12):1–13. https://doi.org/10.1177/0300060520976477.
70. Xie F, Hu Q, Cai Q, Yao R, Ouyang S. IL35 inhibited Th17 response in children with allergic rhinitis. ORL J Otorhinolaryngol Relat Spec. 2020;82(1):47–52. https://doi.org/10.1159/000504197.
71. Rosskopf S, Jahn-Schmid B, Schmetterer KG, Ziabinger GJ, Steinberger P. PD-1 has a unique capacity to inhibit allergen-specific human CD4+ T cell responses. Sci Rep. 2018;8:13543. https://doi.org/10.1038/s41598-018-31757-z.
72. Viganò S, Perreau M, Pantaleo G, Harari A. Positive and negative regulation of cellular immune responses in physiologic conditions and diseases. Clin Dev Immunol. 2012;2012:485781. https://doi.org/10.1155/2012/485781.
73. Acosta GS, Kinaciyan T, Kitzmüller C, Möbs C, Pfützner W, Bohle B. IgE-blocking antibodies following SLIT with recombinant *Mal d 1* accord with improved apple allergy. J Allergy Clin Immunol. 2020;146(4):894–900.e2. https://doi.org/10.1016/j.jaci.2020.03.015.
74. Huber S, Lang R, Steiner M, Aglas L, Ferreira F, Wallner M, et al. Does clinical outcome of birch pollen immunotherapy relate to induction of blocking antibodies preventing IgE from allergen binding? A pilot study monitoring responses during first year of AIT. Clin Transl Allergy. 2018;8:39. https://doi.org/10.1186/s13601-018-0226-7.
75. Hoh RA, Joshi SA, Liu Y, Wang C, Roskin KM, Lee J-Y, et al. Single B-cell deconvolution of peanut-specific antibody responses in allergic patients. J Allergy Clin Immunol. 2016;137(1):157–67. https://doi.org/10.1016/j.jaci.2015.05.029.
76. Clemente JC, Ursell LK, Parfey WL, Knight R. The impact of the gut microbiota on human health: an integrative view. Cell. 2012;148(6):1258–70. https://doi.org/10.1016/j.cell.2012.01.035.
77. Swiatczak B, Cohen IR. Gut feelings of safety: tolerance to the microbiota mediated by innate immune receptors. Microbiol Immunol. 2015;59:573–85. https://doi.org/10.1111/1348-0421.12318.

78. Pascal M, Perez-Gordo M, Caballero T, Escribese MM, Longo MNL, Luengo O, et al. Microbiome and allergic diseases. Front Immunol. 2018;9:1584. https://doi.org/10.3389/fimmu.2018.01584.
79. Asarat M, Apostolopoulos V, Vasiljevoc T, Donkor O. Short-chain fatty acids regulate cytokines and Th17/Treg cells in human peripheral blood mononuclear cells in vitro. Immunol Invest. 2016;45(2):205–22. https://doi.org/10.3109/08820139.2015.1122613.
80. Palm NW, de Zoete MR, Flavell RA. Immune-microbiota interactions in health and disease. Clin Immunol. 2015;159(2):122–7. https://doi.org/10.1016/j.clim.2015.05.014.
81. Satitsuksanoa P, Jansen K, Globinska A, van den Veen W, Akdis M. Regulatory immune mechanisms in tolerance to food allergy. Front Immunol. 2018;9:2939. https://doi.org/10.3389/fimmu.2018.02939.
82. Mangalam AK, Ochoa-Reparaz JO. Editorial: the role of the gut microbiota in health and inflammatory diseases. Front Immunol. 2020;11:565305. https://doi.org/10.3389/fimmu.2020.565305.
83. Coates M, Lee MJ, Norton D, MacLeod AS. The skin and intestinal microbiota and their specific innate immune systems. Front Immunol. 2019;10:2950. https://doi.org/10.3389/fimmu.2019.02950.
84. Sommariva M, Le Noci V, Bianchi F, Camelliti S, Balsari A, Tagliabue E, Sfondrini L. The lung microbiota: role in maintaining pulmonary immune homeostasis and its implications in cancer development and therapy. Cell Mol Life Sci. 2020;77(14):2739–49. https://doi.org/10.1007/s00018-020-03452-8.
85. Evsyutina Y, Komkova I, Zolnikova O, Tkachenko P, Ivashkin V. Lung microbiome in healthy and diseased individuals. World J Respirol. 2017;7(2):39–47. https://doi.org/10.5320/wjr.v7.i2.39.
86. Scharschmidt TC. Establishing tolerance to commensal skin bacteria: timing is everything. Dermatol Clin. 2017;35(1):1–9. https://doi.org/10.1016/j.det.2016.07.007.
87. Byrd AL, Belkaid Y, Serge JA. The human skin microbiome. Nat Rev Microbiol. 2018;16:143–55. https://doi.org/10.1038/nrmicro.2017.157.
88. Al-Nasiry S, Ambrosino E, Schlaepfer M, Morré SA, Wieten L, Willem J, et al. The interplay between reproductive tract microbiota and immunological system in human reproduction. Front Immunol. 2020;11:378. https://doi.org/10.3389/fimmu.2020.00378.
89. Aldunate M, Srbinovski D, Hearps A, Latham CF, Ramsland PA, Gugasyan R, Cone RA, Tachedjian G. Antimicrobial and immune modulatory effects of lactic acid and short chain fatty acids produced by vaginal microbiota associated with eubiosis and bacterial vaginosis. Front Physiol. 2015;6:164. https://doi.org/10.3389/fphys.2015.00164.
90. Onywera H, Williamson A-L, Ponomarenko J, Meiring TL. The penile microbiota in uncircumcised and circumcised men: relationships with HIV and Human Papillomavirus infections and cervicovaginal microbiota. Front Med. 2020;7:383. https://doi.org/10.3389/fmed.2020.00383.
91. Pohl HG, Groah SL, Petez-Losada M, Ljungberg I, Spraque BM, Crandal N, Caldovic L, Hsieh M. The urine microbiome of healthy men and women differs by urine collection method. Int Neurourol J. 2020;24(1):41–51. https://doi.org/10.5213/inj.1938244.122.
92. Krystel-Whittemore M, Dileepan KN, Wood JG. Mast cell: a multi-functional master cell. Front Immunol. 2016;6:620. https://doi.org/10.3389/fimmu.2015.00620.
93. Huber M, Cato ACB, Ainooson GK, Freichel M, Tsvilovskyy V, Jessberger R, et al. Regulation of the pleiotropic effects of tissue-resident mast cells. J Allergy Clin Immunol. 2019;144:S31–45. https://doi.org/10.1016/j.jaci.2019.02.004.
94. Varricchi G, Rossi FW, Galdiero MR, Granata F, Criscuolo G, Spadaro G, et al. Physiological roles of mast cells: Collegium Internationale Allergologicum Update 2019. Int Arch Allergy Immunol. 2019;179:247–61. https://doi.org/10.1159/000500088.
95. da Silva EZM, Jamur MC, Oliver C. Mast cell function: a new vision of an old cell. J Histochem Cytochem. 2014;62(10):698–738. https://doi.org/10.1369/0022155414545334.
96. Komi DEA, Wöhrl S, Bielory L. Mast cell biology at molecular level: a comprehensive review. Clin Rev Allergy Immunol. 2020;58(3):342–65. https://doi.org/10.1007/s12016-019-08769-2.

97. Beck SC, Wilding T, Buka RJ, Baretto RL, Huissoon AP, Krishna MT. Biomarkers in human anaphylaxis: a critical appraisal of current evidence and perspectives. Front Immunol. 2019;10:494. https://doi.org/10.3389/fimmu.2019.00494.
98. Varricchi G, Raap U, Rivellese F, Marone G, Gibbs BF. Human mast cells and basophils-how are they similar how are they different? Immunol Rev. 2018;282:8–34. https://doi.org/10.1111/imr.12627.
99. Wang Y-H. Developing food allergy: a potential immunologic pathway linking skin barrier to gut. F1000Res. 2016;5(F1000 Faculty Rev):2660. https://doi.org/10.12688/f1000research.9497.1.
100. Griffith JW, Sokol CL, Luster AD. Chemokines and chemokine receptors: positioning cells for host defense and immunity. Annu Rev Immunol. 2014;32:659–702.
101. Sibilano R, Frossi B, Pucillo CE. Mast cell activation: a complex interplay of positive and negative signaling pathways. Eur J Immunol. 2014;44:2558–66. https://doi.org/10.1002/eji.201444546.
102. Green DP, Limjunyawong N, Gour N, Pundir P, Dong X. A mast-cell-specific receptor mediates neurogenic inflammation and pain. Neuron. 2019;101:412–20. https://doi.org/10.1016/j.neuron.2019.01.012.
103. Porebski G, Kwiecien K, Pawica M, Kwitniewski M. Mas-related G protein-coupled receptor-X2 (MRGPRX2) in drug hypersensitivity reactions. Front Immunol. 2018;9:3027. https://doi.org/10.3389/fimmu.2018.03027.
104. Xu H, Shi X, Li X, Zou J, Zhou C, Liu W, et al. Neurotransmitter and neuropeptide regulation of mast cell function: a systematic review. J Neuroinflammation. 2020;17:356. https://doi.org/10.1186/s12974-020-02029-3.
105. Mack EA, Pear WS. Transcription factor and cytokine regulation of eosinophil lineage commitment. Curr Opin Hematol. 2020;27(1):27–33. https://doi.org/10.1097/MOH.0000000000000552.
106. Bochner BS. The eosinophil: for better or worse, in sickness and in health. Ann Allergy Asthma Immunol. 2018;121(2):150–5. https://doi.org/10.1016/j.anai.2018.02.031.
107. Ramirez GA, Yacoub M-R, Ripa M, Mannina D, Gariddi A, Saporiti N, et al. Eosinophils from physiology to disease: a comprehensive review. Biomed Res Int. 2018;2018:9095275.
108. Fettrelet T, Gigon L, Karaulov A, Yousefi S, Simon H-U. The enigma of eosinophil degranulation. Int J Mol Sci. 2021;22:7091. https://doi.org/10.3390/ijms22137091.
109. Su J. A brief history of Charcot-Leyden crystal protein/galectin-10 research. Molecules. 2018;23(11):2931. https://doi.org/10.3390/molecules23112931.
110. Guida G, Antonelli A. Eosinophilic phenotype: the lesson from research models to severe asthma. In: Fucs O, Athari SS, editors. Cells of the immune system. London: IntechOpen; 2020. p. 1–22. https://doi.org/10.5772/intechopen.92123.
111. Becker S, Rasp J, Eder K, Berghaus A, Kraner MF, Gröger M. Non-allergic rhinitis with eosinophilia syndrome is not associated with local production of specific IgE in nasal mucosa. Eur Arch Otorhinolaryngol. 2016;273(6):1469–75. https://doi.org/10.1007/s00405-015-3769-4.
112. Nadif R, Zerimech F, Bouzigon E, Matran R. The role of eosinophils and basophils in allergic diseases considering genetic findings. Curr Opin Allergy Clin Immunol. 2013;13(5):507–13. https://doi.org/10.1097/ACI.0b013e328364e9c0.
113. Zheng H, Zhang Y, Pan J, Liu N, Qin L, Liu M, Wang T. The role of type 2 innate lymphoid cells in allergic diseases. Front Immunol. 2021;12:586078. https://doi.org/10.3389/fimmu.2021.586078.
114. Wallrapp A, Riesenfeld SJ, Burkett PR, Abdulnour RE, Nyman J, Dionne D, et al. The neuropeptide NMU amplifies ILC2-driven allergic lung inflammation. Nature. 2017;549:351–6. https://doi.org/10.1038/nature24029.
115. Pasha MA, Patel G, Hopp R, Yang Q. Role of innate lymphoid cells in allergic diseases. Allergy Asthma Proc. 2019;40(3):138–45. https://doi.org/10.2500/aap.2019.40.4217.
116. Yamauchi K, Ogasawara M. The role of histamine in the pathophysiology of asthma and the clinical efficacy of antihistamines in asthma therapy. Int J Mol Sci. 2019;20:1733. https://doi.org/10.3390/ijms20071733.

117. Voisin T, Bouvier A, Chiu IV. Neuro-immune interactions in allergic diseases: novel targets for therapeutics. Int Immunol. 2017;29(6):247–61. https://doi.org/10.1093/intimm/dxx040.
118. Rosales C. Neutrophil: a cell with many roles in inflammation or several cell types? Front Immunol. 2018;9:113. https://doi.org/10.3389/fphys.2018.00113.
119. Hellebrekers P, Vrisekoop N, Koenderman L. Neutrophil phenotypes in health and disease. Eur J Clin Investig. 2018;48(Suppl 2):e12943. https://doi.org/10.1111/eci.12943.
120. Capucetti A, Albano F, Bonecchi R. Multiple roles for chemokines in neutrophil biology. Front Immunol. 2020;11:1259. https://doi.org/10.3389/fimmu.2020;01259.
121. Hawkins PT, Stephens LR, Suire S, Wilson M. PI3K signaling in neutrophils. Curr Top Microbiol Immunol. 2010;346:183–202. https://doi.org/10.1007/82_2010_40.
122. Takami M, Terry V, Petruzzelli L. Signaling pathways involved in IL-8-dependent activation of adhesion through Mac-1. J Immunol. 2002;168(9):4559–66. https://doi.org/10.4049/jimmunol.168.9.4559.
123. Futosi K, Fodor S, Mócsai A. Neutrophil cell surface receptors and their intracellular signal transduction pathways. Int Immunopharmacol. 2013;17(3):638–50. https://doi.org/10.1016/j.intimp.2013.06.034.
124. Polak D, Hafner C, Briza P, Kitzmuller C, Elbe-Burger A, Samadi N, Gschwandtner M, Pfutzner W, Zlabinger GJ, Jahn-Schmid B, Bohle B. A novel role for neutrophils in IgE-mediated allergy: evidence for antigen presentation in late-phase reactions. J Allergy Clin Immunol. 2019;143(3):1143–52. https://doi.org/10.1016/j.jaci.2018.06.005.
125. Takashima A, Yao Y. Neutrophil plasticity: acquisition of phenotype and functionality of antigen-presenting cell. J Leukoc Biol. 2015;98:489–96. http://refhub.elsevier.com/S0091-6749(18)30858-3/sref43
126. Trizzino M, Zucco A, Deliard S, Wang F, Barbieri E, Veglia F, et al. EGR1 is a gatekeeper of inflammatory enhancers in human macrophages. Sci Adv. 2021;7(3):eaaz8836. https://doi.org/10.1126/sciadv.aaz8836.
127. Murray PJ. Macrophage polarization. Annu Rev Physiol. 2016;79:541–66. https://doi.org/10.1146/annurev-physiol-022516-034339.
128. Ivashkiv LB. IFNγ: signalling, epigenetics and roles in immunity, metabolism, disease and cancer immunotherapy. Nat Rev Immunol. 2018;18(9):545–58. https://doi.org/10.1038/s41577-018-0029-z.
129. Tang-Huau TL, Segura E. Human in vivo-differentiated monocyte-derived dendritic cells. Semin Cell Dev Biol. 2019;86:44–9. https://doi.org/10.1016/j.semcdb.2018.02.018.
130. Mosmann TR, Coffman RL. Th1 and Th2 cells: different patterns of lymphokine secretion lead to different functional properties. Annu Rev Immunol. 1989;7:145–73. https://doi.org/10.1146/annurev.iy.07.040189.001045.
131. Zlotnik A. Perspective: insights on the nomenclature of cytokines and chemokines. Front Immunol. 2020;11:908. https://doi.org/10.3389/fimmu.2020.00908.
132. Castan L, Magnan A, Bouchaud G. Chemokine receptors in allergic diseases. Allergy. 2017;72:682–90. https://doi.org/10.1111/all.13089.
133. Pali-Schöll I, Jensen-Jarolim E. The concept of allergen-associated molecular patterns (AAMP). Curr Opin Immunol. 2016;42:113–8. https://doi.org/10.1016/j.coi.2016.08.004.
134. Botos I, Segal DM, Davies DR. The structural biology of toll-like receptors. Structure. 2011;19(4):447–59. https://doi.org/10.1016/j.str.2011.02.004.
135. Peters K, Peters M. The role of lectin receptors and their ligands in controlling allergic inflammation. Front Immunol. 2021;12:635411. https://doi.org/10.3389/fimmu.2021.635411.
136. Drickamer K, Taylor ME. Recent insights into structures and functions of C-type lectins in the immune system. Curr Opin Struct Biol. 2015;34:26–34. https://doi.org/10.1016/j.sbi.2015.06.003.
137. Tontini C, Bulfone-Paus S. Novel approaches in the inhibition of IgE-induced mast cell reactivity in food allergy. Front Immunol. 2021;12:613461. https://doi.org/10.3389/fimmu.2021.613461.

The Role of the Neuroimmune Network in Allergic Inflammation

4

Contents

Didactics

Knowledge. Upon successful completion of this chapter, students should be able to:

1. Describe the neuroimmune system.
2. Distinguish between neurotransmitters and neuropeptides.
3. Name and describe two types of neurotransmitter receptors.
4. List pro-tolerogenic neuro molecules.
5. List pro-immunogenic neuro molecules.
6. List critical neuro molecules.

Supplementary Information The online version contains supplementary material available at [https://doi.org/10.1007/978-3-031-04309-3_4].

V. V. Klimov, *Textbook of Allergen Tolerance*,
https://doi.org/10.1007/978-3-031-04309-3_4

7. Give examples of mutations in genes encoding neuropeptides and enzymes necessary for neurotransmitter synthesis.
8. Describe the role of neurotransmitters in neurologic and mental pathology.
9. Describe the innervation of target organs.
10. Explain the principles of "neurogenic inflammation."
11. Describe the role of neuro molecules in allergen tolerance breakdown.

Acquired Skills. Upon successful completion of this chapter, students should demonstrate the following skills:

1. Interpret the knowledge related to the neuroimmune system.
2. Critically evaluate the scientific literature about neuro molecules.
3. Discuss the scientific articles from the current research literature to criticize experimental data and formulate new hypotheses in allergy.

Attitude and Professional Behaviors. Students should be able to:

1. Have the readiness to be hard-working.
2. Behave professionally at all times.
3. Recognize the importance of studying and demonstrate a commitment.

4.1 Introduction

In the past, due to the compartmentalization of disciplines, biology and biomedical sciences long developed in isolation from each other. In particular, immunology was isolated from neuroscience. Nowadays, there is clear evidence for the production and use of immune factors by the central nervous system and the production and use of neuroendocrine mediators by the immune system. So far, more than 120 such neuro molecules either with pro-immunogenic, or pro-tolerogenic, or immunomodulatory effects, are known. Alterations in communication pathways between these two systems can account for many pathological conditions initially strictly considered organ disorders [1, 2]. The participation of neuro molecules in the pathogenesis of allergic inflammation, including conventional and local endotypes of atopic diseases in the unified airway [3], made this problem very relevant. Some mutations of neuropeptide genes, the genes of enzymes required for neurotransmitter synthesis, and their receptors and transporters' genes may be one more crucial pathologic challenge for allergists and other clinicians [4].

4.2 Innervation of the Allergic Target Organs

The allergic target organs are innervated differently and consequently undergo the effects of a distinct set of synaptic transmission neuro molecules [5] (see Table 4.1).

Table 4.1 Types of synaptic transmission neuro molecules

Category	Characterization of signal transmission	Impact on immune system in the context of allergen tolerance/ allergic inflammation	Molecules
Excitatory neurotransmitters	For a short time, they have managed to increase the electrical excitability on the postsynaptic membrane due to ion flow that leads to the facilitation of signal transmission	Pro-immunogenic, pro-inflammatory (except norepinephrine)	Acetylcholine Norepinephrine Dopamine[a] L-glutamate Histamine
Inhibitory neurotransmitters	For a short time, they have managed to decrease the electrical excitability on the postsynaptic membrane due to ion flow that results in the reduction of signal transmission	Pro-tolerogenic, anti-inflammatory	Serotonin γ aminobutyric acid (GABA) Glycine
Modulatory neurotransmitters	They spend a long time in the cerebrospinal fluid that affects the activity of other neurons, and target cells	Immunomodulatory	Acetylcholine Norepinephrine Dopamine L-glutamate Serotonin
Neurohormones	They act in the whole body	Immunomodulatory, pro-immunogenic	Oxytocin Vasopressin Melatonin
Neuropeptides	They are slow-onset long-lasting modulatory synaptic neuro molecules packaged in large granular vesicles	Pro-immunogenic, pro-inflammatory Pro-tolerogenic, anti-inflammatory	Substance P (SP) Neuromedin U Calcitonin-gene-related peptide (CGRP)[a] Vasoactive intestinal peptide (VIP)[a]
Atypical neurotransmitters (neurochemicals)	They are synthesized “on-demand” and released from the postsynaptic membrane	Immunomodulatory, pro-tolerogenic	Gaseous[a] Endocannabinoids Adenosine, ATP
Nonclassified neurotransmitters	Neuropeptides	Pro-tolerogenic	Endorphins

[a]Also ambivalent effects

The *skin* is innervated by the somatosensory nervous system, which includes a complex of sensory neurons and receptors subtypes such as nociceptors, pruriceptors, thermoreceptors, mechanoreceptors, and chemoreceptors. Neuronal cell bodies are located in the dorsal root ganglia having the central projections to the brainstem and spinal cord [5].

The *gastrointestinal tract* is provided with:

1. Dorsal root ganglia-derived sensory neurons of the somatosensory nervous system.
2. A vegetative nervous system (VNS), which consists of the parasympathetic (vagus nerve) fibers, whose cell bodies reside in the nodose and jugular ganglia, and brainstem, and sympathetic neurons, whose cell bodies reside in the paravertebral ganglia.
3. Its own autonomic, the self-contained nervous system called the enteric nervous system (ENS), which consists of submucosal and myenteric plexuses including intrinsic neurons responsible for gut secretions, nutrient absorption, local blood flow, smooth muscle contractions, and interneurons. The bodies of extrinsic (sympathetic and vagal neurons), associated with the ENS are outside the gut [5–8]. The maintenance of gut homeostasis depends on the coordinated functioning of the ENS and intestinal immune system. These systems appear to control allergen tolerance in the gut due to a prevalence of pro-tolerogenic neurotransmitters and neuropeptides.

In contrast to the skin and gastrointestinal tract, the *unified airway's* innervation is characterized by a distinctive peculiarity [9, 10]. These organs are innervated by

1. Somatosensory neurons having their cell bodies in the jugular/nodose ganglia and thoracic dorsal root ganglia.
2. The vegetative nervous system (VNS) via parasympathetic, whose cell bodies reside in the petrosal ganglion and brainstem, and sympathetic fibers, whose cell bodies reside in the paravertebral ganglia.

However, the unified airway has no own autonomic, self-contained nervous system [5], but the VNS appears to be important for the development of local forms of allergy such as local asthma [11, 12], local allergic rhinitis [13, 14], "dual" allergic rhinitis [15, 16], and local allergic conjunctivitis [17].

4.3 Functional Organization of the Neuroimmune Network

The neuroimmune network's neuronal counterpart consists of neurons and their bodies in the central nervous system, spinal cord, various ganglia, somatosensory, sympathetic, parasympathetic, enteric nerve fibers, and neuro molecules (see Table 4.1). There are also non-neuronal cells, neuroglia, which do not produce electrical impulses, but maintain homeostasis of neurons, supply nutrients and oxygen to neurons, play a specific role in synaptic transmission, and form myelin. The neuroimmune network's neuroendocrine counterpart comprises the hypothalamic-pituitary-adrenal (HPA) axis described by H. Selye (see Fig. 4.1). Neurons of all types of the nervous systems, neuroendocrine cells, non-neuronal cells, and microbiota produce different neuro molecules, which act on the neurons themselves and target organs and cells of the immune system [18, 19].

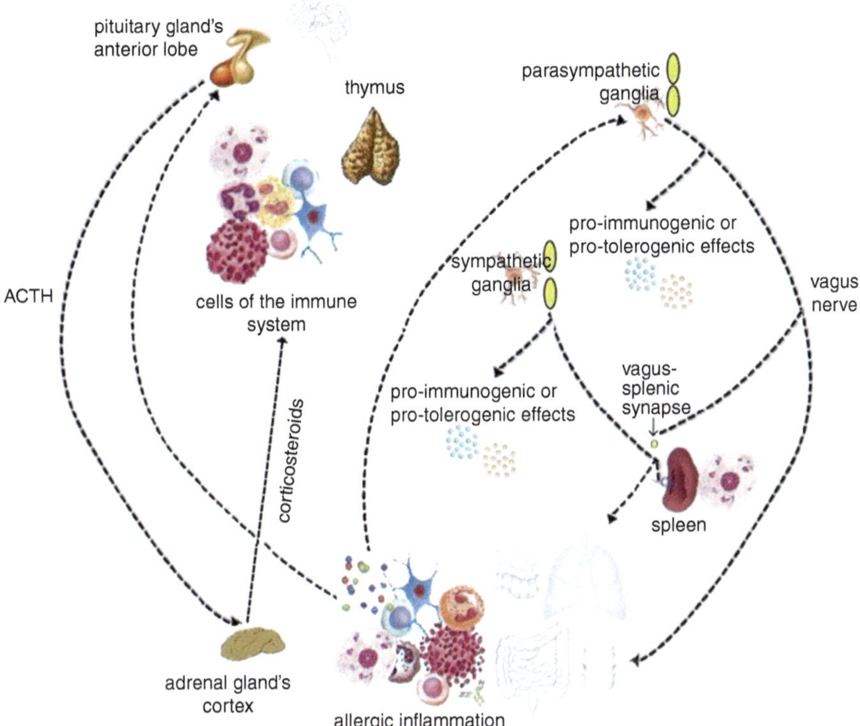

Fig. 4.1 The neuroimmune network. When an allergen enters the body, the hypothalamic-pituitary-adrenal (HPA) axis, a part of the neuroimmune network starts to respond. The pituitary gland's anterior lobe releases adrenocorticotropic (ACTH) hormone upregulating the adrenal cortex to synthesize corticosteroids. The corticosteroids engage immune cells and biomolecules and polarize their activity toward inflammatory or protective non-inflamed phenotypes. The corticosteroids themselves exert a pro-tolerogenic effect, whereas the vagus nerve through pro-immunogenic neurotransmitter acetylcholine more frequently displays a pro-immunogenic action. However, the vagus nerve forms a synapse at the celiac ganglion with the splenic adrenergic nerve allowing the so-called cholinergic anti-inflammatory pathway. ACTH adrenocorticotropic hormone

Following physiologic or pathologic stress, including environmental allergens entry into the body, the pituitary gland's anterior lobe releases adrenocorticotropic (ACTH) hormone stimulating the adrenal cortex to synthesize corticosteroids, which involve different types of the immune system's cells and cytokines, and respectively polarize the activity of immune system to inflammatory or tissue-protective non-inflamed phenotypes [20]. Eventually, corticosteroids exert a pro-tolerogenic effect concerning adaptive immunity. Also, a feedback circuit exists between allergic inflammation and HPA.

The neuroimmune network allows a different modality of immune activity depending on pathologic circumstances. The vagus nerve forms a synapse at the celiac ganglion with the splenic adrenergic nerve, which comes in contact with lymphocytes expressing β_2 adrenergic receptor (β_2AR) that facilitates the synthesis of acetylcholine from lymphocytes. Signal transduction following acetylcholine-induced activation of a nicotinic receptor (a7nAchR) inhibits inflammasome activity to reduce the production of inflammatory cytokines. This neuronal reflex circuit through the afferent vagus nerve, called the cholinergic anti-inflammatory pathway, can attenuate the exacerbated "non-resolving inflammation" by suppressing the accumulation of neutrophils and acting on macrophages, DCs, and lymphocytes [20]. Thus, within the neuro-immune framework, cells of the immune cells acquire more functional plasticity. On the other hand, all neuronal activity types are modulated by cells of the immune system and modified depending on the expressed target cell receptors [21].

A new model for the unified airway, the respiratory tract *neuroimmune unit*, has been supposed to analyze and generalize COVID-19-linked acute respiratory distress syndrome and "cytokine storm" in the lung [10]. In the review, Godinho-Silva et al. [8] have discussed a new paradigm on neuroimmune cell units at discrete anatomical sites and described neuroimmune inputs in the functioning of the gut, lung, skin, adipose tissue, mucosal barriers, and separate cell lineages.

Neuroendocrine (NEC) cells, sometimes called "diffuse neuroendocrine system," are specialized epithelial cells frequently associated with intraepithelial nerve fibers and scattered throughout the body, particularly in the endocrine glands and allergic target organs. They can receive signals from neurons and respond, releasing neuro molecules, hormones, and enzymes [22, 23]. NECs regulate many functions at the systemic and regional levels due to the production of neurotransmitters (GABA, serotonin, norepinephrine, histamine, acetylcholine, etc.) and neuropeptides (CGRP, VIP, etc.) [24, 25]. However, NECs have been reported as cells promoting allergic inflammation though [21]. In particular, CGRP and GABA released from the NECs can exert a pro-immunogenic activity in a controversial manner [25].

4.4 Types of Synaptic Transmission Neuro Molecules

A neurotransmitter must meet some criteria: (1) It must be produced by neurons; (2) It will be present in the first neuron's (i.e., axon's) presynaptic membrane and released in amounts sufficient to exert a defined action on the second neuron's post-synaptic membrane or target cells in effector organs; (3) Exogenous administration should mimic the action of the endogenously synthesized neurotransmitter; and (4) Intrinsic mechanisms must exist to remove neurotransmitters from their site of action [26, 27]. Neurotransmitters are packaged in small synaptic vesicles and found in the blood and target organs, whereas neuropeptides are formed in large synaptic vesicles. On the one hand, neurotransmitters influence innate and adaptive immune responses. But on the other hand, immune cells send signals to the brain through cytokines and are present in the brain to impact neural responses [21].

Some of the neuro molecules, including dopamine, L-glutamate, serotonin, and substance P, are critical in the classical neuroimmune network, closely associated with the hypothalamic-pituitary-adrenal (HPA) axis, vagus nerve, sympathetic nervous system, and vagus-splenic synapse [20]. Depending on their defined action, all neurotransmitters may be categorized as excitatory (*pro-immunogenic*), inhibitory (*pro-tolerogenic*), and modulatory (*immunomodulatory*) (see Table 4.1). Destroyed bidirectional communication between the nervous and immune systems is a common feature in immunopathological disorders [20, 28].

The brain also synthesizes molecules, neurochemicals, neurohormones, and neuropeptides, which act on various receptors of the immune system's cells but do not fulfill the criteria for neurotransmitters [29–32]. So far, only 12 small-molecule neurotransmitters and over 100 neuropeptides have been identified [18]. During crosstalk between the nervous system and immune system, most neuro molecules exploit membrane vesicles, ligand-gated, voltage-gated and stretch-activated ion channels, transporters for extracellular transport and entry into cells, as well as G-protein-coupled receptors in the signaling process [20].

4.4.1 Neurotransmitter Receptors

Neurotransmitter receptors expressed on both sides of the synaptic cleft are (1) *ionotropic* and (2) *metabotropic*. Ionotropic receptors have transmembrane ion channels divided into (1) ligand-gated, (2) voltage-gated, and (3) stretch-activated ion channels. The functioning of these receptors carries out directly and depends on binding to neurotransmitters as ligands, changing the presynaptic membrane's action potentials or mechanical stretching of the cell's membrane. Ionotropic receptors are permeable to sodium, potassium, calcium, chloride, and bicarbonate ions. Opening and closing the ion channels are triggered by changing the charge gradient between the sides of the synaptic cleft. Metabotropic receptors or transmembrane G-protein-coupled receptors do not have channels but, in contrast with ionotropic receptors, engage second messengers and various signaling pathways inside the cell acting indirectly [33, 34]. Neurotransmitter *transporters* are proteins that move neuro molecules through membranes and inside involved neurons and target cells (see Fig. 4.2).

Neurotransmitter recognition occurs at the postsynaptic membrane's exterior side and affects the receptor on the receiving neuron or target cell. The activated receptor can return to its resting state once the neurotransmitter has been removed by enzymatic hydrolysis or uptake into the presynaptic neuron's ending or surrounding glial cells.

From a clinical viewpoint, deviations from functioning neuro molecules and their receptors and transporters predominantly concern nervous and mental disorders [26, 35] (see Table 4.2). However, some genetic alterations show associations with the susceptibility to allergic conditions (see Sect. 4.8).

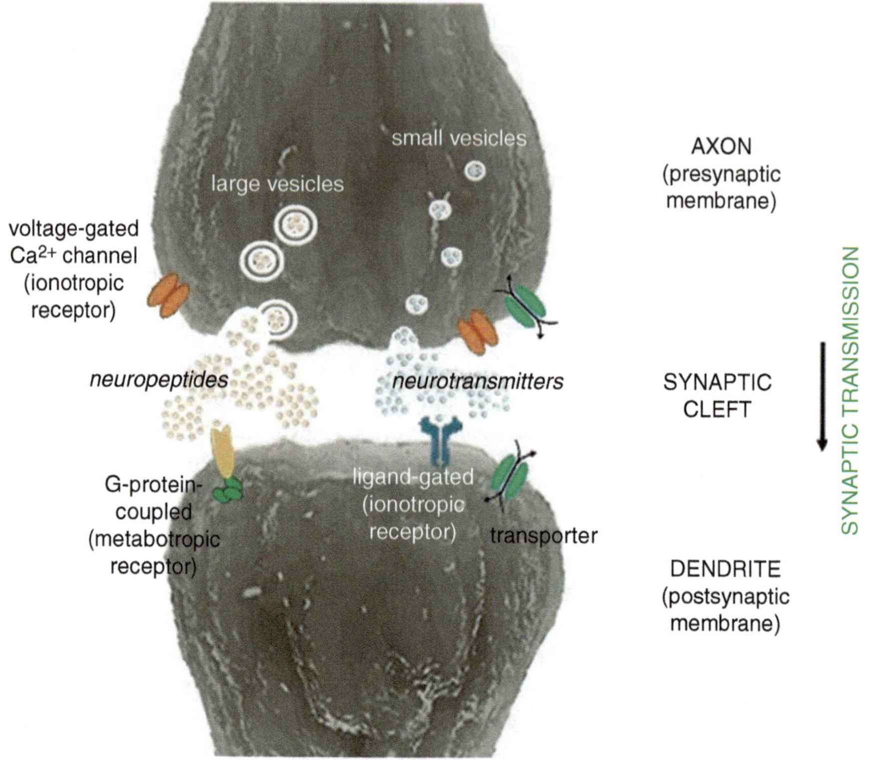

Fig. 4.2 Neurotransmitter and neuropeptide receptors.
The synapse consists of the presynaptic membrane, synaptic cleft, and postsynaptic membrane. Neurotransmitters are established and released from the small vesicles in the axon's terminal, whereas neuropeptides are formed and secreted from the large vesicles. Neuro molecules' receptors expressed on both sides of the synapse are divided into inotropic and metabotropic. The ionotropic receptors have ion channels, and metabotropic receptors use various signaling pathways. Transporters help neuro molecules move through the membranes

4.4.2 Place of Neuro Molecules in Allergen Tolerance Maintenance and Breakdown

Most mechanisms of allergic inflammation wherever they proceed cannot be explained only by the participation of immune cells and molecules [9]. Allergen tolerance maintenance is the case. To a more significant extent, allergen tolerance breakdown especially requires neuronal influence since it destroys established homeostasis in target organs and the whole body. Each target organ has a specific innervation, which provides neurons of distinct nerves, including the vagus nerve, sympathetic nerves, somatosensory fibers, and the enteric nervous system, only in the gut [5]. Neurotransmitters and neuropeptides synthesized in the nervous tissue and non-neuronal cells have short-term life but frequently long-term effects sharing

Table 4.2 Changes of neurotransmitters in nervous and mental disorders

Main neurotransmitter	Location	↓ ↑	Nervous/mental disorder
Acetylcholine	Brain's cortex and hippocampus	↓	Alzheimer's disease
Acetylcholine	Peripheral synapses between parasympathetic neurons and muscles	↓	Miasthenia gravis
Norepinephrine	Brain's locus coeruleus and limbic system	↓	Depression
Dopamine	Dopaminergic neurons of brain's substantia nigra	↓	Parkinson's disease
Dopamine	Brain's frontal lobes	↑	Schizophrenia
Dopamine	Mesolimbic pathway between the ventral tegmental area (midbrain) and ventral striatum of basal ganglia (forebrain)	↓	Depression
L-glutamate	Myelin covers of cerebral and spinal neurons	↑	Multiple sclerosis
L-glutamate	Cerebral and spinal motor neurons	↑	Amyotrophic lateral sclerosis
Serotonin	Brainstem, reticular formation, many regions of the brain, gastrointestinal tract	↓	Depression, anxiety
Serotonin	Brainstem, reticular formation, many regions of the brain, gastrointestinal tract	↓	Obsessive-compulsive disorder
GABA	Many regions of the brain	↓	Epilepsy
GABA	Many regions of the brain	↓	Amyotrophic lateral sclerosis

with the immune system and constituting the mutual neuroimmune system. On the other hand, if "neurogenic inflammation" occurs [36], neurons innervating the target organs can damage them using neurotransmitters and neuropeptides as a tool. In this context, the role of neuro molecules in allergen tolerance-related processes is essential and must not be underestimated.

The neuro molecules possess multidirectional effects and different forms of interaction that can be controversial or counteractive. We divided all molecules into pro-immunogenic and pro-tolerogenic in a logically grouped manner and according to references, considering their participation in the mechanisms of allergen tolerance.

Neuro molecules may be categorized as conventional neurotransmitters, atypical neurotransmitters, neuropeptides, neurohormones (or peptide hormones), and nonclassified neurotransmitters. They are the tool with which the neuroimmune system [20, 21] operates in the body, at the systemic level and regional level, including the participation in the pathogenesis of allergic inflammation. Besides, the neuro molecules are factors of "neurogenic inflammation" [36].

For more information about allergic inflammation in the context of participation of neuro molecules, see Fig. 4.3. However, some contradictory data are not reflected here.

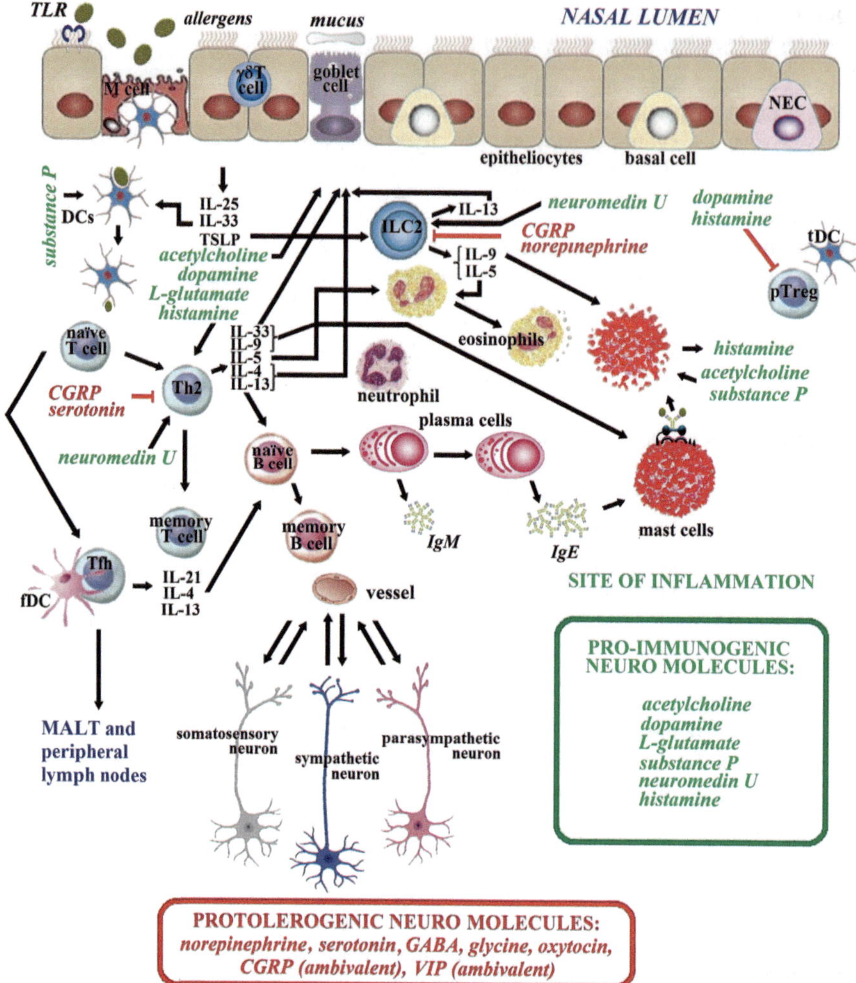

Fig. 4.3 Allergen tolerance breakdown in allergic rhinitis in the context of participation of neuro molecules.
Neuro molecules exert different effects during allergen tolerance breakdown. Acetylcholine stimulates the goblet cells to secrete mucus, and along with dopamine, L-glutamate, and histamine, upregulates Th2-dependent immune response. Conversely, pro-tolerogenic calcitonin-gene-related peptide (CGRP) and serotonin suppress Th2 response. Neuromedin U activates ILC2, but CGRP and norepinephrine inhibit these cells. Acetylcholine and substance P upregulate the degranulation of mast cells, dopamine and histamine downregulate pTregs. So, pro-immunogenic neuro molecules are predominated. DC dendritic cell, TSLP thymic stromal lymphopoietin, Tfh follicular helper T cell, fDC follicular dendritic cell, tDC tolerogenic dendritic cell, ILC2 group 2 innate lymphoid cell, pTreg peripheral regulatory T cell, NEC neuroendocrine cell, CGRP calcitonin-gene-related peptide, GABA γ aminobutyric acid, TLR toll-like receptors

4.5 Prevalent Pro-Immunogenic Neuro Molecules

Acetylcholine is the main neurotransmitter of the parasympathetic nervous system synthesized in neurons and non-neuronal cells, including immune cells from choline and acetyl-coenzyme A by the enzyme choline acetyltransferase. Immune cells such as T cells and monocytes can interact with cholinergic nerves associated with lymph vessels or with acetylcholine synthesized by immune cells themselves [26]. Acetylcholine can bind the muscarinic receptors (M1AchR, M2AchR) and nicotinic receptor (a7nAchR) on ciliated epitheliocytes, promoting Th2 cells growth, mucus secretion, degranulation of mast cells, and basophils [37]. Acetylcholine stimulates in cell cultures Th2 cell proliferation and production of IL-4, IL-5, IL-13, CCL17 (TARC), and CCL22 (MDC) through the activation of dendritic cells obtained from monocytes [38].

Released acetylcholine can act re-switching via vagus-splenic synapse toward the sympathetic nervous system temporarily and paradoxically acquiring the pro-tolerogenic activity called the cholinergic anti-inflammatory pathway [20]. For example, it downregulates ILC2 proliferation and upregulates regulatory T (pTregs) cells. However, acetylcholine is a predominant pro-immunogenic and pro-inflammatory neurotransmitter. A decrease in acetylcholine in target organs causes a reduction in cholinergic promotion of allergic inflammation [37]. The nasal cavity's solitary chemosensory cells can use cholinergic neurotransmission leading to the neurogenic inflammatory pathway [39].

Dopamine is a critical neurotransmitter, a catecholamine, linked with emotions, the brain's pleasure, reward system, and gambling. Dopamine is synthesized in the brain and peripheral sympathetic neurons [26] from (1) L-tyrosine by tyrosine hydroxylase, (2) phenylalanine by phenylalanine hydroxylase, and (3) L-DOPA by aromatic amino acid decarboxylase. It has been identified in cells of the immune system such as pTregs, macrophages, granulocytes, dendritic cells, T cells, and B cells. It functions via D_1–D_5 receptors, but immune effects mediated by dopamine may be ambivalent, mainly pro-immunogenic, and, to a smaller extent, pro-tolerogenic [20]. D_1 expressed on DCs provides Th2 and Th17 differentiation, whereas expression on pTregs leads to decreased functionality of these regulatory cells. Signaling through D_3 upregulates chemotactic migration of naïve CD8+ T cells; signaling through D_4 promotes Th2 differentiation; D_5 facilitates secretions of counteractive cytokines, TNF-α, and IL-10. Signaling through D_2 receptors is usually pro-tolerogenic [20].

Notably, the communication between dopamine and CD4+ T cells provides an age-related mechanism underlying susceptibility to Th2-mediated allergic inflammation at an early age [40]. During B cell-mediated responses, the activity of dopamine in the brain is markedly elevated. Besides, dopamine released from T cells can enhance intracellular reactive oxygen species (ROS) production, leading to oxidative stress and apoptosis in peripheral lymphocytes [41, 42]. Moreover, dopamine can damage the nervous tissue possessing a potency to neurotoxicity, including neurons in which it is produced, and predisposing to Parkinson's disease [40].

From a clinical viewpoint, dopamine is used as a medication for intravenous injections to achieve peripheral effects as it does not pass the blood-brain barrier. In addition, dopamine agonists and levodopa are used as medications for Parkinson's disease.

l-*glutamate*, a critical neurotransmitter, a precursor of GABA, is synthesized from glutamine in the brain by the glutaminase and from α-ketoglutaric acid in the citric acid cycle. It is present in almost all organs and tissues of the body. L-glutamate influences learning and memory and impacts the functioning nervous and immune systems through two groups of receptors, mGluRs (metabotropic) and iGluRs (ionotropic) [20]. Through iGluRs, L-glutamate promotes T cell migration, IL-2 secretion, IL-2 receptor expression, and via mGluRs, it prevents apoptosis in activated T cells, facilitates TCR signaling, and upregulates Th1 cells differentiation [20]. The neurotransmitter possesses a potency to neurotoxicity [26]; therefore, this substance may be harmful as a dietary supplement. L-glutamate from dietary supplements can cause human brain damage and the development of neurodegenerative diseases, obesity, and infertility. It acquires excitotoxic properties in the extracellular form [43].

In the experiment, glutamine metabolism was studied in mice with airway inflammation induced by house dust mites and lipopolysaccharide. This model allowed the abundant proliferation of IL-4 and IL-17-producing T cells. Administration of glutaminase, an inhibitor of glutamine, decreased eosinophilia, T cell cytokine production, and airway hyperresponsiveness [44]. A significant increase in L-glutamate concentration in the nasal mucosa has been shown in allergic rhinitis [45]. In addition, L-glutamate provides mast cells with communication between neurons and mast cells [46]. Mast cell-neuronal interactions contribute to pain and itch in which "neurogenic inflammation" is central, but specific mediators released by mast cells are necessary to promote this process [47].

Histamine is produced by histidine decarboxylase from histidine in the brain, mast cells, basophils, and a neosynthesis process in T cells [48]. It exploits H_1–H_4 receptors. H_1 and H_4 receptors are expressed in many cells, including mast cells and basophils, and engaged in IgE-dependent reactions. H_2 receptors are involved in the Th1 response and H_3 receptors take part in the functioning of the blood-brain barrier [49]. Histamine controls sleep/wake behavior in the brain and, paradoxically, the release of the inhibitory neurotransmitter GABA [50].

In the periphery, histamine, mainly through H_1 and H_2 receptors, upregulates antigen-presenting DCs, polarizes immune responses toward Th1 and Th2 pathways, induces IL-31 production promoting skin itch, enhances the production of inflammatory chemokines [5], and downregulates pTreg cells [48, 49]. Some recent studies demonstrated the participation of H_4 receptors in the pathogenesis of itch that implies the requirement in changing therapeutic strategy in chronic allergic dermatitis [5].

From a clinical viewpoint, not only H_1 and H_2 blockers but also H_4 antagonists should be included in the therapy for allergic inflammation.

Vasopressin is a posterior pituitary gland's neurohormone encoded by the *VP gene*, functioning as the factor responsible for restoring the HPA axis's homeostasis, upregulating adaptive and innate immunity, and healing [51]. Besides, vasopressin impacts social behavior, sexual motivation, prolactin secretion, circadian rhythm, water reabsorption, and increased blood pressure [52]. The immunostimulatory action of vasopressin on the immune system exerts itself in the neuroimmune system and HPA axis.

In the experiment, the major pro-inflammatory mediators produced in response to peripheral inflammation induced by lipopolysaccharide (LPS), prostaglandin E_2, IL-1β, IL-6, and TNF-α excited vasopressin neurons in rats. These effects occurred in 30 min and were sustained for more than 6 h. In contrast, brain injection of anti-IL-6 antibodies prevented the LPS induced-activation of vasopressin neurons [53].

Melatonin, the pineal gland (or epiphysis) hormone, a biorhythmic regulator, proved to focus on research as a potential factor, modulating many immune processes taken as stress reactions. Regarding the immune system, melatonin is a pro-immunogenic factor, which can particularly limit cancerous cell growth. Also, it exerts pro-inflammatory ability in asthma, leading to bronchial constriction [54]. In asthma, the effects of melatonin appear to be controversial [55]. However, it prevents inflammasome NLRP3 activation [56] and limits radical oxygen species (ROS) production.

In the experiment, it has been found that concentrations of Th1, Th2, and Th17-related cytokines in peripheral blood were lower in mice that had undergone pinealectomy, compared with normal mice. The expression of signaling molecules of T cell and B cell activation pathways were downregulated in the pinealectomy group, compared with the control group. Melatonin administration resulted in the upregulation of these molecules in the pinealectomy group being significantly higher than that of the control group. So, melatonin upregulated the activation of T cells and B cells [57].

Substance P, a critical neuroimmune network's neuropeptide, is released from the terminals of specific somatosensory nerves in the brain, regulating emotion and functions of lots of immune cells. It is encoded by the *TAC1 gene* and synthesized in many immune cells [20, 26, 58]. Substance P exerts its biological activity through neurokinin receptors found in close association with cells containing serotonin and norepinephrine. The experiment with a murine model demonstrated the ability of substance P to induce Th2-linked inflammation [1].

It has been reported that this neuropeptide upregulated mast cells and basophils and their degranulation in chronic urticaria and chronic spontaneous urticaria. Mean serum substance P level was significantly higher in the whole group of atopic persons and in the subgroup of patients with allergic rhinitis [59]. Substance P stimulates proximally located mDC-2 via the Mas-related G-protein-coupled receptor A1 (MRGPRA1) that initiates Th2-response to allergens [60]. Substance P amplifies the polarization of Th1- and Th17-mediated responses depending on the microenvironment [20, 58], secretion of pro-inflammatory cytokines by T cells and macrophages [20], production of chemokines CCL2 (MCP-1), CCL4 (MIP-1β), CCL5 (RANTES), and CXCL2 (MIP-2α), angiogenesis [26], and degranulation of mast cells and basophils [1]. On the other hand, substance P inhibits IL-10 synthesis, CD8+ T cells migration, and cytotoxicity of NK cells [20].

Neuromedin U is found in somatosensory neurons of the hypothalamus, spinal cord, and allergic target organs, such as the unified airway and gastrointestinal tract, and other organs. It recognizes two receptors, peripheral NMUR1 and central NMUR2 [61]. Via NMRU2, neuromedin U responds to stress stimuli, inhibits appetite, and promotes an increase in epinephrine but not norepinephrine in serum, leading to enhanced blood pressure and heart rate. Through NMUR1, neuromedin U promotes Th2 cell proliferation, contracts smooth muscles, including airflow restriction, promotes mucosal edema, attracts eosinophils to the site of allergic inflammation [62]. Neuromedin U also triggers ILC2 proliferation and expression of type 2 cytokines, including IL-5 and IL-13 [1, 7, 8, 26, 61, 62]. So far, two ILC2-mediated inflammatory pathways, IgE-dependent and IgE-independent, have been described [4].

The specific role neuromedin U plays in asthma. Human Th2 cells express a higher level of NMUR1, whereas neuromedin U induces Th2 cytokine production in these cells, suggesting a possible meaning in allergic asthma [63]. Asthmatic patients have a denser network of sensory neurons around small airways and a low threshold for their activation in response to airborne irritants. Neuromedin U is involved in nociceptive reflexes in the lung, participating in the nociceptor activation upon allergen exposure at the beginning of allergic inflammation [62].

Thus, neuromedin U exerts marked pro-immunogenic and pro-inflammatory effects.

Quiz A

Reading a question, please choose only one right answer.

Question 1

The neuroimmune system does not include:

1. The enteric nervous system (ENS).
2. The stomach.
3. The parasympathetic nervous system.
4. Hypothalamic-pituitary-adrenal (HPA) axis.

Question 2

The unified airway is innervated by:

1. Somatosensory neurons and vegetative nervous system.
2. Sympathetic and parasympathetic nervous systems.
3. Somatosensory neurons and enteric nervous system.
4. Enteric nervous system and vagus nerve.

Question 3

Neuropeptides are released into the synapse from:

1. The large vesicles.
2. The vessels.
3. The small vesicles.
4. The epithelial cells.

Question 4
Neurotransmitters are released into the synapse from:

1. The connective tissue.
2. The small vesicles.
3. The vessels.
4. The large vesicles.

Question 5
Atypical neurotransmitters are released:

1. From the neuron's presynaptic membrane.
2. From endocrine glands.
3. From the neuron's postsynaptic membrane.
4. From salivary glands.

Question 6
These neurotransmitters can exert neurotoxicity:

1. Acetylcholine and histamine.
2. Substance P.
3. Neuromedin U.
4. 4. L-glutamate and dopamine.

Question 7
The target organ, which has its own autonomic self-contained nervous system, is:

1. The skin.
2. The genitourinary tract.
3. The unified airway.
4. The gastrointestinal tract.

Question 8
The enteric nervous system secretes more:

1. Pro-tolerogenic neuro molecules.
2. Pro-immunogenic neuro molecules.
3. Pro-inflammatory neuro molecules.
4. Corticosteroids.

Question 9
Histamine's receptors involved in IgE-dependent inflammation are:

1. H_3.
2. H_1 and H_4.
3. H_2 and H_3.
4. H_2.

Question 10

Ionotropic receptors for neurotransmitters do not include:

1. Ligand-gated ion channels.
2. Voltage-gated receptors.
3. Metabotropic receptors.
4. Stretch-activated ion channels.

Question 11

These neurotransmitters inhibit pTreg cells:

1. Acetylcholine and substance P.
2. Melatonin and vasopressin.
3. Neuromedin U and substance P.
4. Dopamine and histamine.

Question 12

This neuro molecule activates ILC2 cells:

1. Substance P.
2. Neuromedin U.
3. Acetylcholine.
4. Dopamine.

Question 13

A critical pro-immunogenic neurotransmitter:

1. Acetylcholine.
2. 2. L-glutamate.
3. Histamine.
4. Vasopressin.

Question 14

Dopamine is formed in:

1. The parasympathetic nervous system.
2. Dopaminergic neurons of the brain and sympathetic nervous system.
3. Enterochromaffin tissue of the gut.
4. An anterior pituitary gland.

Question 15

Acetylcholine uses the following receptors:

1. M1AchR, M2AchR, and a7nAchR.
2. D_1–D_5.
3. mGluRs and iGluRs.
4. H_1–H_4.

Question 16
Substance P upregulates:

1. Proliferation of Th2 cells.
2. Differentiation of allergen-specific B cells.
3. Degranulation of mast cells.
4. Differentiation of Th2 cells.

4.6 Predominant Pro-Tolerogenic Neuro Molecules

Norepinephrine (noradrenaline), a stress-mobilizing sympathetic neurotransmitter, catecholamine, is produced in the brainstem neurons, by sympathetic nerves, adrenal medulla (neuroendocrine cells), and Merkel cells in the skin [26, 42]. Adrenergic receptors like β_2AR are expressed in immune cells, including T cells, B cells, macrophages, and NK cells [26, 64]. This neurotransmitter influences the immune system as an immunomodulatory factor. Notably, noradrenaline mainly inhibits the activity of immune cells, such as neutrophils, NK cells, and monocytes, but these effects execute depending on norepinephrine concentration in the biological fluids, the local environment, receptor expression, and costimulation [21].

Norepinephrine upregulates the production of IL-10 [26], promotes a tissue-protective phenotype in ENS muscular macrophages [8], limits ILC2-dependent type 2 inflammation, and counteracts the effects of neuromedin U to activate ILC2s [65]. Interestingly, norepinephrine can promote inflammation in the initial phase of immune reactions (innate immunity), whereas it downregulates inflammation in the later phase (adaptive immunity) [26, 64].

A little-known phenotype of the nose's innervation dysfunction has been described, which is accompanied by sinonasal symptoms: nasal obstruction, discharge, sneezing, polyp growth, and facial pain. It is supposed that this dysfunction may be associated with the adrenergic imbalance of the nose's neuroimmune system characterized by downregulation of adrenoreceptors and destroyed release of norepinephrine [66].

Serotonin (5-hydroxytryptamine, 5-HT) is a critical neurotransmitter synthesized (1) from L-tryptophan by 5-tryptophan hydroxylase and (2) 5-hydroxy-L-tryptophan by tryptophan decarboxylase, and a variety of other subsequent enzymes in the gastrointestinal tract's enterochromaffin cells, enteric neurons, neuroendocrine epithelial cells, and neurons of the central nervous system, and actively taken up by platelets, basophils, and mast cells [20, 67]. Serotonin functions through 5-HT$_1$-5-HT$_7$ receptors and serotonin transporter (SERT) as the potent pro-tolerogenic neurotransmitter, mainly derived from peripheral non-neuronal sources. Serotonin receptors are expressed on many cells, including immune cells, depending on the cell lineage. On the one hand, serotonin transmission between neurons in the brain is responsible for mood, feelings of pleasure, sleep, appetite, and, on the other hand, it predominantly promotes pro-tolerogenic effects [67, 68]. Serotonin upregulates the differentiation of tolerogenic DCs and IL-10 synthesis by Th2 cells [20, 69].

In an experiment, it was found that the activation of serotonin by selective 5-HT_2 agonist alleviated airways hyperresponsiveness, mucus overproduction, lung eosinophilia, suppressed Th2 proliferation, and IL-5 and IL-13 production in mice with ovalbumin-induced asthma [70]. Another experiment has shown the downregulating effect of serotonin on IL-4 in basophils and IgE due to Th2 response in mice. The same results were noted in cell cultures in humans [71].

The pro-tolerogenic effects are also mediated by inhibiting the production of pro-inflammatory cytokines such as TNF-α and IL-12 and downregulating the maturation of inflammatory DCs [20]. Serotonin functions within the enteric nervous system (ENS) as a crucial pro-tolerogenic neurotransmitter, which creates a zone of allergen tolerance in the gut [6].

γ Aminobutyric acid (GABA) is the major inhibitory neurotransmitter in the central nervous system displaying anti-anxiety effects. GABA is produced from L-glutamate by glutamic acid decarboxylase in the brain and spinal cord neurons and other cells (e.g., T cells, macrophages, and dendritic cells) in many places, including the unified airway [72–74]. There are two main GABA receptors, $GABA_A$ (ionotropic) and $GABA_B$ (metabotropic), which mediate this neurotransmitter's activity [72, 73, 75]. To date, GABAergic mechanisms have been demonstrated throughout the body, including the synthesis in neuroendocrine epithelial cells. As for the immune system, GABA exhibits pro-tolerogenic effects inhibiting T cell proliferation and IL-6 and IL-12 production in macrophages [26, 73].

In the experiment, the agonist of $GABA_A$, Honokiol, was administered to ovalbumin-sensitized mice, which developed allergic asthma. There were decreased TNF-α, IL-6, Th1 and Th17 cytokines compared to increased Th2 cytokines, IL-10, TGF-β, and FoxP3+ cells in the lung. Honokiol therapy led to a reduction in airway hyperresponsiveness and lung eosinophilia despite enhanced Th2 cytokines [76].

GABA inhalations significantly decreased bronchial hyperresponsiveness in humans with asthma [77].

From a clinical viewpoint, persons with atopic allergies sometimes suffer from anxiety disorders. GABA-based medications do not pass through the blood-brain barrier. Penetrating the blood-brain barrier benzodiazepines are used medically to get GABA-like effects because their receptors are associated with GABA receptors. However, benzodiazepines can induce drug dependence.

Glycine is synthesized from choline, serine, hydroxyproline, and threonine through the liver, kidneys, and other organs' metabolism by different enzymes. It is an inhibitory neurotransmitter in the central nervous system's caudal part, responsible for supporting the growth, quality of sleep, pain signaling, and well-being [78, 79]. In the periphery, glycine via glycine (GlyRs) receptors exerts hepatoprotective, antioxidant, and pro-tolerogenic effects stimulating the secretion of IL-10 and limiting the clonal expansion of T cells and B cells, production of pro-inflammatory cytokines (IL-1β and TNF-α) by macrophages, generation of the reactive oxygen species (ROS) in neutrophils [79, 80].

Glycine can play an essential role as an immunomodulator through effects on signaling in parenchymal, vascular, and inflammatory cells separate from the cytoprotection it provides. However, it can combine with cytoprotection against cell death in vivo and in vitro, sometimes in the same cells, to suppress tissue damage during various diseases [81].

From a clinical viewpoint, glycine-based medications are used medically in mild forms of insomnia and anxiety disorder.

Oxytocin is the posterior pituitary neurohormone mediating anti-stress, well-being, social interaction, growth, feelings of love, childbirth, and regeneration. It uses one known G-protein-coupled oxytocin receptor [82]. Oxytocin is synthesized as an inactive precursor protein encoded by the *OXT gene*, progressively hydrolyzed by a series of enzymes, and degraded to active fragments, which are released into the bloodstream [82]. Under control of the HPA axis, oxytocin plays a pivotal role in the functioning of the immune system, exerting pro-tolerogenic properties in the context of inhibiting inflammation. Notably, intrathymic oxytocin is known to promote central immune self-tolerance of T cells [83].

Oxytocin establishes the oxytocin-secreting system in the brain as a part of the neuroimmune system that includes oxytocin neurons recognizing various signals from the peripheral tissues and subsequently integrating them to release oxytocin into the bloodstream. In the periphery, oxytocin suppresses the production of pro-inflammatory cytokines, recruits inflammatory cells in the uterus, specifically during human labor, and activates the generation of regulatory CD4+CD25+FoxP3+ T cells [84].

Calcitonin-gene-related peptide (CGRP) exists in two isoforms, α and β [26], encoded by separate genes and synthesized due to alternative splicing. α-CGRP is released from sensory neurons of the central nervous system, spinal cord, and trigeminal ganglion. In contrast, β-CGRP is mainly produced by the immune cells, neuroendocrine epithelial cells, and the gut. CGRP uses calcitonin-like (CLR) receptors throughout the body, suggesting that the neuropeptide may modulate a wide range of physiological functions and pathology [26]. CGRP promotes the transmission of pain (migraine), decreases appetite, and increases heart rate. Also, CGRP inhibits the activation of ILC2 and the differentiation of Th2 cells [85, 86].

The serum level of CGRP as an angiogenic, vasodilating, and immune-modulating peptide was measured in patients with severe COVID-19 acute respiratory distress syndrome. Low CGRP levels were revealed compared with the control that negatively correlated with patients' condition due to vasoconstriction, improper angiogenesis, less epithelial repair, and faulty immune responses [87].

CGRP is a bivalent neurotransmitter, which can cause pro-immunogenic effects. However, CGRP preferentially plays a role as a pro-tolerogenic and anti-inflammatory mediator responsible for preventing tissue damage during allergic inflammation and other types of inflammation [26].

Vasoactive intestinal peptide (VIP) is related to the glucagon/secretin family and encoded by the *VIP gene*. This cholinergic neuron-derived neuropeptide functions through the two main receptors, VPAC1 and VPAC2, and many other receptors, closely linked with the nociceptive neurons and autonomic enteric nervous system (ENS) [88]. VIP is a releasing factor in the hypothalamus that influences social behaviors, promoting the secretion of some neurohormones in the pituitary's anterior lobe and causing the spasmolytic action to smooth muscles and vasodilatory effect throughout the body, in particular in the gut [89]. Particularly, VIP is a transmitter of parasympathetic neurons, which relax smooth muscle cells in the lung compared to cholinergic postganglionic neurons [9].

Intestinal group 3 innate lymphoid (ILC3s) cells have a high expression of the VPAC2 receptor for VIP, and its activation by VIP markedly increases the production of IL-22 by ILC3 and the barrier function of the intestinal epithelium. Destruction of signaling through VPAC2 led to impaired production of IL-22 and enhanced susceptibility to inflammation in the gut [7, 9].

VIP as a neurotransmitter shows ambivalent actions since it limits the differentiation of Th1 and Th17 cells and the release of pro-inflammatory cytokines and chemokines but promotes the Th2 cells differentiation, survival, and migration [21, 88]. At the same time, VIP induces the generation of tolerogenic DCs and CD4+CD25+FoxP3+ pTregs, the important cells of allergen tolerance [8, 90]. Despite its contraversial properties, VIP mainly demonstrates the prevalent pro-tolerogenic action in a tissue-specific manner [88].

Endocannabinoids are bioactive lipids, atypical neurotransmitters functioning due to an abundance of cannabinoid receptors CB1 and CB2 on neurons, immune cells, endocrine cells, and other cells, but they undergo rapid degradation [26, 91]. In the brain, receptor CB1 is predominantly present in the hippocampus, amygdala, and hypothalamus, whereas CB2 is expressed in the immune system's cells.

Many lipid neurotransmitters, including anandamide and 2-arachidonyl glycerol, constitute the endocannabinoid system. Anandamide alleviates physical pain and helps patients with posttraumatic stress disorder. 2-arachidonyl glycerol is a full agonist of CB1 and CB2 receptors, which play an important role in the downregulation of inflammation due to immunosuppressive action [91].

In total, the endocannabinoid system is responsible for tissue homeostasis and apoptosis, pro-tolerogenic, and anti-metastatic effects. This system is generally anti-proliferative through CB2 activation, but it can become proliferative upon low-level activation and even low-level toxic upon the influence of L-glutamate [91]. Besides, endocannabinoids promote pTreg cells, inhibit autoreactive lymphocytes and T cells' functional activity [26, 92].

From a clinical viewpoint, cannabis's phytocannabinoids can mimic endocannabinoids' action and is used medically as a safer alternative to opioids and benzodiazepines.

Endorphins are neuropeptides acting as endogenous opioids. There are three families of classical endogenous opioid peptides: endorphins, enkephalins, and dynorphins. Well-studied β-endorphin is synthesized in the pituitary gland and lymphocytes, contributing to analgesia at sites of inflammation [26]. The opioid G-protein-coupled receptors, μ (morphine), δ, and κ, are distributed in the brain, spinal cord, gastrointestinal tract, and immune cells. β-endorphin is an endogenous ligand for μ receptors, enkephalins exploit δ receptors, and dynorphins use κ receptors [93]. Endorphins binding to their receptors leads to analgesia, anti-stress and anti-inflammatory action, and well-being [94]. The effect of endorphins on the immune system is mainly pro-tolerogenic and anti-inflammatory [26, 93].

It has been reported that endorphins inhibit the conversion of Th1 polarization to Th2 deviation, diminish Th17 cells involved in chronic inflammation, prevent tissue damage, and promote Tregs that lead to tolerance and immune homeostasis [95]. In another report, the β-endorphin concentration was significantly decreased in patients with allergic rhinitis than in healthy persons, and was no association between the concentrations of β-endorphin and serum total IgE [96].

From a clinical viewpoint, persons addicted to drugs such as heroin have abnormally stimulated their opiate receptors. So, due to the processes of downregulation and exhaustion, they have a less active endorphin system.

Gaseous neurotransmitters are related to atypical neurotransmitters, acting in the brain and throughout the body and in the course of the regulation of the HPA axis [97]. They are also termed *gasotransmitters* [98]. This group includes nitric oxide, carbon monoxide, hydrogen sulfide, and some other gases whose either anti-inflammatory or pro-inflammatory action depends on gases' concentrations and the nature of the tissue where they operate. These gases can even damage various tissues, exerting a potency to neurotoxicity and exitotoxicity [29]. In the periphery, particularly in the enteric nervous system, gasotransmitters are produced by the human symbiotic microbiota exerting a wide variety of effects: vasodilatation, smooth muscle cell growth, reactive oxygen species (ROS) generation, platelet aggregation, monocyte adhesion, etc. [99].

In an experiment, the nitric oxide-producing cells inhibited T cell activation, involved Treg cells in the lung, and downregulated airway hyperresponsiveness in ovalbumin-sensitized mice [100]. In another experiment, nitric oxide synthase 2-knockout mice were more sensitive to ovalbumin-induced airway inflammation and demonstrated enhanced total cells number in lung lavage and increased airway hyperresponsiveness [101].

Adenosine, atypical neurotransmitter, can actively be released by various cells into the tissue environment and be produced through the degradation of extracellular ATP [31]. ATP is related to a group of damage-associated molecular patterns (DAMPs), ligands for PRRs. Adenosine may degrade, and its products also have biological activity. There are four G-protein-coupled receptors: A1, A2A, A2B, and A3, but A1 and A2A adenosine receptors have a higher affinity for adenosine than A2B and A3 receptors [102]. Besides, there are the purinergic receptors, P1, P2X, and P2Y, which are used by ATP.

Adenosine is an ambivalent neurotransmitter exerting both pro-tolerogenic and pro-immunogenic activity depending on the study model and involved receptor. Still, most studies reported anti-inflammatory activity of the A2A receptor. Through the A2A receptor, during allergen sensitization, adenosine decreased IFN-γ and the accumulation of eosinophils, neutrophils, and lymphocytes in bronchoalveolar lavage, inhibited the release of histamine from mast cells and basophils [26, 102, 103], and promoted the proliferation of tolerogenic DCs. The main pro-tolerogenic function of adenosine is to suppress immunogenic DCs during adaptive responses [31]. However, its role in asthma and urticaria is controversial [102]. This neurotransmitter also plays a neuroprotective role in the course of the initial phases of ischemic preconditioning.

4.7 Prevalent Neuro Molecules in the Target Organs

See sets of prevalent neuro molecules in the target organs in Table 4.3.

Table 4.3 Sets of prevalent neuro molecules in the target organs

Target organ		Neuro molecules	Reference
	Skin	Acetylcholine, norepinephrine, dopamine, histamine, and substance P	[104]
	Lung	Acetylcholine, serotonin, CGRP, nitric oxide, and substance P	[10]
	Gut	Serotonin, GABA, CGRP, norepinephrine, and dopamine	[6, 19, 105, 106]
	Genitourinary tract (females and males)	Dopamine, serotonin, norepinephrine, GABA, opioids, vasopressin, and oxytocin	[107, 108]

4.8 Polymorphisms and Mutations in Some Neuro Molecules Genes, and Related Genes, Which May Concern Allergies

Over the last two decades, the area has been developing actively. For example, the *histamine N-methyl transferase (HNMT) gene* (located on 2q22.1) encoded the principal enzyme metabolizing histamine is responsible for the biotransformation in bronchial epithelium and smooth muscle contraction in the unified airway [109]. Genetic alteration of the *HNMT gene* results in high susceptibility to asthma and mental retardation. Organic cation transporter-3 (OCT-3) is capable of reuptaking dopamine and other neurotransmitters (*OCT-3 gene* is located on 6q25.3). Some *OCT-3 gene* polymorphisms may be relevant to severe asthma [110, 111]. The genetic alteration of the *histidine decarboxylase (HDC) gene* (located on 15q21.2) required for histamine synthesis leads to a decrease in the number of mast cells, downregulation of allergic inflammation, and social behavior deviation [112].

The genetic alteration of the *NMUR1 gene* (located on 2q37.1) results in the loss of neuromedin U—NMUR1 signaling, the disorder of ILC2 activation and mast cell degranulation, limitation of allergic inflammation following allergen challenge in vivo [61].

DOPA decarboxylase is an enzyme important for synthesizing both dopamine and serotonin. Mutation in the *DDC gene* (located on 7p12.2-p12.1) leads to the metabolic disturbance of these two neurotransmitters, aromatic L-amino acid decarboxylase deficiency, linked with chronic nasal congestion, developmental delay, and other associated disorders in children [113].

5-tryptophan hydroxylase-2 is the main enzyme required for serotonin synthesis. Mutation in the *TPH2 gene* (located on 12q21.1) reduces serotonin synthesis, resulting in increased susceptibility to attention deficit hyperactivity disorder [114]. Wang et al. [115] described the syndrome's association with a low level of serotonin and almost all forms of atopic allergic diseases.

4.9 "Neurogenic Inflammation"

▶ **Definition** "Neurogenic inflammation" is a new phenomenon joining inflamed components of the immune system and neurons, including immune mediators and neuro molecules, and playing a role in the different forms of allergen tolerance breakdown in specific target organs.

The accumulation of knowledge on nociceptive primary afferents and synaptic transmission neuro molecules led to the concept that neuronal signaling can establish "neurogenic inflammation" [36]. It has become clear that neuronal regulation of immunity plays an essential role in the context of allergic inflammation [5]. Nociceptive primary afferents express many neuro molecules exerting impact on the immune system's cells, modify nociceptive input before it reaches the central nervous system, and damage the tissue they innervate [36]. Mast cells, which take part in inflammation, are in close contact with nerves in the nasal mucosa [116]. Eosinophils, another key innate effector cell type in allergic reactions, have also been found to localize close to cholinergic nerves in allergic rhinitis [117]. Allergic inflammation in the allergic target organs involves complex crosstalk between neurons and immune cells that could play a critical role in mediating disease progression. The nervous system could be a novel and exciting target for these conditions [5]. These bidirectional neuroimmune interactions occur early and significantly impact the onset and development of allergic inflammation. On the whole, the molecular mechanisms of the phenomenon of "neurogenic inflammation" are not completely understood. In the presence of allergic inflammation, the neuronal function can also be chronically upregulated depending on the stimulation of nociceptive sensory nerves and neurotrophins such as nerve growth factor (NGF) [118].

The 1986 Nobel Laureates R. Levi-Montalcini and S. Cohen first identified the nerve growth factor (NGF). NGF is responsible for the survival of somatosensory and sympathetic neurons, the pain perception in many types of inflammatory processes playing a multifunctional role in the nociceptive transmission and "neurogenic inflammation," and regulation of innate and adaptive immunity. NGF is released from mast cells upon degranulation in allergic inflammation. Besides, it is associated with autoimmune diseases like type 1 diabetes mellitus [119].

In the context of allergic inflammation linked to the neuroimmune network, we considered the potential neuro molecules with predominant pro-immunogenic action and exerting pro-tolerogenic effects. Under certain conditions, some of them (L-glutamate, dopamine, and gasotransmitters) exhibit the ability to excitotoxicity and neurotoxicity which is important from a clinical viewpoint.

Key Points

1. Most mechanisms of allergic inflammation cannot be explained only by the participation of immune cells and molecules. Allergen tolerance especially requires neuronal influence since it corresponds to established homeostasis in target

organs. In the neuroimmune framework, the bidirectional crosstalk is provided with many of the neurotransmitters and neuropeptides produced by somatosensory, sympathetic, parasympathetic, and autonomic enteric neurons in the gut, non-neuronal cells, and microbiota.
2. These functional plasticity neuro molecules can mediate either pro-immunogenic or pro-tolerogenic effects depending on the expressed receptors on the immune system's target cells and local microenvironment in the inflammatory site.
3. In the context of allergen tolerance and allergic inflammation, there are neuro molecules with predominant pro-immunogenic effects, such as acetylcholine, dopamine, L-glutamate, melatonin, vasopressin, substance P, and neuromedin U, and displaying potential pro-tolerogenic action, such as serotonin, GABA, norepinephrine, oxytocin, CGRP, and VIP.
4. Under certain conditions, some neurotransmitters (L-glutamate, dopamine, and gasotransmitters) exert a potency to neurotoxicity and match the concept of "neurogenic inflammation."

Take-Home Messages

1. Write an essay about the neuroimmune system.
2. Write a paragraph about the vagus-splenic synapse.
3. Describe the innervation of target organs.
4. List pro-immunogenic neurotransmitters and neuropeptides.
5. List pro-tolerogenic neurotransmitters and neuropeptides.
6. Make a slide presentation about neuro molecules.
7. Name the critical neurotransmitters.
8. Write a paragraph about neurotransmitter receptors.
9. Name "alarmins."
10. Describe "neurogenic inflammation."
11. Give an example of a mutation in the gene of neuropeptide or enzyme required to synthesize a neurotransmitter.
12. Name the target cells for neuromedin U.

Quiz B

Reading a question, please choose only one right answer.

Question 1

The target organ, which has its own autonomic self-contained nervous system, is:

1. The unified airway.
2. The gastrointestinal tract.
3. The skin.
4. The genitourinary tract.

Question 2
Neurotransmitters are released into the synapse from:

1. The large vesicles.
2. The vessels.
3. The small vesicles.
4. The epithelial cells.

Question 3
Neuropeptides are released into the synapse from:

1. The small vesicles.
2. The vessels.
3. The large vesicles.
4. The epithelial cells.

Question 4
Acetylcholine is formed in:

1. The parasympathetic nervous system.
2. The sympathetic nervous system.
3. Nociceptive neurons.
4. Somatosensory neurons.

Question 5
Acetylcholine is:

1. Pro-tolerogenic neurotransmitter.
2. Pro-tolerogenic neuropeptide.
3. Pro-immunogenic neurotransmitter.
4. Anti-inflammatory neuropeptide.

Question 6
Can L-glutamate exert neurotoxicity:

1. No.
2. Yes.
3. Never.
4. No way.

Question 7
Dopamine through D_1 expressed on DCs provides:

1. Differentiation of Th2 and Th17 cells.
2. Upregulation of tDCs.

3. Upregulation of pTregs.
4. Proliferation of MDSCs.

Question 8
Histamine's receptors involved in IgE-dependent inflammation are:

1. H_2.
2. H_1 and H_4.
3. H_2 and H_3.
4. H_3.

Question 9
Substance P does not induce:

1. Th2-linked inflammation.
2. Degranulation of mast cells and basophils.
3. Differentiation of Th1 and Th17 cells.
4. Proliferation of pTregs.

Question 10
Neuromedin U impacting ILC2 can trigger:

1. IgE-independent inflammatory pathway.
2. Establishment of allergen tolerance.
3. Production of IgG antibodies.
4. Production of IL-1, TNF-α, and IL-6.

Question 11
A neurotransmitter, which can stimulate the goblet cells to produce mucus:

1. Serotonin.
2. Glycine.
3. Acetylcholine.
4. Norepinephrine.

Question 12
Neuro molecules upregulating Th2 cells are:

1. CGLP and serotonin.
2. Neuromedin U and CGRP.
3. Norepinephrine and glycine.
4. Dopamine and histamine.

Question 13
The critical pro-tolerogenic neurotransmitter is:

1. Serotonin.
2. Dopamin.
3. 3. L-glutamate.
4. Substance P.

Question 14
A critical pro-immunogenic neurotransmitter:

1. Norepinephrine.
2. Dopamine.
3. Serotonin.
4. GABA.

Question 15
CGRP inhibits:

1. Vasodilatation.
2. Angiogenesis.
3. Activation of ILC2.
4. Transmission of pain.

Question 16
"Neurogenic inflammation":

1. Is not linked with allergic inflammation.
2. Does not impact the immune system.
3. Can promote damage of innervated tissues, where it develops.
4. Can lead to allergen tolerance maintenance.

References

1. Chen C-S, Barnoud C, Scheiermann C. Peripheral neurotransmitters in the immune system. Curr Opin Physiol. 2021;19:73–9. https://doi.org/10.1016/j.cophys.2020.09.009.
2. Dantzer R. Neuroimmune interactions: from the brain to the immune system and vice versa. Physiol Rev. 2018;98:477–504. https://doi.org/10.1152/physrev.00039.2016.
3. Klimov AV, Isaev PYu, Klimov VV, Sviridova VS. Endotypes of allergic rhinitis and asthma accompanying food allergy. Bull Sib Med. 2019;18(2):287-289. https://doi.org/10.20538/1682-0363-2019-2-287-289.
4. Yamauchi K, Ogasawara M. The role of histamine in the pathophysiology of asthma and the clinical efficacy of antihistamines in asthma therapy. Int J Mol Sci. 2019;20:1733. https://doi.org/10.3390/ijms20071733.

5. Voisin T, Bouvier A, Chiu IV. Neuro-immune interactions in allergic diseases: novel targets for therapeutics. Int Immunol. 2017;29(6):247–61. https://doi.org/10.1093/intimm/dxx040.
6. Mittal R, Debs LH, Patel AP, Nguyen D, Patel K, O'Connor G, et al. Neurotransmitters: the critical modulators regulating gut-brain axis. J Cell Physiol. 2017;232(9):2359–72. https://doi.org/10.1002/jcp.25518.
7. Klose CSN, Veiga-Fernandes H. Neuroimmune interactions in peripheral tissues. Eur J Immunol. 2021;51:1602–14. https://doi.org/10.1002/eji.202048812.
8. Godinho-Silva C, Cardoso F, Veiga-Fernandes H. Neuro-immune cell units: a new paradigm in physiology. Annu Rev Immunol. 2019;37:19–46. https://doi.org/10.1146/annurev-immunol-042718-041812.
9. Audrit KJ, Delventhal L, Aydin O, Nassenstein C. The nervous system of airways and its remodeling in inflammatory lung diseases. Cell Tissue Res. 2017;367:571–90. https://doi.org/10.1007/s00441-016-2559-7.
10. De Virgillis F, Di Giovanni S. Lung innervation in the eye of a cytokine storm: neuroimmune interactions and COVID-19. Nat Rev Neurol. 2020;16:645–52. https://doi.org/10.1038/s41582-020-0402-y.
11. Campo P, Eguiluz-Gracia I, Salas M, Rodriguez MJ, Perez-Sanchez N, Gonzalez M, Molina A, Mayorga C, Torres MJ, Rondón C. Bronchial asthma triggered by house dust mites in patients with local allergic rhinitis. Allergy. 2019;74(8):1502–10. https://doi.org/10.1111/all.13775.
12. Kılıç E, Kutlu A, Hastalıkları G, Hastanesi KD, Servisi AI, Hastanesi KD, et al. Does local allergy (entopy) exists in asthma? J Clin Anal Med. 2016. Letters to Editors from 01.02.2016; https://doi.org/10.4328/JCAM.3272.
13. Campo P, Eguiluz-Gracia I, Bogas G, Salas M, Plaza Seron C, Perez N, Mayorga C, Torres MJ, Shamji MH, Rondón C. Local allergic rhinitis: implications for management. Clin Exp Allergy. 2019;49(1):6–16. https://doi.org/10.1111/cea.13192.
14. Klimov AV, Kalyuzhin OV, Klimov VV, Sviridova VS. Allergic rhinitis and the phenomenon of entopy. Bull Sib Med. 2020;3:137–43. https://doi.org/10.20538/1682-0363-2020-3-137-143.
15. Eguiluz-Gracia I, Fernandez-Santamaria R, Testera-Montes A, Ariza A, Campo P, Prieto A, Perez-Sanchez N, Salas M, Mayorga C, Rondon C. Coexistence of nasal reactivity to allergens with and without IgE sensitization in patients with allergic rhinitis. Allergy. 2020;1:1689–98. https://doi.org/10.1111/all.14206.
16. Maoz-Segal R, Machnes-Maayan D, Veksler-Offengenden I, Frizinsky S, Hajyahia S, Agmon-Levin N. Local allergic rhinitis: an old story but a new entity. In: Gendeh BS, Turkalj M, editors. Rhinosinusitis. London: IntechOpen; 2019. p. 1–9. https://doi.org/10.5772/intechopen.86212.
17. Yamana Y, Fukuda K, Ko R, Uchio E. Local allergic conjunctivitis: a phenotype of allergic conjunctivitis. Int Ophthalmol. 2019;39:2539–44. https://doi.org/10.1007/s10792-019-01101-z.
18. Cuevas J. Neurotransmitters and their life cycle. 2019. Access: http://www.sciencedirect.com/science/article/pii/B9780128012383113182.; https://doi.org/10.1016/B978-0-12-801238-3.11318-2.
19. Ortiz GG, Loera-Rodriguez LH, Cruz-Serrano JA, Torres-Sanchez ED, Mora-Navarro MA, Delgado-Lara DLC, et al. Gut-brain axis: role of microbiota in Parkinson's disease and multiple sclerosis. In: Artis AS, editor. Eat, learn, remember. London: IntechOpen; 2018. p. 11–30. https://doi.org/10.5772/intechopen.79493.
20. Hodo TW, de Aquino MTP, Shimamoto A, Shanker A. Critical neurotransmitters in the neuroimmune network. Front Immunol. 2020;11:1869. https://doi.org/10.3389/fimmu.2020.01869.
21. Kabata H, Artis D. Neuro-immune crosstalk and allergic inflammation. J Clin Invest. 2019;129(4):1475–82. https://doi.org/10.1172/JCI124609.
22. Niezgoda M, Kasacka I. Gastrointestinal neuroendocrine cells in various types of hypertension – a review. Prog Health Sci. 2017;7(2):117–25. https://doi.org/10.5604/01.3001.0010.7860.

23. Noguchi M, Furukawa KT, Morimoto M. Pulmonary neuroendocrine cells: physiology, tissue homeostasis and disease. Dis Model Mech. 2020;13(12):dmm046920. https://doi.org/10.1242/dmm.046920.
24. Modasia A, Parker A, Jones E, Stentz R, Brion A, Goldson A, et al. Regulation of enteroendocrine cell networks by the major human gut symbiont Bacteroides thetaiotaomicron. Front Microbiol. 2020;11:575595. https://doi.org/10.3389/fmicb.2020.575595.
25. Bankova LG, Barrett NA. Epithelial cell function and remodeling in nasal polyposis. Ann Allergy Asthma Immunol. 2020;124:333–41. https://doi.org/10.1016/j.anai.2020.01.018.
26. Kerage D, Sloan EK, Mattarollo SR, McCombe PA. Interaction of neurotransmitters and neurochemicals with lymphocytes. J Neuroimmunol. 2019;332:99–111. https://doi.org/10.1016/j.jneuroim.2019.04.006.
27. Hampel L, Lau T. Neurobiological principles: neurotransmitters. In: Riederer P, Laux G, Mulsant B, Le W, Nagatsu T, editors. NeuroPsychopharmacotherapy. Cham: Springer; 2020. p. 1–21. https://doi.org/10.1007/978-3-319-56015-1_365-1.
28. Wilkinson M, Brown R. Neurotransmitters. In: An introduction to neuroendocrinology. Cambridge: Cambridge University Press; 2015. p. 78–119. https://doi.org/10.1017/CBO9781139045803.006.
29. Meriney SD, Fanselow EE. Gaseous neurotransmitters. In: Meriney SD, Fanselow EE, editors. Synaptic transmission, Chapter 20. Cambridge: Academic Press; 2019. p. 435–47. https://doi.org/10.1016/B978-0-12-815320-8.00020-X.
30. Elphick MR, Mirabeau O, Larhammar D. Evolution of neuropeptide signalling systems. J Exp Biol. 2018;221(3):1–27. https://doi.org/10.1242/jeb.151092.
31. Silva-Vilches C, Ring S, Mahnke K. ATP and its metabolite adenosine as regulators of dendritic cell activity. Front Immunol. 2018;9:2581. https://doi.org/10.3389/fimmu.2018.02581.
32. Fogaça MV, Lisboa SF, Aguilar DC, Moreira FA, Gomes FV, Casarotto PC, Guimarães FS. Fine-tuning of defensive behaviors in the dorsal periaqueductal gray by atypical neurotransmitters. Braz J Med Biol Res. 2011;45(4):357–65. https://doi.org/10.1590/S0100-879X2012007500029.
33. McEnery MW, Siegal RE. Neurotransmitter receptors. In: Aminoff MJ, Daroff RB, editors. Encyclopedia of the neurological sciences. Oxford: Elsevier/Academic Press; 2014. p. 552–64. https://doi.org/10.1016/B978-0-12-385157-4.00044-0.
34. Catterall WA. Ion channel voltage sensors: structure, function, and pathophysiology. Neuron. 2010;67(6):915–28. https://doi.org/10.1016/j.neuron.2010.08.021.
35. Choudhury A, Sahu T, Ramanujam PL, Banerjee AK, Chakraborty I, Kumar AR, Arora N. Neurochemicals, behaviours and psychiatric perspectives of neurological diseases. Neuropsychiatry. 2018;8(1):395–424. https://doi.org/10.4172/Neuropsychiatry.1000361.
36. Carlton SM. Nociceptive primary afferents: they have a mind of their own. J Physiol. 2014;592(16):3403–11. https://doi.org/10.1113/jphysiol.2013.269654.
37. Bosmans G, Bassi GS, Florens M, Gonzalez-Dominguez E, Matteoli G, Boeckxstaens GE. Cholinergic modulation of type 2 immune responses. Front Immunol. 2017;8:1873. https://doi.org/10.3389/fimmu.2017.01873.
38. Gori S, Vermeulen M, Remes-Lenicov F, Jancic C, Scordo W, Caballos A, et al. Acetylcholine polarizes dendritic cells toward a Th2-promoting profile. Allergy. 2017;72(2):221–31. https://doi.org/10.1111/all.12926.
39. Saunders CJ, Christensen M, Finger TE, Tizzano M. Cholinergic neurotransmission links solitary chemosensory cells to nasal inflammation. PNAS. 2014;111(16):6075–80. https://doi.org/10.1073/pnas.1402251111.
40. Wang W, Cohen JA, Wallrapp A, Trieu KG, Barrios J, Shao F, et al. Age-related dopaminergic innervation augments T helper 2-type allergic inflammation in the postnatal lung. Immunity. 2019;51:1102–1118.e7. https://doi.org/10.1016/j.immuni.2019.10.002.
41. Weng M, Xie X, Liu C, Lim K-L, Zhang C-W, Li L. The sources of reactive oxygen species and its possible role in the pathogenesis of Parkinson's disease. Parkinsons Dis. 2018;2018:9163040. https://doi.org/10.1155/2018/9163040.
42. Klimov VV. Adaptive immune responses. In: From basic to clinical immunology. Cham: Springer; 2019. https://doi.org/10.1007/978-3-030-03323-6.

43. Samuels A. Dose dependent toxicity of glutamic acid: a review. Int J Food Prop. 2020;23(1):412–9. https://doi.org/10.1080/10942912.2020.1733016.
44. Contreras Healey DC, Cephus JY, Barone SM, Chowdhury NU, Dahunsi DO, Madden MZ, et al. Targeting in vivo metabolic vulnerabilities of Th2 and Th17 cells reduces airway inflammation. J Immunol. 2021;206(6):1127–39. https://doi.org/10.4049/jimmunol.2001029.
45. Lee H-S, Goh E-K, Wang S-G, Chon K-M, Kim H-K, Roh H-J. Detection of amino acids in human nasal mucosa using microdialysis technique: increased glutamate in allergic rhinitis. Asian Pac J Allergy. 2006;23(4):213–9. Access: https://www.researchgate.net/publication/7206172
46. Alim MA, Grujic M, Ackerman PW, Kristiansson P, Eliasson P, Peterson M, Pejler G. Glutamate triggers the expression of functional ionotropic and metabotropic glutamate receptors in mast cells. Cell Mol Immunol. 2020;17(10):1117. https://doi.org/10.1038/s41423-020-0421-z.
47. Gupta K, Harvima IT. Mast cell-neural interactions contribute to pain and itch. Immunol Rev. 2018;282(1):168–87. https://doi.org/10.1111/imr.12622.
48. Saeki M, Nishimura T, Kaminuma O, Ohtsu H, Mori A, Hiroi T. Crosstalk between histamine and T cells in allergic diseases. Curr Immunol Rev. 2016;12(1):10–3. https://doi.org/10.2174/1573395511666150706180936.
49. Thangam EB, Jemima EA, Singh H, Baig MS, Khan M, Mathias CB, et al. The role of histamine and histamine receptors in mast cell-mediated allergy and inflammation: the hunt for new therapeutic targets. Front Immunol. 2018;9:1873. https://doi.org/10.3389/fimmu.2018.01873.
50. Scammell TE, Jackson AC, Franks NP, Wisden W, Dauvilliers Y. Histamine: neural circuits and new medications. Sleep. 2019;42(1):1–8. https://doi.org/10.1093/sleep/zsy183.
51. Bérczi I, Stephano A. Vasopressin, the acute phase response and healing. In: Insights to neuroimmune biology. Elsevier; 2016. p. 185–99. https://doi.org/10.1016/B978-0-12-801770-8.00008-2.
52. Quintanar-Stephano A, Campos-Rodríges R, Kovacs K. Vasopressin and immune function. Adv Neuroimmune Biol. 2011;1(2):143–56. https://doi.org/10.3233/NIB-2011-029.
53. Palin K, Moreau ML, Sauvant J, Orcel H, Nadjar A, Rabié A, Show FM. Interleukin-6 activates arginine vasopressin neurons in the supraoptic nucleus during immune challenge in rats. Am J Physiol Endocrinol Metab. 2009;296(6):E1289–99. https://doi.org/10.1152/ajpendo.90489.2008.
54. Marseglia L, D'Angelo G, Manti S, Salpietro C, Arrigo T, Barberi I, et al. Melatonin and atopy: role in atopic dermatitis and asthma. Int J Mol Sci. 2014;15(8):13482–93. https://doi.org/10.3390/ijms150813482.
55. Guan R, Malkani RG. Melatonin, sleep, and allergy. In: Fishbein A, Sheldon S, editors. Allergy and sleep. Cham: Springer; 2019. p. 367–84. https://doi.org/10.1007/978-3-030-14738-9_272019.
56. Hardeland R. Melatonin and inflammation - story of a double-edged blade. J Pineal Res. 2018;65(4):e12525. https://doi.org/10.1111/jpi.12525.
57. Luo J, Zhang Z, Sun H, Song J, Chen X, Huang J, Lin X, Zhou R. Effect of melatonin on T/B cell activation and immune regulation in pinealectomy mice. Life Sci. 2020;242:117191. https://doi.org/10.1016/j.lfs.2019.117191.
58. Mashaghi A, Marmalidou A, Tehrani M, Grace PT, Pothoulakis C, Dana R. Neuropeptide substance P and the immune response. Cell Mol Life Sci. 2016;73(22):4249–64. https://doi.org/10.1007/s00018-016-2293-z.
59. Vena GA, Cassano N, Di Leo E, Calogiuri GF, Nettis E. Focus on the role of substance P in chronic urticaria. Clin Mol Allergy. 2018;16:24. https://doi.org/10.1186/s12948-018-0101-z.
60. Perner C, Flayer CH, Zhu X, Aderhold PA, ZNA D, Voisin T, et al. Substance P release by sensory neurons triggers dendritic cell migration and initiates the type-2 immune response to allergens. Immunity. 2020;53(5):1063–77.e7. https://doi.org/10.1016/j.immuni.2020.10.001.
61. Wallrapp A, Riesenfeld SJ, Burkett PR, Abdulnour RE, Nyman J, Dionne D, et al. The neuropeptide NMU amplifies ILC2-driven allergic lung inflammation. Nature. 2017;549:351–6. https://doi.org/10.1038/nature24029.

62. Ren X, Dong F, Zhuang Y, Wang Y, Ma W. Effect of neuromedin U on allergic airway inflammation in an asthma model (review). Exp Ther Med. 2020;19(2):809–16. https://doi.org/10.3892/etm.2019.8283.
63. Ye Y, Hue L. The potential role of neuromedin U in human type-2 immunity. Eur Respir J. 2019;54(Suppl 63):OA1626. https://doi.org/10.1183/13993003.congress-2019.OA1626.
64. Pongratz G, Straub RH. The sympathetic nervous response in inflammation. Arthritis Res Ther. 2014;16(6):504. http://arthritis-research.com/content/16/6/504.
65. Moriyama S, Brestoff JR, Flamar AL, Moeller JB, Klose CSN, Rankin LC, et al. Beta2-adrenergic receptor-mediated negative regulation of group 2 innate lymphoid cell responses. Science. 2018;359:1056–61. https://doi.org/10.1126/science.aan4829.
66. Yao A, Wilson JA, Ball SL. Autonomic nervous system dysfunction and sinonasal symptoms. Allergy Rhinol (Providence). 2018;9:1–9. https://doi.org/10.1177/2152656718764233.
67. Herr N, Bode C, Duerschmied D. The effects of serotonin in immune cells. Front Cardiovasc Med. 2017;4:48. https://doi.org/10.3389/fcvm.2017.00048.
68. Shajib MS, Khan WI. The role of serotonin and its receptors in activation of immune responses and inflammation. Acta Physiol (Oxford). 2015;213:561–74. https://doi.org/10.1111/apha.12430.
69. Švajger U, Rožman P. Induction of tolerogenic dendritic cells by endogenous biomolecules: an update. Front Immunol. 2018;9:2482. https://doi.org/10.3389/fimmu.2018.02482.
70. Nau F, Miller J, Saravia J, Ahlert T, Yu B, Happel K, Cormier S, Nichols C. Serotonin 5-HT2 receptor activation prevents allergic asthma in a mouse model. Am J Physiol Lung Cell Mol Physiol. 2015;308(2):L191–8. https://doi.org/10.1152/ajplung.00138.2013.
71. Schneider E, Machavoine F, Bricard-Rignault R, Levasseur M, Petit-Bertron AF, Gautron S, et al. Downregulation of basophil-derived IL-4 and in vivo T(H)2 IgE responses by serotonin and other organic cation transporter 3 ligands. J Allergy Clin Immunol. 2011;128(4):864–71.e2. https://doi.org/10.1016/j.jaci.2011.04.043.
72. Dionisio L, De Rosa MJ, Bouzat C, MDC E. An intrinsic GABAergic system in human lymphocytes. Neuropharmacology. 2011;60(2–3):513–9. https://doi.org/10.1016/j.neuropharm.2010.11.007.
73. Jin Z, Mendu SK, Birnir B. GABA is an effective immunomodulatory molecule. Amino Acids. 2013;45(1):87–94. https://doi.org/10.1007/s00726-011-1193-7.
74. Xiang Y-Y, Wang S, Liu M, Hirota JA, Li J, Ju W, et al. A GABAergic system in airway epithelium is essential for mucus overproduction in asthma. Nat Med. 2007;13(7):862–7. https://doi.org/10.1038/nm1604.
75. Barragan A, Weidner JM, Jin Z, Korpi ER, Birnir B. GABAergic signalling in the immune system. Acta Physiol. 2015;213(4):819–27. https://doi.org/10.1111/apha.12467.
76. Munroe ME, Businga TR, Kline JN, Dishop GA. Anti-inflammatory effects of the neurotransmitter agonist honokiol in a mouse model of allergic asthma. J Immunol. 2010;185:5586–97. https://doi.org/10.4049/jimmunol.1000630.
77. Dimić D, Timotijevic L, Nicolic I, Zdravkovic A, Nikcevic L, Dimic N, Simeunovic I. Effects of GABA on lung function in asthmatics after methacholine inhalation. Eur Respir J. 2017;50(Suppl 61):PA3574. https://doi.org/10.1183/1393003.congress-2017.PA3574.
78. Razak MA, Begum PS, Viswanath B, Rajagopal S. Multifarious beneficial effect of non-essential amino acid, glycine: a review. Oxidative Med Cell Longev. 2017;2017:1716701. https://doi.org/10.1155/2017/1716701.
79. Breitinger U, Breitinger H-G. Modulators of the inhibitory glycine receptor. ACS Chem Neurosci. 2020;11(12):1706–25. https://doi.org/10.1021/acschemneuro.0c00054.
80. den Eynden JV, Ali SS, Horwood N, Carmans S, Brône B, Hellings N, et al. Glycine and glycine receptor signalling in non-neuronal cells. Front Mol Neurosci. 2009;2:9. https://doi.org/10.3389/neuro.02.009.2009.
81. Weinberg JM, Venkatachalam MA, Bienholz A. The role of glycine in regulated cell death. Cell Mol Life Sci. 2016;73(11–12):2285–308. https://doi.org/10.1007/s00018-016-2201-6.
82. Moberg KU, Handlin L, Kendall-Tackett K, Petersson M. Oxytocin is a principal hormone that exerts part of its effects by active fragments. Med Hypotheses. 2019;133:1–9. https://doi.org/10.1016/j.mehy.2019.109394.

83. Li T, Wang P, Wang SC, Wang Y-F. Approaches mediating oxytocin regulation of the immune system. Front Immunol. 2017;7:693. https://doi.org/10.3389/fimmu.2016.00693.
84. Wang Y-F. Center role of the oxytocin-secreting system in neuroendocrine-immune network revisited. J Clin Exp Neuroimmunol. 2016;1(1):102.
85. Wallrapp A, Burkett PR, Riesenfeld SJ, Kim SJ, Christian E, Abdulnour RE, et al. Calcitonin gene-related peptide negatively regulates alarmin-driven type 2 innate lymphoid cell responses. Immunity. 2019;51:709–23.e6. https://doi.org/10.1016/j.immuni.2019.09.005.
86. Nagashima H, Mahlakoiv T, Shih HY, Davis FP, Meylan F, Huang Y, et al. Neuropeptide CGRP limits group 2 innate lymphoid cell responses and constrains type 2 inflammation. Immunity. 2019;51:682–95.e6. https://doi.org/10.1016/j.immuni.2019.06.009.
87. Ochoa-Callejero L, Garcia-Sanmartin J, Villoslada-Blanco P, Iniguez M, Perez-Matute P, Pujadas E, et al. Circulating levels of calcitonin gene-related peptide are lower in COVID-19 patients. J Endocr Soc. 2021;5(3):199. https://doi.org/10.1210/jendso/bvaa199.
88. Iwasaki M, Akiba Y, Kaunitz JD. Recent advances in vasoactive intestinal peptide physiology and pathophysiology: focus on the gastrointestinal system. F1000Res. 2019;8:1629. https://doi.org/10.12688/f1000research.18039.1.
89. Watanabe J. Vasoactive intestinal peptide. In: Takei Y, Ando H, Tsutsui K, editors. Handbook of hormones. Oxford: Academic Press; 2016. p. 150–2. https://doi.org/10.1016/B978-0-12-801028-0.00146-X.
90. Raker VK, Domogalla MP, Steinbrink K. Tolerogenic dendritic cells for regulatory T cell induction in man. Front Immunol. 2015;6:569. https://doi.org/10.3389/fimmu.2015.00569.
91. Sallaberry CA, Astern L. The endocannabinoid system, our universal regulator. J Young Investig. 2018;34(6):48–55. https://doi.org/10.22186/jyi.34.5.48-55.
92. Dhital S, Stokes JV, Park N, Seo KS, Kaplan BLF. Cannabidiol (CBD) induces functional Tregs in response to low-level T cell activation. Cell Immunol. 2017;312:25–34. https://doi.org/10.1016/j.cellimm.2016.11.006.
93. Liang X, Liu R, Chen C, Ji F, Li T. Opioid system modulates the immune function: a review. Transl Perioper Pain Med. 2016;1(1):5–13. Access: https://www.ncbi.nlm.nih.gov/pmc/articles/PMC4790459/.
94. Ironside M, Kumar P, Kang M-S, Pizzagalli DA. Brain mechanisms mediating effects of stress on reward sensitivity. Curr Opin Behav Sci. 2018;22:106–13. https://doi.org/10.1016/j.cobeha.2018.01.016.
95. Shrihari TG. Endorphins – a natural healer. J Cancer Prev Curr Res. 2018;9(5):223–34.
96. Sha J, Meng C, Li L, Xiu Q, Zhu D. Correlation of serum b-endorphin and the quality of life in allergic rhinitis. Dis Markers. 2016:2025418. https://doi.org/10.1155/2016/2025418.
97. Mancuso C, Navarra P, Preziosi P. Roles of nitric oxide, carbon monoxide, and hydrogen sulfide in the regulation of the hypothalamic–pituitary–adrenal axis. J Neurochem. 2010;113:563–75. https://doi.org/10.1111/j.1471-4159.2010.06606.x.
98. Fagone P, Mazzon E, Bramanti P, Bendtzen K, Nicoletti F. Gasotransmitters and the immune system: mode of action and novel therapeutic targets. Eur J Pharmacol. 2018;834:92–102. https://doi.org/10.1016/j.ejphar.2018.07.026.
99. Oleskin AV, Shenderov BA. Neuromodulatory effects and targets of the SCFAs and gasotransmitters produced by the human symbiotic microbiota. Microb Ecol Health Dis. 2016;27:30971. https://doi.org/10.3402/mehd.v27.30971.
100. Deshane J, Zmijewski JW, Luther R, Gaggar A, Deshane R, Lai J-F, et al. Free radical-producing myeloid-derived regulatory cells: potent activators and suppressors of lung inflammation and airway hyperresponsiveness. Mucosal Immunol. 2011;4:503–18. https://doi.org/10.1038/mi.2011.16.
101. Bratt JM, Franzi LM, Linderholm AL, Last MS, Kenyon NJ, Last JA. Arginase enzymes in isolated airways from normal and nitric oxide synthase 2-knockout mice exposed to ovalbumin. Toxicol Appl Pharmacol. 2009;234(3):273–80. https://doi.org/10.1016/j.taap.2008.10.007.
102. Garcia-Garcia L, Olle L, Martin M, Roca-Ferrer J, Munoz-Cano R. Adenosine signaling in mast cells and allergic diseases. Int J Mol Sci. 2021;22:5203. https://doi.org/10.3390/ijms22105203.

103. Matsuo Y, Yanase Y, Irifuku R, Ishii K, Kawaguchi T, Takahagi S, Hide I, Hide M. The role of adenosine for IgE receptor-dependent degranulation of human peripheral basophils and skin mast cells. Allergol Int. 2018;67:524–6. https://doi.org/10.1016/j.alit.2018.03.007.
104. Pondeljak N, Lugović-Mihić L. Stress-induced interaction of skin immune cells, hormones, and neurotransmitters. Clin Ther. 2020;42(5):757–70. https://doi.org/10.1016/j.clinthera.2020.03.008.
105. Assas BM, Pennock JI, Miyan JA. Calcitonin gene-related peptide is a key neurotransmitter in the neuro-immune axis. Front Neurosci. 2014;8:23. https://doi.org/10.3389/fnins.2014.00023.
106. Auteri M, Zizzo MG, Serio R. GABA and GABA receptors in the gastrointestinal tract: from motility to inflammation. Pharmacol Res. 2015;93:11–21. https://doi.org/10.1016/j.phrs.2014.12.001.
107. Graziottin A, Giraldi A. Anatomy and physiology of women's sexual function. In: Porst H, Buvat J, editors. Standard practice in Sexual Medicine, Chapter 19. Oxford: Blackwell; 2006. p. 289–304.
108. Calabrò RS, Cacciola A, Bruschetta D, Milardi D, Quattrini F, Sciarrone F, et al. Neuroanatomy and function of human sexual bahavior: a neglected or unknown issue? Brain Behav. 2019;9:e01389. https://doi.org/10.1002/brb3.1389.
109. Anvari S, Vyhlidal CA, Dai H, Jones BL. Genetic variation along the histamine pathway in children with allergic versus nonallergic asthma. Am J Respir Cell Mol Biol. 2015;53:802–9. https://doi.org/10.1165/rcmb.2014-0493OC.
110. Yamauchi K, Shikanai T, Nakamura Y, Kobayashi H, Ogasawara M, Maeyama K. Roles of histamine in the pathogenesis of bronchial asthma and reevaluation of the clinical usefulness of antihistamines. Yakugaku Zasshi. 2011;131:185–91. https://doi.org/10.1248/yakushi.131.185.
111. Chen L, Hong C, Chen EC, Yee SW, Xu L, Almof EU, et al. Genetics and epigenetic regulation of the organic cation transporter 3, LC22A3. Pharm J. 2013;13:110–20. https://doi.org/10.1038/tpj.2011.60.
112. Ohtsu H, Tanaka S, Terui T, Hori Y, Makabe-Kobayashi Y, Pejler G, et al. Mice lacking histidine decarboxylase exhibit abnormal mast cells. FEBS Lett. 2001;502:53–6. https://doi.org/10.1016/S0014-5793(01)02663-1.
113. Wen Y, Wang J, Zhang Q, Chen Y, Bao X. The genetic and clinical characteristics of aromatic L-amino acid decarboxylase deficiency in mainland China. J Hum Genet. 2020;65:759–69. https://doi.org/10.1038/s10038-020-0770-6.
114. McKinney J, Johansson S, Halmoy A, Dramsdahl M, Winge I, Knappskog PM, et al. A loss-of-function mutation in tryptophan hydroxylase 2 segregating with attention-deficit/hyperactivity disorder. Mol Psychiatry. 2008;13:365–7. https://doi.org/10.1038/sj.mp.4002152.
115. Wang L-J, Yu Y-H, Fu M-L, Yeh W-T, Hsu J-L, Yang Y-H, et al. Attention deficit–hyperactivity disorder is associated with allergic symptoms and low levels of hemoglobin and serotonin. Sci Rep. 2018;8:10229. https://doi.org/10.1038/s41598-018-28702-5.
116. Le DD, Schmit D, Heck S, Omlor AJ, Sester M, Herr C, et al. Increase of mast cell-nerve association and neuropeptide receptor expression on mast cells in perennial allergic rhinitis. Neuroimmunomodulation. 2016;23:261–70. https://doi.org/10.1159/000453068.
117. Thornton MA, Akasheh N, Walsh MT, Moloney M, Sheahan PO, Smyth CM, et al. Eosinophil recruitment to nasal nerves after allergen challenge in allergic rhinitis. Clin Immunol. 2013;147:50–7. https://doi.org/10.1016/j.clim.2013.02.008.
118. Sarin S, Undem B, Sanico A, Togias A. The role of the nervous system in rhinitis. J Allergy Clin Immunol. 2006;118(5):999–1014. https://doi.org/10.1016/j.jaci.2006.09.013.
119. Skaper SD. Nerve growth factor: a neuroimmune crosstalk mediator for all seasons. Immunology. 2017;151(1):1–15. https://doi.org/10.1111/imm.12717.

Conventional Atopic Diseases

5

Contents

Didactics

Knowledge. Upon successful completion of this chapter, students should be able to:

1. List the groups of conventional atopic diseases.
2. Be familiar with the interpretation of patient's history, clinical, component resolved data for diagnosis, and results of skin prick testing (SPT).
3. Differentiate roles of various allergology methods of investigation.
4. Draw clinical symptoms of atopic disorders.

Supplementary Information The online version contains supplementary material available at [https://doi.org/10.1007/978-3-031-04309-3_5].

V. V. Klimov, *Textbook of Allergen Tolerance*,
https://doi.org/10.1007/978-3-031-04309-3_5

5. Define allergen tolerance maintenance and breakdown of atopic conditions. Distinguish between allergic asthma and allergic rhinitis.
6. Describe the pathology and clinical symptoms of atopic dermatitis.
7. Define toxico-allergic and systemic disorders, including urticaria and anaphylaxis.

Acquired Skills. Upon successful completion of this chapter, students should demonstrate the following skills:

1. Interpret the knowledge related to routine allergology.
2. Critically evaluate the clinical literature about atopic diseases.
3. Discuss the scientific articles from the current research literature to criticize experimental and clinical data and formulate new hypotheses in allergy.
4. Obtain a patient's history, including the history of present illness, past medical history, social, family, and occupational history, and review of systems.
5. Perform a patient's physical examination thoroughly.
6. Execute and read SPT and intradermal test using the simulator.
7. Explain the rationale for the choice of diagnosis of allergy in a patient.
8. Have a clear perception of the presented allergology definitions expressed orally and in written form.
9. Formulate the presented immunology and allergy terms.
10. Correctly answer the quiz questions.

Attitude and Professional Behaviors. Students should be able to:

1. Have the readiness to be hard-working.
2. Behave professionally at all times.
3. Recognize the importance of studying and demonstrate their commitment.
4. Demonstrate the consideration for the patient's feelings, ethnic, religious, cultural, and social background, and display empathy.

5.1 Introduction

From a clinical viewpoint, any allergist should determine the atopic disorder in patients with different allergic diseases. The atopy is the "queen" of all types of allergies and pseudo allergies. In predisposed atopic individuals, the term "*atopic march*" means consistent involvement of allergic target organs in the following order: the skin, nose/conjunctive, and bronchi [1] or the progression from atopic dermatitis to the development of other allergic disorders such as IgE-mediated food allergies, allergic rhinitis, and asthma in later childhood [2]. Some elderly patients may simultaneously develop all atopic conditions. Also, any allergist should be aware that allergen-specific immunotherapy (AIT) may only be used as a high-effective approach in atopic individuals. The development of atopic dermatitis in infancy and subsequent allergic rhinitis and asthma in later childhood is known as the atopic march. However, the discovery of filaggrin mutations [3] demonstrated the idea of a causal link between atopic dermatitis and later onset atopic disorders. These studies suggest such a skin barrier serves as a site for allergen entry and colonization of bacterial pathogens. It may induce systemic Th2 immunity that predisposes patients to allergy in the unified airway [4]. Despite arisen doubt concerning "atopic march" due to *filaggrin gene* mutations, this phenomenon exists. Many other gene mutations and epigenetic modifications complicate the course of atopic diseases [5].

5.2 Allergologic Investigations

5.2.1 Patient's Current and Past Medical History and Physical Examination

All medical evaluations of patients suffering from allergies begin with a history (or anamnesis) and physical examination.

In history, it is especially important to document:

- The history of the present disease (general complaints; type of onset and signs; which factors seem to be provocative; link with a certain period of the year; which therapy seems to be effective, etc.)
- The family history (in particular, atopic heredity)
- The past medical history (the age at which the first allergic signs occurred; type and sites of allergic signs; which therapy was effective; associated diseases; etc.)
- The social and occupational (in adults) history

In the physical examination, look particularly for:

- The vital signs (pulse, respiratory rate, blood pressure)
- The state of the skin (which morphological lesions and their sites, itching, secondary infections, etc.)
- The presence of edema and redness of the conjunctive
- Nasal obstruction, type, and values of discharge and sputum
- Wheezing, dry rale, expiratory dyspnea

5.2.2 Component Resolved Diagnosis (CRD)

Since 1988, cDNA encoding allergens was cloned for the first time from insect venom, birch, and HDM. This achievement, *component resolved diagnosis (CRD)*, marked the beginning of molecular allergology, and, in addition, substantial global datasets facilitated routine allergist's work in the face of the omics revolution [6]. Therefore, the precision of diagnostic procedures in allergology has improved significantly by producing recombinant and purified allergenic molecules. It also increased the analytic sensitivity and diagnostic specificity and decreased potential risks, possible cross-reactivity versus primary (species-specific and genuine) sensitization. The list of required allergenic molecules cloned or purified and introduced for medical use rapidly enhances but is still insufficient. Especially in polysensitized patients with seasonal allergies, clinicians often face a complex setting for the decision on AIT prescription [7].

There are some approaches to fulfilling CRD. Serologic analyses based on biotechnologically engineered allergens can be performed in singleplex assays testing one allergen at a time or in a multiplex approach, allowing IgE's simultaneous determination toward many molecules. The singleplex assays (ImmunoCAP, Thermo Fisher Scientific/Phadia, Uppsala, Sweden) might be favorable because they are much cheaper and do not provide potentially unnecessary information [8]. Multiplex (ImmunoCAP Immuno Solid-phase Allergen Chip [ISAC]) has been the preferred version for the last decade.

An intermediate option between singleplex assays and microarrays or macro arrays are the customized allergen profiles (Euroline; Euroimmun, Lübeck, Germany), which combine allergen extracts and a set of the most relevant related allergenic molecules to distinguish cross-reactivity, genuine sensitization, and possibly assess the risk profile [9].

$$\text{Positive CRD result} > 0.35\,\text{kU} / \text{L}.$$

During the transition time, allergists can operate with two allergen generations, allergen extracts, and allergenic molecules. There is a problem, which allergen generation, extracts, or molecules, must preferentially be considered for the reliable assessment of sensitization. A carried out study included the measurement of specific IgE to allergen extracts of peanuts and peaches and four allergenic molecules of peanut and three peaches in 943 Sicilian persons suffering from food allergies and suspected food allergies to these products. The results demonstrated 25.9% of patients suspected of peanut sensitization were positive to peanut extracts and only 1.5% to allergenic molecules; 2.8% of persons suspected of peach allergy were positive to peach extracts and 1.3% to allergenic molecules. The results may reflect a situation in which some required allergenic molecules are lacking [10].

Component resolved diagnosis (CRD) marked the beginning of molecular era in allergology and coincided with the omics revolution [6, 7].

5.2.3 Debates in Allergic Skin Tests

Skin prick testing (SPT) is an essential test procedure to confirm sensitization in IgE-mediated allergic disease in atopic subjects *in vivo*. Position papers include international standards for allergic skin tests' performing and assessing protocols [11]. The first publication about SPT was made by Ebruster in 1959 [12], who discovered this diagnostic test as a primary diagnostic tool to detect IgE-dependent atopic pathology. Even though molecular allergology is an innovative and promising area, allergic skin testing should be considered a complementary, more selective, third-line diagnostic modality reserved for particular cases, such as complex allergies and polysensitization [13]. Diagnostic reliability to confirm allergic sensitization is associated with physiologic and biochemical properties of IgE, namely, the cytophilic feature to bind to mast cells/basophils in the tissues [14]. Accordingly, it is imperative to emphasize that these tests should always be considered obligatory in a careful medical history compilation and physical examination.

The discovery of the local atopic diseases in the unified airway makes physicians use SPT modifications as local allergen challenge [15] and *intradermal tests*. In contrast with SPT, intradermal tests with indoor allergens display a higher sensitivity [16, 17]. Unfortunately, there is no explanation for this fact yet. Detection of nasal specific IgE using CRD does not demonstrate a higher sensitivity compared with the nasal allergen provocation test (NAPT) in local allergic rhinitis [18].

Nowadays, SPT and CRD are the subjects of dispute among allergists. There are two typical viewpoints as follows: (1) Is it time to arrive at the age of molecular allergy diagnosis in daily patient care? [19] and (2) Allergy skin testing cannot be replaced by molecular diagnosis soon [13].

Execution of allergic skin testing (see Figs. 5.1 and 5.2) Absolute or relative contraindications to SPT include uncontrolled asthma, severe or unstable cardiovascular disease, concurrent β-blocker therapy, and pregnancy. A trained nurse executes allergic skin tests in the allergist's office. Before the tests, it is necessary to discontinue medications such as antihistamines, membrane stabilizers, and anti-leukotrienes according to their half-life elimination. When performing a prick or scratch test, a tiny drop of a possible allergen is pricked or scratched onto a certain area of the epidermis on the volar forearm, whereas for an intradermal test, a small amount of the potential allergen is injected by a thin needle inside a particular area of the epidermis. A prick/scratch test is assessed after 20 min, taking into account the diameter of the wheal. The diameter of the papule evaluates an intradermal test after 20 min (early phase) and 4–6 h (late phase). In both cases, histamine uses as a positive control to assess the wheal reaction of the skin before testing.

Reading the results of allergic skin testing (see Fig. 5.3; Table 5.1).

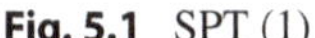

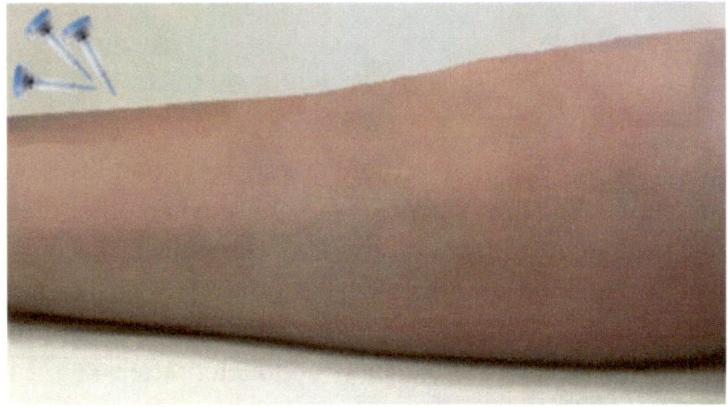

Fig. 5.1 SPT (1)

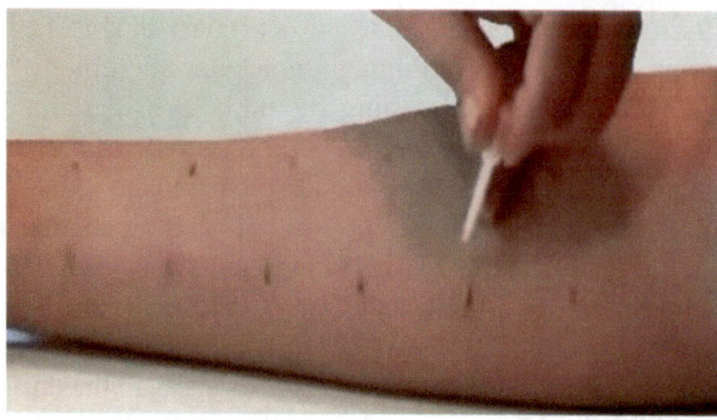

Fig. 5.2 SPT (2)

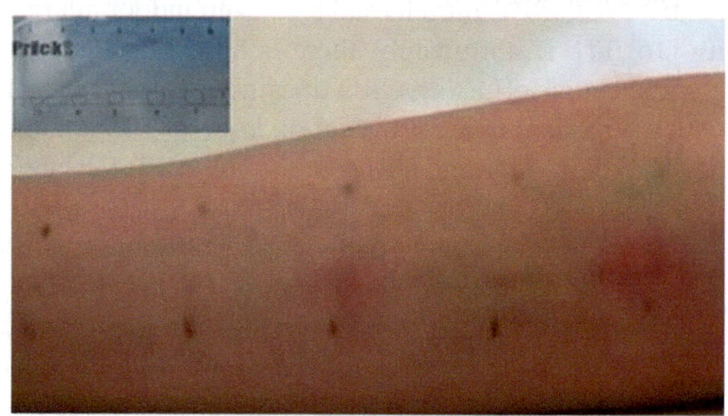

Fig. 5.3 SPT (3)

Table 5.1 Reading the allergic skin tests

Type hypersensitivity	Reading	Skin lesions	Size	Degree
Type I (atopy), early phase (SPT, intradermal testing)	In 20 min	Itching wheal, erythema, pseudopodia	2–3 mm	+
			4–5 mm	++
			6–10 mm	+++
			>10 mm	++++
Type I (atopy), late phase (intradermal testing)	In 4–6 h	Papule, erythema, pseudopodia	5–7 mm	+
			8–14 mm	++
			15–20 mm	+++
			>20 mm	++++
Type IV (intradermal testing)	In 48–72 h	Papule (infiltrate)	5–7 mm	+
			8–14 mm	++
			15–20 mm	+++
			>20 mm	++++

Atopy patch tests are indicated in IgE conditions such as food allergies, atopic dermatitis, and polyvalent sensitization when other diagnostic approaches are negative, and are conducted rarely. The technique resembles the application of skin tests, which carry out in type IV allergic disorders like contact allergic dermatitis but allergens triggering type I hypersensitivity are used (e.g., HDM, pollen, and food products). Reading the tests is conducted after 48–72 h by erythema, papules, and vesicles [20].

5.3 Allergic Asthma

▶ **Definition** Allergic asthma is a recurrent atopic inflammatory disease of lower airways caused by indoor and other allergens, and characterized by obstruction of the lower airways, bronchospasms, wheezing, and coughing.

Asthma is caused by well-known allergens like HDM (see Fig. 5.4), pet dander, cockroaches, mold, and pollens in susceptible atopic individuals. The *filaggrin gene*-deficient mutations are important not only for the atopic dermatitis pathogenesis. These mutations in airway epitheliocytes can increase epithelial permeability, promoting inhaled allergen entry into the lung [21]. Chronic asthma symptoms such as wheeze, shortness of breath, chest tightness, and cough are linked with changes in the structure of the large and small airways and airway remodeling [22]. The airway remodeling is characterized by goblet cell hyperplasia with an excess of mucus secretion, smooth muscle cell hyperplasia with bronchoconstriction, and airway hyperresponsiveness with combined symptoms. Mast cells, eosinophils, and neutrophils play an important role in the pathogenesis of allergic inflammation in

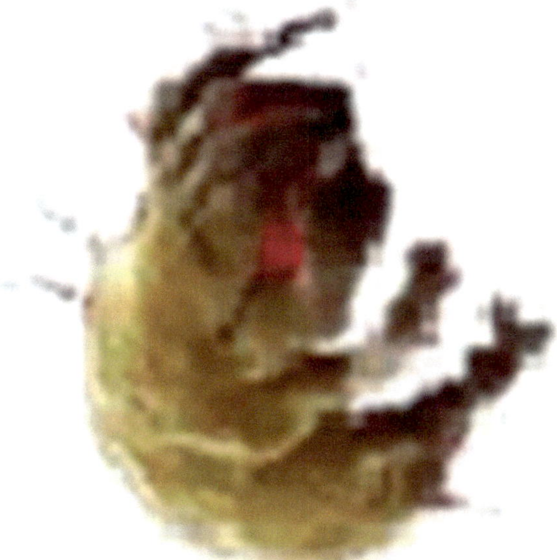

Fig. 5.4 *Dermatophagoides pteronissinus*—European HDM Classically, asthma has been categorized as either atopic/extrinsic or nonatopic/intrinsic [24]. According to international position papers on allergies and asthma [16, 25], the classification divides asthma severity into four groups: intermittent, persistent-mild, persistent-moderate, and persistent-severe. Severe asthma is a distinct disease form, in contrast to mild and moderate asthma. Also, asthma may be controlled and uncontrolled. An additional approach takes into consideration the phenotypes and endotypes of the disease [26]. Phenotype is characterized by clinical features with no direct relationship to disease mechanisms and treatment, whereas endotype is a disease subgroup with particular cellular and molecular mechanisms or treatment response [24, 26, 27].

asthma. Neurotransmitter histamine triggers airway obstruction via smooth muscle contraction, bronchial secretion, and airway mucosal edema [5]. Accumulating evidence indicates that allergen-specific Th2 cells and their cytokines such as IL-4, IL-5, IL-13, and IL-33 orchestrate these pathognomonic features of asthma [23].

There is a growing body of experimental data on the contribution of neutrophils or neutrophil-derived products to allergic asthma pathogenesis [28]. The asthmatic patient subpopulation has been described, preferentially with adult-onset asthma, associated with "neutrophil inflammation" and IL-8 (CXCL8), IL-17, TNF-α, etc., and resembles, but not identical to *chronic obstructive pulmonary disease (COPD)* [29]. The Th2-low/Th17/neutrophilic endotype of asthma and high IL-17 level respectively correlate with the severity of the disease. These patients are particularly elderly persons with metabolic comorbidities, including obesity, metabolic syndrome, and diabetes mellitus. Conversely, children and younger adult individuals frequently develop the Th2-high/eosinophilic endotype of asthma, and the disease is inherent in a milder course. However, late onset persistent eosinophilic asthma also exists [30].

Recent studies clearly show that not only Th2 cytokines but also other T cell-related cytokines (for example, of Th9, Th17, and Th22 profiles) and epithelium-derived cytokines, so-called alarmins IL-25, IL-33, and thymic stromal lymphopoietin (TSLP), are involved in the pathogenesis of asthma [31]. Furthermore, cytokines and chemokines may serve as predictive biomarkers of future asthma in children since there is evidence that the earliest cytokine and chemokine signals will come from bronchial epithelial cells [32]. Surprisingly, group 2 innate lymphoid (ILC2) cells can induce allergic inflammation in asthma without allergen-specific IgE [31].

As a rule, asthma may begin at the age of 4 years and older, having a significant long-term impact on the quality of life for patients. Asthmatic attacks can be triggered not only by causative allergens but also by respiratory infection, physical exercise, cold air, drugs like aspirin, or pollutants like sulfur dioxide, phthalates, etc. Exposure to air pollutants induces oxidative stress in the lung. Failure to detoxify air pollutants results in the release of the neutrophil chemokine IL-8, chemokine CCL20 (MIP-3α), and pro-inflammatory cytokines IL-1β, IL-6, and TNF-α promoting Th17 cells generation. Alarmins, epithelial cell-derived IL-25, IL-33, and TSLP, can be released following cellular damage resulting from oxidative stress, exposure to pollutants, and proteolytic allergens. The allergens (e.g., *Der p 2*) can also bind to pathogen-associated molecular pattern (PAMP) receptors like TLR4 and activate ILC2 cells to release IL-13 driving mucus production, and IL-5 recruiting eosinophils [33].

See allergen tolerance breakdown in asthma in Fig. 5.5.

Asthma often coexists with other atopic diseases like allergic rhinitis and atopic dermatitis. Commonly, asthma associated with food allergies affects 14% of school-age children in the United States [34]. Compared with children without food allergies, children with clinical food sensitization are two to four times more likely to have asthma. There is a strong link between food sensitization or food allergies and poor asthma control, including increased asthma-related healthcare hospitalization

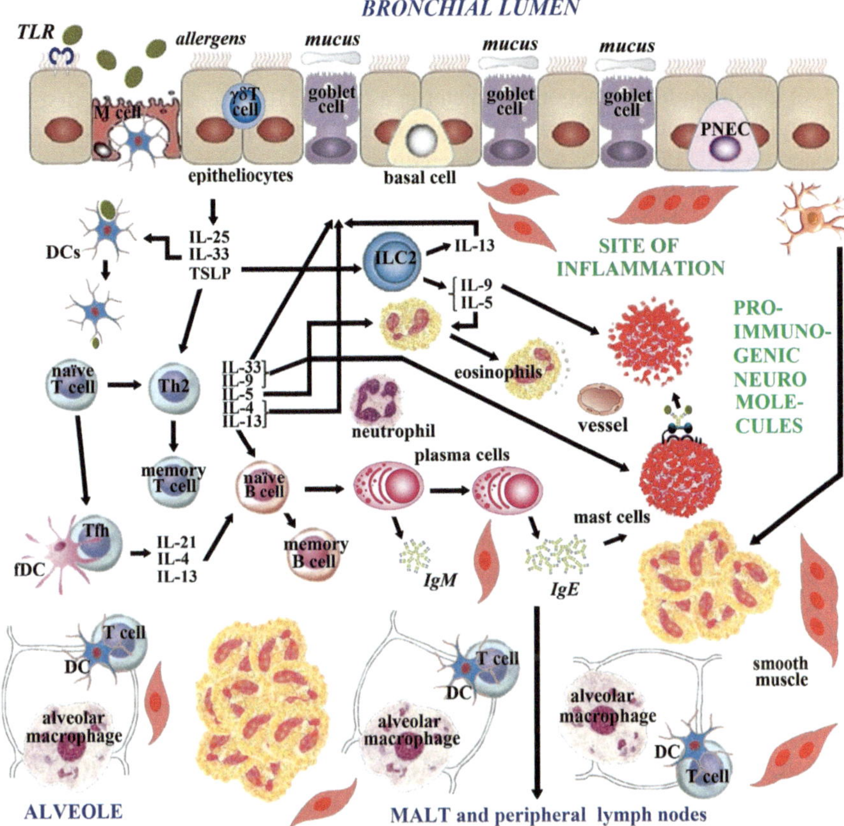

Fig. 5.5 Allergen tolerance breakdown in asthma. Allergen tolerance breakdown resembles the initial IgE-dependent response (see the description in Fig. 1.1), and overcoming the system of allergen tolerance maintenance also occurs. Due to the entry of recent causative allergens and a new wave of IgE-dependent response, allergic inflammation in lower airways gets novel portions of IgE antibodies and activated eosinophils, neutrophils, and monocytes depending on asthma's endotype. The influence of pro-immunogenic neurotransmitters predominates in the process. DCs dendritic cells, fDC follicular DC, Tfh follicular helper T cell, TSLP thymic stromal lymphopoietin, TLR toll-like receptors, PNEC pulmonary neuroendocrine cell

and emergency medication use. On the other hand, asthma is a risk factor for more severe and sometimes fatal anaphylactic reactions in associated food allergies [34]. Children with cosensitized food and inhalant allergens have more severe clinical symptoms and abnormal laboratory findings in allergic rhinitis and asthma [35]. Ingestion of snails in patients allergic to HDM can exacerbate the severe asthma course, and airborne allergens from occupational sources such as wheat, fish, and seafood may induce asthmatic symptoms like so-called "food-induced asthma" [36]. In addition, exposure to airborne food particles on flights is also important in asthmatic attacks manifestation [37].

Recently, local asthma was described after discovering local allergic rhinitis and local allergic conjunctivitis [38, 39]. All local atopic diseases may be linked with the peculiarities of the unified airway innervation [40]. See Chap. 6.

An important lung function parameter in asthma [25] is the ratio of the first second forced expiratory volume (FEV_1) to forced vital capacity (FVC) or slow vital capacity (CVC) (*Tiffeneau Index*), which diminishes in cases of bronchial obstruction: lower 0.75–0.80 in adults and 0.90 in children. *Fractional exhaled nitric oxide (FeNO)* is a widely exploited parameter assessing the level of chronic allergic inflammation in asthma. In addition, the measurement of nitric oxide, an atypical gasotransmitter, enables the prediction of response to inhaled corticosteroids (if FeNO > 35 ppb) and the reversibility of bronchial obstruction [41].

A biomarker is a specific biological indicator providing an objective measure of health/disease status. For example, biomarkers for asthma can be measured in different biological specimens such as blood, sputum, bronchoalveolar lavage, exhaled breath condensate, bronchial biopsy, and urine [41]. A suitable biomarker allows the definition of the specific phenotype/endotype of asthma useful in the monitoring and prognosis of the disease. Conventional biomarkers, including fractional exhaled nitric oxide, blood, sputum eosinophilia, and serum total IgE provide high specificity but poor sensitivity in the Th2-high/eosinophilic endotype asthma [42, 43].

Asthma is inherent in heterogeneity and complexity in clinical and immunologic features and division into some endotypes. As mentioned above, both two main endotypes, T2 (Th2-high/eosinophilic) and non-T2 (Th2-low/Th17/neutrophilic), include patients with mild, moderate, and severe asthma [44]. Well-known immunologic markers of Th2-high/eosinophilic asthma are a high level of type 2 cytokines: IL-5, IL-4, IL-13, IL-25, IL-33, and TSLP [30, 45, 46] as well as eosinophil cationic protein (ECP), eosinophil-derived neurotoxin (EDN), and urinary cysteinyl leukotriene E4 metabolite. Besides, levels of periostin, a matricellular protein, may serve as a biomarker of eosinophilic airway inflammation, fixed airflow limitation, and induction of anti-IL-13 biological therapy [45, 46].

Phenotypes/endotypes are the product of gene and environment interplay, and these processes can be expressed as measurable markers—metabolomes. Currently, six gene expression markers in Th2-high/eosinophilic asthma are known: alkaline phosphatase, tissue-nonspecific isozyme (ALPL), Charcot–Leyden crystal (CLC) protein [47], carboxypeptidase A3 (CPA3), CXCR2, and deoxyribonuclease l-like 3 (DNASElL3). Expression of these genes is associated with a better response to inhaled corticosteroids and can help distinguish asthma endotypes [45, 48]. In addition, new biomarkers, several small microRNA molecules involved in the gene regulation are assessed by genome-wide association studies. They may be used in distinguishing asthma from COPD or their overlap and reliable establishing asthma remission [45, 46].

In a study, patients with severe asthma who reduced treatment according to conventional biomarker-directed therapy showed no evidence of clinical exacerbation, despite being on lower corticosteroid doses. Also, no significant difference has been found in the proportion of patients who had a reduced corticosteroid dose between those who were assigned to the Th2/eosinophilic asthma biomarker strategy compared with those committed to standard care [49]. In another study, clinical evidence has reported that conventional type 2 biomarkers for severe asthma are insufficient to evaluate asthma severity. Besides, biomarkers for nonatopic severe asthma require further research [50].

So far, asthma biomarkers with Th2-low/Th17/neutrophilic endotype and other rare endotypes (paucigranulocytic, mixed granulocytic, nonallergic eosinophilic, and nonallergic non-eosinophilic asthma) are characterized poorly. They are cytokines and enzymes, such as IL-1β, IL-6, IL-8, IL-17, TNF-α, myeloperoxidase, neutrophil elastase, and increased expression of inflammasome NLRP3 [45, 46].

In overweight patients with adult-onset asthma, biomarkers may be low levels of blood eosinophils, transforming growth factor-α (TGF-α), and high levels of IL-6 and CCL5 (RANTES) [51].

A limited number of biomarkers are currently available in the pediatric population, including blood and sputum eosinophils, serum IgE, periostin, and fractional exhaled nitric oxide, mainly reflecting different molecular components of Th2-high/eosinophilic endotype of airway inflammation [41].

Management for asthma therapy includes education, allergen avoidance, pharmacotherapy, and allergen-specific immunotherapy (AIT). Before treatment, patients must make an informed decision about the therapy through discussion with healthcare professionals. Treatment of allergic asthma consists of many therapeutic options [25]: inhaled corticosteroids, leukotriene receptor antagonists, anti-IgE, anti-cytokine, anti-cytokine-receptor-based monoclonal antibodies (biologics), β-agonists, H_1-antihistamines, chemoattractant receptor-homologous molecule expressed on Th2 cells (CRTH2) antagonists [46, 52], and allergen-specific immunotherapy (AIT).

5.4 Allergic Rhinitis (Rhinoconjunctivitis)

▶ **Definition** Allergic rhinitis is the recurrent atopic inflammatory disease of upper airways caused by indoor and other allergens, and characterized by nasal obstruction, rhinorrhea, sneezing, coughing, and often conjunctival symptoms.

Allergic rhinitis is a global health problem [53–55] frequently associated with allergic asthma. Allergic rhinitis is a classical atopic disease associated with Th2-mediated sensitization, overproduction of IgE antibodies, and chronic allergic inflammation. Its combined classification takes into consideration: (1) the season (perennial and seasonal), (2) symptom recurrence (intermittent or persistent), and (3) severity (mild or moderate-to-severe) [16, 53, 55]. Allergic rhinitis (rhinoconjunctivitis) develops by atopic individuals in two phenotypes: (1) perennial or (2) seasonal rhinitis (rhinoconjunctivitis) [56, 57]. Nowadays, both phenotypes of allergic rhinitis, in particular perennial rhinitis, are a source of considerable morbidity and the manifestation of asthma for atopic individuals, impacting the quality of life,

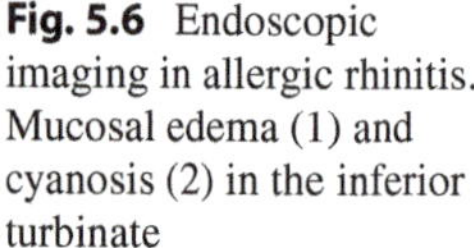

Fig. 5.6 Endoscopic imaging in allergic rhinitis. Mucosal edema (1) and cyanosis (2) in the inferior turbinate

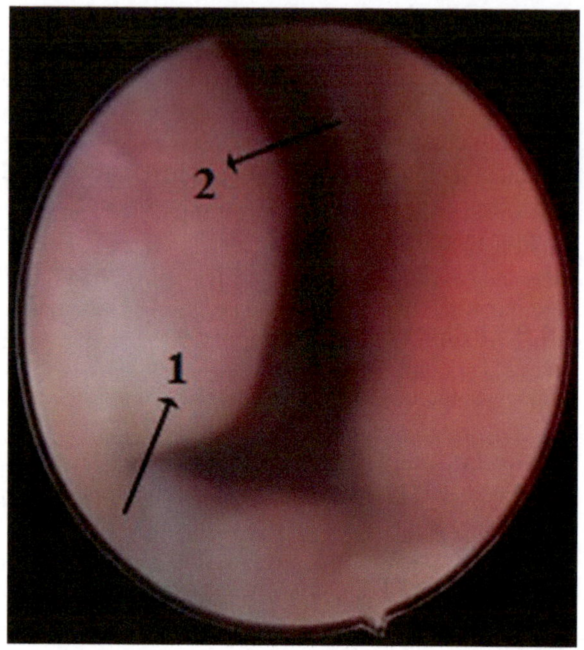

productivity, sleep, exercise tolerance, and social functioning, and creating a significant financial burden on healthcare systems throughout the world [54, 56, 58].

In allergic rhinitis, patients complain of chronic symptoms of nasal obstruction, itching, rhinorrhea, paroxysmal sneezing, and sometimes loss of smell, snoring, and conjunctival redness and swelling [54, 59]. Clinically, phenotypes of "nonallergic rhinitis" almost do not differ from phenotypes of allergic rhinitis [16, 60]. A confirmatory diagnosis of allergic rhinitis is more likely when rhinitis is seasonal, or with a family history of atopy [61]. As a rule, examination and investigation include a patient's history (family, past medical, social, occupational, etc.), allergic skin tests, serum/nasal secretion IgE assays (component resolved diagnosis), nasal secretion cytology, video rhinoscopy, acoustic rhinometry, tests for asthma, etc. [61, 62]. Video rhinoscopic picture of the lower turbinate in allergic rhinitis is specific (see Fig. 5.6).

Perennial rhinitis commonly starts at the age of 3–5 years. It manifests itself as these symptoms all year round and sometimes throughout life, being persistent and complicated by nasal polyps, sinusitis, and asthma, or conversely mild and subtle. Allergens of *Dermatophagoides* house dust mites, cats, and other pets, feathers, cockroaches, and molds are the main culprit proteins for IgE-dependent sensitization in persons with perennial rhinitis [63]. In seasonal rhinitis or "pollinosis," the pathology caused by plant pollens may commence at any age across large areas of both hemispheres during specific periods of the year when gramineous plants and trees pollinate. Allergenic pollens of birch, timothy, ragweed, and a wide variety of plants evoke type I hypersensitivity (IgE-dependent sensitization) [14, 64, 65].

The peculiarities of each pollination season depend on the climate, geography zone, hemisphere, and other factors. Traditionally, pollination in the Northern hemisphere is divided into three waves (see Figs. 5.7, 5.8, 5.9, and 5.10):

1. *Spring season*, when there are flowering trees and shrubbery (birch, oak, elm, ash, poplar, maple, hazelnut, etc.);
2. *Summer season*, when meadow grasses (timothy, orchard, rye, bluegrasses, wheatgrass, fescue, etc.) pollinate; and
3. *Fall season*, when there is the pollination of weeds (ragweed, sagebrush, goosefoot, nettle, pigweed, etc.).

Nowadays, pollination, each species pollen's structure, pollen concentration in the atmosphere depending on the season, weather, and climate-changing are an arduous purpose of modern investigation [64, 65].

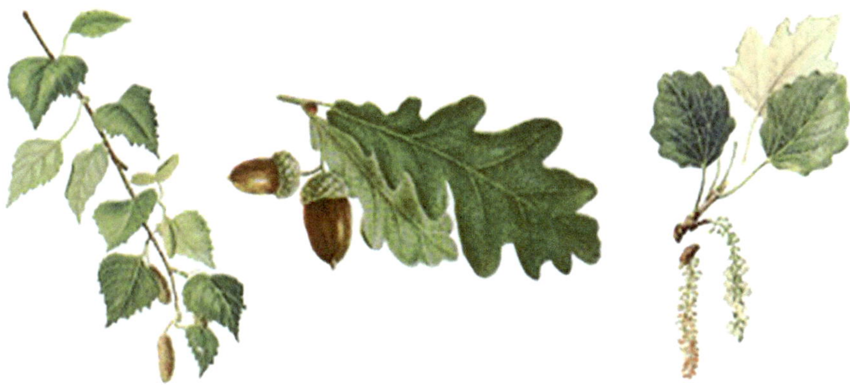

Fig. 5.7 Spring pollination (1): birch, oak, poplar

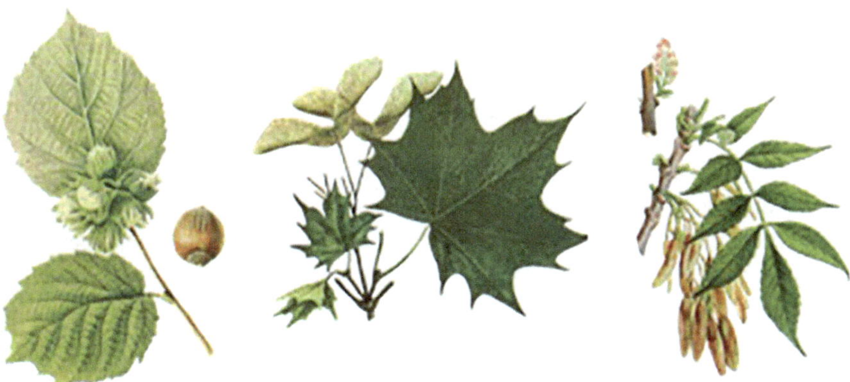

Fig. 5.8 Spring pollination (2): hazelnut, maple, ash

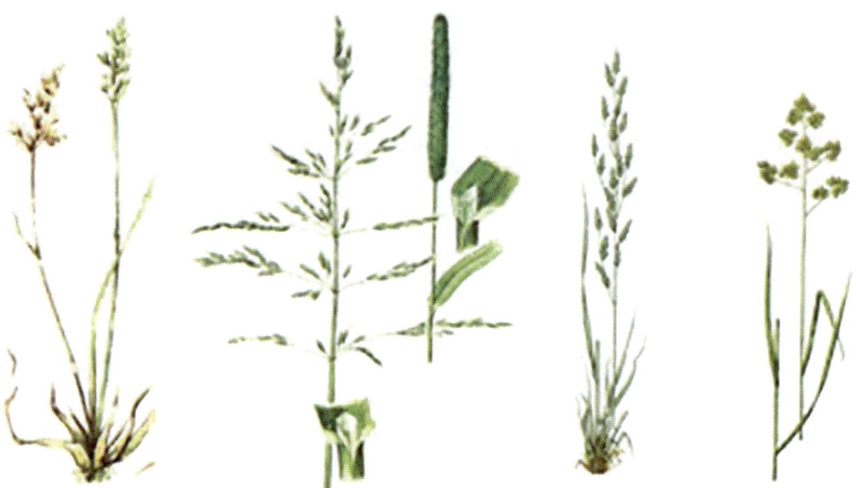

Fig. 5.9 Summer pollination: bluegrasses, ryegrass, timothy, fescue, orchard

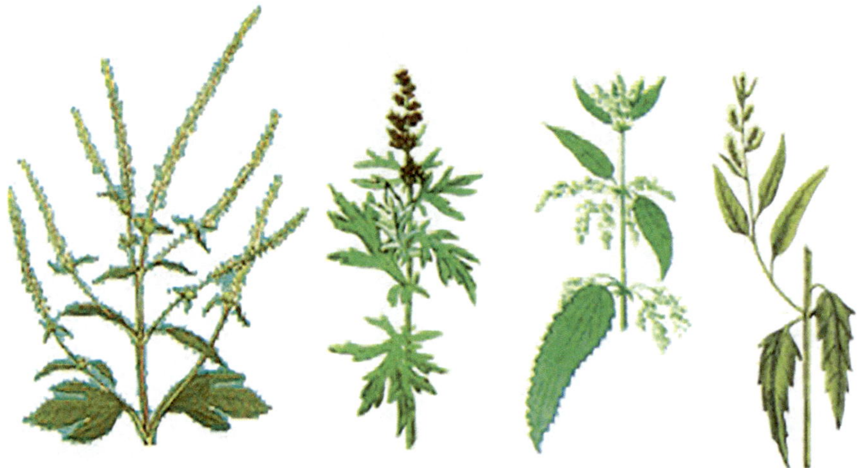

Fig. 5.10 Fall pollination: ragweed, sagebrush, nettle, goose-foot

New biomarkers in allergic rhinitis, particularly based on nasal mucus proteome, are currently in development. The nasal mucus proteome contains various components; proteomic techniques can facilitate the investigation of the nasal secretome and its role as potential biomarker for new diagnostic or therapeutic approaches. Using classical ELISA, elevated levels of IgE, kallikrein, eosinophilic cationic protein (ECP), substance P, VIP, and other proteins have been found in allergic rhinitis. In allergic rhinitis, by applying a new proteomic approach (mass spectrometry), the nasal mucus proteome displayed the inflammatory and alteration features that could be used as biomarkers in the disease [66]. Over the last decade, several other clinical phenotypes and endotypes, including local and "dual" allergic rhinitis, were consistently described in various research studies [67, 68], whereas endotyping and confirmatory biomarkers showed a more perspective impact on management and personalized therapy for patients of allergic rhinitis [69, 70].

Management for allergic rhinitis treatment consists of education, allergen avoidance, pharmacotherapy, and allergen-specific immunotherapy (AIT). Initially, patients must make an informed decision about therapy through discussion with healthcare professionals. Therapy for the disease includes H_1-antihistamines, intranasal corticosteroids, leukotriene receptor antagonists, and allergen-specific immunotherapy (AIT). Biologics may be prescribed in stratified patients with very severe allergic rhinitis [58].

Quiz A

Reading a question, please choose only one right answer.

Question 1

Allergological method taking into account the cytophilic property of IgE:

1. Basophil activation test.
2. Video rhinoscopy.
3. Allergic skin testing.
4. Component resolved diagnosis (CRD).

Question 2

In skin prick testing (SPT), histamine is used as:

1. A positive control.
2. A negative control.
3. A visual assessment.
4. A provocation test.

Question 3

An endotype of asthma is characterized by a more severe course:

1. Th2/eosinophilic asthma's endotype.
2. Th1/Th17/neutrophilic asthma's endotype.
3. Asthma induced by physical exercise.
4. Asthma with other atopic conditions.

Question 4

Endoscopic imaging in allergic rhinitis includes:

1. Mucosal cyanosis.
2. Ulceration.
3. Septal deviation.
4. Papillomatosis.

Question 5

Skin lesions by which SPT assesses a reaction:

1. Vesicle.
2. Ulcer.
3. Wheal.
4. Papule.

Question 6

Allergic inflammation in the lung may be associated with the IgE-independent pathway due to:

1. ILC2 activation.
2. Th2 participation.
3. Eosinophils.
4. Neutrophils.

Question 7

ILC2 cells secrete:

1. IFN-α, IFN-β, and IL-18.
2. IL-5, IL-9, and IL-13.
3. IFN-γ, IL-2, and TNF-β.
4. IL-4, IL-6, IL10, and IL-13.

Question 8

Alarmins activate:

1. Th2, ILC2, and DCs.
2. Allergen-specific memory B cells.
3. Th1, Th17, and Th22.
4. Mast cells and basophils.

Question 9

ILC2 cells are activated by:

1. CGRP.
2. Norepinephrine.
3. Alarmins: IL-25, IL-33, and TSLP.
4. Serotonin.

Question 10

Method assessing the nasal obstruction:

1. Video rhinoscopy.
2. Rhinomanometry.

3. Radiology.
4. Nasal cytology and histology.

Question 11
The classical endotype of allergic rhinitis is:

1. Conventional.
2. Local.
3. "Dual."
4. Nonallergic.

Question 12
Allergic response leads to the formation of:

1. IgM antibodies.
2. IgA antibodies.
3. Allergen-specific T cells and B cells.
4. CD4+ dependent immune inflammation.

Question 13
Sensitization and allergic response are the same processes:

1. They are different processes.
2. Surely but clarification requires.
3. They resemble each other but are slightly different.
4. They resemble each other but are too different.

Question 14
This disease is not related to atopic conditions:

1. Allergic asthma.
2. Allergic contact dermatitis.
3. Allergic rhinitis.
4. Atopic dermatitis.

Question 15
These allergens are not relevant to seasonal allergic rhinitis:

1. Birch.
2. Timothy.
3. Ragweed.
4. Latex.

Question 16
The fall season of pollination of allergen plants includes:

1. Goose-foot.
2. Birch.
3. Orchard.
4. Fescue.

5.5 Atopic Dermatitis

▶ **Definition** Atopic dermatitis (eczema) is the chronic allergic inflammation of the skin in children and adults, which is characterized by itch, dryness, various skin lesions, and lichenification.

Atopic dermatitis is a chronic inflammatory skin disease, characterized by epidermal disorders based on Th2/Th22-predominant inflammation, with variable increases in Th1 and Th17 [71], and mutations in the *filaggrin gene* [3, 21]. In predisposed persons or atopic individuals, HDM allergens and other allergens are inhaled, ingested, and enter the skin (so-called *transcutaneous sensitization*), and trigger advanced B cell-mediated immune response to the predominant formation of IgE antibodies, which are carried to the skin to be bound to FcεRIs on mast cells and turn on the allergic inflammation. Sometimes, infectious complications caused by *S. aureus*, *C. albicans*, *Herpes simplex*, etc., may occur. The disease usually starts in childhood, turning on atopic march [2] but often persists into adulthood. The extent and localization of skin lesions vary with age and race or ethnic group [72]. Repeated exposure to these allergens results in chronic skin inflammation with various skin lesions and severe itching that can significantly impact the quality of life for patients, particularly if the skin lesions are extensive.

Multiple somatosensory neuron-derived receptors such as nociceptors, pruriceptors, thermoreceptors, mechanoreceptors, and chemoreceptors [40] allow the skin sensing of many external and internal stimuli, including those going from the inflammatory sites.

Children with atopic dermatitis are estimated to be six times more likely to develop food allergies than their healthy peers. Furthermore, the risk of developing IgE-mediating food allergy is nearly 40% in children with moderate-to-severe atopic dermatitis. However, elimination diets are not known to cure atopic dermatitis. They may have unfavorable consequences such as nutritional deficiencies, growth failure, and reduced quality of life for the patient and family [73].

In some cases, immunologic tolerance to causative allergens is restored to lead to the long-term remission of the disease. Nevertheless, some patients may develop eczema, secondary bacterial, fungal, viral infections, and rough lichenification as complications of the main allergic inflammatory process. Local atopic dermatitis was not found to correspond to peculiarities of the skin's innervation [40].

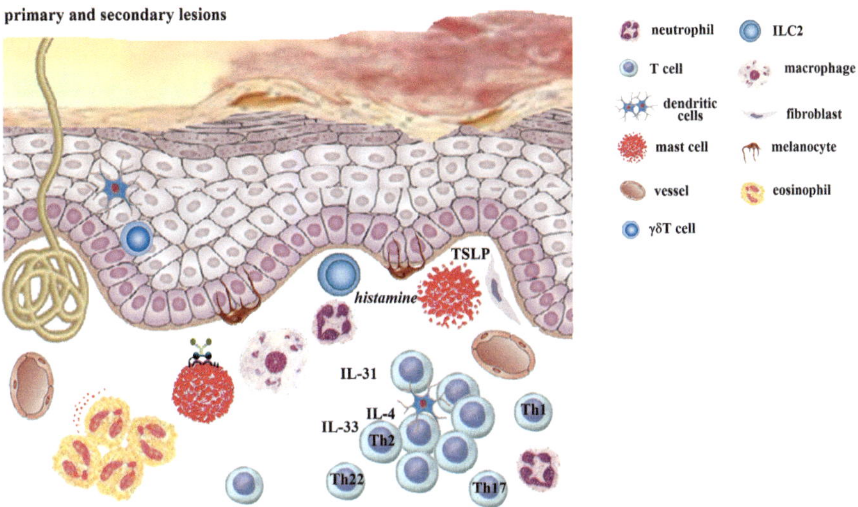

Fig. 5.11 The skin in atopic dermatitis. In atopic dermatitis, repeated exposure to allergens causes a constant IgE-dependent response and chronic allergic skin inflammation. The epidermis is damaged by the primary lesions, macules, papules, vesicles, secondary lesions, crusts, fissures, excoriation, and lichenification. However, specific lesions in atopic dermatitis are unavailable. An itch is frequently a leading symptom on which secondary lesions depend and which has complex pathogenesis linked with histamine, thymic stromal lymphopoietin (TSLP), IL-31, IL-33, and nerve growth factor (NGF), and in summary with "neurogenic inflammation." TSLP thymic stromal lymphopoietin, Th helper T cell

The index ScorAD is the best validating scoring system to evaluate the extent of skin inflammation and concurrent symptoms in atopic dermatitis. The extent can be graded from 0 to 100. The intensity part of the ScorAD consists of some skin pathologic elements: erythema, papulation, excoriations, lichenification, crusts, and dryness. The ScorAD formula is the following:

$$A/5 + 7B/2 + C,$$

where A corresponds to the extent (0–100), B is defined as the intensity (0–18), and C reflects the subjective symptoms (0–20) [74].

The Hanifin and Rajka criteria are the most recognized diagnostic criteria and are widely considered the "gold standard" for atopic dermatitis diagnosis [75]. Recently, some new biomarkers: CD30, IL-12, IL-16, IL-18, IL-31, chemokines CCL17 (TARC), and CCL22 (MDC), were described to correlate with atopic dermatitis severity and skin symptoms. They did not show high sensitivity and specificity for regular diagnostic use. Histamine, an epithelium's products TSLP and IL-33, as well as IL-31 and nerve growth factor (NGF) are recognized as biomolecules, which actively induce skin itch, a sample of "neurogenic inflammation" (see Fig. 5.11) [76]. The cognate receptor for IL-31 is composed of IL-31RA and the oncostatin M receptor, both expressed on pruriceptor sensory neurons that mediate itch and on skin keratinocytes [40].

The prevalent neuro molecules operating in the skin, taking into account their receptors on keratinocytes, are acetylcholine, norepinephrine, dopamine, histamine, and substance P [77].

There are two types of biomarkers in atopic dermatitis, diagnostic and monitoring. Both types use the skin, blood, peripheral blood cells, saliva, tears, and urine as sources for study [78]. The following biomarkers, mainly chemokines, are recommended by the International Eczema Council [79] for patients with atopic dermatitis:

1a. Biomarkers improving differentiation of atopic dermatitis and psoriasis are CCL27 (CTACK) and inducible nitric oxidase synthase (NOS2). CCL27 is expressed on keratinocytes mediating the migration of T cells into the skin, whereas NOS2 via the production of nitric oxide regulates the functional activity of many immune cells in the skin.
1b. Biomarkers correlating with clinical severity are filaggrin, IL-13 (of Th2 profile), IL-22 (of Th22 profile), CCL17 (TARC), CCL18 (PARC), CCL22 (MDC), CCL26 (eotaxin-3), and CCL27 (CTACK).
2. Predictive biomarkers that may help to monitor the efficacy of treatment are CCL17 (TARC) and CCL22 (MDC). CCL17 is responsible for T cell migration and Th2 response, and elevated blood CCL17 level is not specific to atopic dermatitis and can also be found in other skin diseases. CCL22, chemokine upregulating T cell migration and Th2 response, is reported as the best biomarker of disease response using different therapeutic approaches.

There is evolving evidence of systemic immune activation and detectable abnormalities in nonlesional skin in atopic dermatitis. A study found increases in serum cytokines IL-13 and IL-22 and chemokine CCL17 (TARC) in atopic dermatitis versus healthy individuals. ScorAD positively correlated with IL-13 and IL-22, even more strongly, in the nonlesional skin [80]. Another study involved an analysis of a population of infants ($n = 161$) that were at high risk of atopic disease. Researchers used sampled serum, peripheral blood mononuclear cells, and clinical parameters upon entry and 5 years later to assess the correlation of IL-13 and CCL13 (MCP-4) with ScorAD at both time points. Eventually, 33 infant serum analytes were identified as data, which could predict atopic dermatitis severity 5 years later [81]. In the third study, 26 patients aged 18–65 years with atopic dermatitis were examined to characterize the proteomic signature of tape-strips from the patients before and after dupilumab therapy. Significant decreases after dupilumab were observed in immune markers such as CCL13 (MCP-4) and CCL17 (TARC) (of Th2 profile), IL-12B and CXCL1 (GROα) (of Th17/Th22 profiles), and innate immunity (IL-6, IL-8, IL-17C), while the Th1 chemokines CXCL9 (MIG) and CXCL10 (IP-10) remained elevated [82].

Novel approaches to the identification of biomarkers are currently being established due to omics technologies. For example, researchers found skin parameters based on proteomics valuable for moderate-to-severe atopic dermatitis that included IL-13, CCL17 (TARC), CCL20 (MIP-3α), CXCL10 (IP-10), etc. Gene and protein expressions were positively correlated [83]. Small microRNA molecules engaged in gene regulation are examined by genome-wide association studies. Each microRNA may have hundreds of gene targets and modulate the production of a large number of proteins. However, the measurement of microRNAs as biomarkers that allow diagnosis and assessment of disease activity are not yet in clinical use [84]. Tracking biomarkers based on new omics technologies in real-life settings and clinical trials and longitudinal studies of atopic dermatitis and beyond has the potential utility and perspectives [82].

Before the therapy begins, patients must make an informed decision about the treatment through discussion with parents and healthcare professionals. Treatment for atopic dermatitis includes emollients, corticosteroid gels, creams and ointments, antihistamines, dupilumab (antagonist of IL-4Rα, which inhibits IL-4 and IL-13) [85], antimicrobial medications if required, and AIT.

5.6 Urticaria and Anaphylaxis

▶ **Definition** Urticaria is a multifactor, toxico-allergic skin disorder characterized by acute or persisting itching wheal rash. Angioedema is a similar toxico-allergic skin disorder, including hereditary forms, described by the deeper dermis giving larger swollen skin areas. Anaphylaxis is a sudden onset of food-related or toxico-allergic to the whole body, life-threatening syndrome, depicted by a series of skin and systemic symptoms.

Urticaria manifests as either transient short-lasting wheals or sudden angioedema, or both. A wheal is surrounded by red itching erythema, located on different skin areas, and developed within several minutes. As skin-colored, non-itchy, slowly developing, and persisting for several days, angioedema appears. The angioedema in the upper airways may be life-threatening because of the risk of asphyxiation. There is the monogenic hereditary angioedema—C1-INH deficiency [86, 87]. The *C1INH gene* (on 11q12.1) is a member of a large protease inhibitor gene family.

Urticaria may be acute (<6 weeks) and chronic spontaneous (>6 weeks and even more than 5 years). Acute urticaria exerts as IgE-dependent (atopic) or IgG-mediated (toxico-allergic) and occurs in children and adults in association with

1. foodstuffs [88],
2. *Hymenoptera* insect venom (toxin) [89–91], and
3. medication/vaccine administration [92].

Chronic inducible urticaria, a non-IgE-mediated disorder, is caused by some provoking factors such as cold, heat, vibration, solar light, pressure, exercise, emotional stress, chemicals, cosmetics, plant components, and latex. [93].

Chronic urticaria is based on continuous activating and degranulating mast cells and basophils with the release of histamine, bradykinin, prostaglandins, cysteinyl leukotrienes, eosinophilic, and neutrophilic chemotactic factors, and platelet-activating factor. The mast cell factors result in vasodilation and increased vascular permeability with the conclusive formation of wheals and angioedema [94].

Cytokines and chemokines TNF-α, IL-1, IL-4, IL-5, IL-6, IL-8, IL-16, CCL2 (MCP-1), CCL3 (MIP-1α), and CCL5 (RANTES) synthesized by mast cells, Th1, and Th2 cells have been identified in the skin and peripheral blood in patients with chronic urticaria [93]. Cytokines secreted by epithelium IL-33, IL-25, and TSLP (alarmins) for starting via ILC2 immune responses, play an essential role in skin itch [40]. To a large extent, allergen tolerance breakdown in IgE-dependent urticaria and angioedema develops "neurogenic inflammation" [76] derived from skin somatosensory (pruriceptive, nociceptive, etc.) neurons.

Autoimmunity matters much in the pathogenesis of chronic spontaneous (or idiopathic) urticaria evoked either by IgE autoantibodies against self-antigens or IgG autoantibodies directed against the mast cells high-affinity receptor FcεRI or IgE [94]. The concept of autoimmunity originated from the observation that thyroid disorders and thyroid autoantibodies are more prevalent in chronic urticaria [95]. It has been shown that approximately 50% of patients with chronic urticaria have autoantibodies directed against a subunit of the IgE receptor or IgE itself, resulting in the degranulation of mast cells. In some cases, triggering factors may be IgG antibodies, including those directed against toxins.

Drug allergic reactions are not always IgE-dependent. Notably, descriptions have been made of mas-related G protein-coupled receptor X2 (MRGPRX2)-mediated degranulation of mast cells resulting in severe allergic manifestation [96]. Previously so-called "pseudo allergy" reactions exist now in many forms under other names.

Many classical therapeutic approaches are employed in acute and chronic urticaria, which include almost all anti-allergy medications. However, emerging treatment options for chronic urticaria are mainly targeted at mast cell activity using (1) biologics such as omalizumab and ligelizumab, and (2) cyclosporine [97].

In 1913, C.R. Richet won the Nobel Prize for his discovery of anaphylaxis. Anaphylaxis is an IgE-dependent or toxico-allergic condition like urticaria widespread on the whole body because of sudden allergen tolerance breakdown in the ensemble with systemic "neurogenic inflammation." The cardiovascular collapse and respiratory arrest may lead to death if medical assistance does not follow on time. The same pathogenic factors play a role in the anaphylaxis's and urticaria's pathogenesis, yet the condition is not severe and there is no threat to life in the case of urticaria if it is not localized in the larynx and small intestine [98, 99].

There are two pathways for anaphylaxis onset.

1. For anaphylaxis induction by allergen-specific IgE and FcεRI-bearing effector cells, a small amount of allergen requires (concentration of allergen-specific IgG is low).
2. For anaphylaxis induction by allergen-specific IgG and FcγR-bearing effector cells, more allergen and a large concentration of IgG require.

Table 5.2 Emergency procedures in acute allergic reactions

Clinical signs	Treatment
Urticaria, angioedema	1. Antihistamines: diphenhydramine (Benadryl®)—adults: 25 mg *per os* in 6 h for 2–5 days; children: 1 mg/kg *per os* in 8 h for 2–5 days
	2. Corticosteroids: prednisone—adults: 20–80 mg *per os* daily for 2–5 days; children: 0.5–1 mg/kg *per os* daily for 2–5 days
Anaphylaxis	1. Epinephrine 0.25–0.5 mL of the 10 times diluted standard solution slowly intravenously, possibly repeated at intervals of 2–3 min
	2. Corticosteroids, e.g., prednisone 250–1000 mg intravenously
	3. Volume replacement, preferentially with a 5% human albumin solution
Fall in blood pressure (<90 systolic)	Epinephrine 0.25–0.5 mL of the 10 times diluted standard solution 1–2 times/h 0.25–0.5 mL subcutaneously
Bronchospasms	Inhalation of β_2-adrenergic agonists such as albuterol

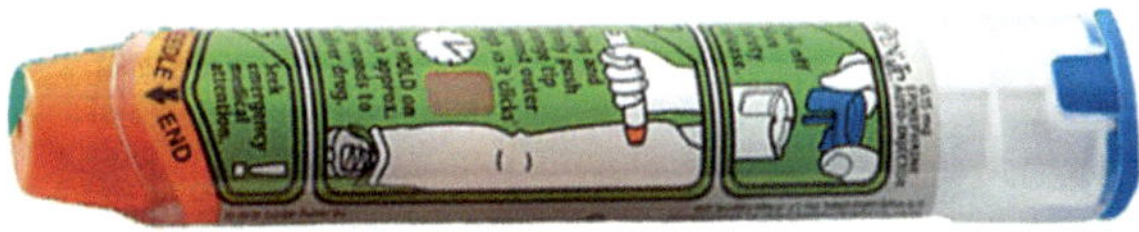

Fig. 5.12 Epinephrine auto-injector (EAI). Here and further, there are pictures of demonstration items

In some cases, both pathways are involved in anaphylaxis manifestation [100].

Food anaphylaxis from genetic, epigenetic, and pathogenic viewpoints is described in Chap. 7. See medical procedures indicated for acute allergic reactions in Table 5.2 and Fig. 5.12.

5.7 Medication Therapy for Allergies

▶ **Definition** Medication therapy is one of two possible approaches to the treatment of allergic disorders.

Pharmacotherapy and allergen-specific immunotherapy (AIT) are prescribed according to international position papers in therapy for allergy [16, 25]. Pharmacotherapy is carried out according to medical personnel's experience, numerous options for oral or systemic use, topical intranasal and inhalant application, and some alternative techniques.

From a clinical viewpoint, the purpose of anti-allergy therapy for allergic diseases and syndromes is the prevention of emergency department visits and hospitalizations, decrease in allergic signs and symptoms, achievement of long-term control of these common chronic conditions, and quality of life maintenance.

There are two treatment modalities, which may be used only for individuals with atopic allergic conditions:

1. medication therapy, including biologics, and
2. AIT by some routes of allergen administration.

Medication therapy includes several various drugs with different mechanisms of action.

5.7.1 Antihistamines

The 1957 Nobel Laureate, D. Bovet, developed *antihistamines* in 1937, blocking the neurotransmitter histamine (see Fig. 5.13) and widely exploiting allergy therapy. Antihistamines are probably the best-known type of allergy remedies, and most are readily available from a pharmacy without a prescription.

Antihistamines act on the tissues through histamine receptors. There are four types of histamine receptors (see Table 5.3 and Chap. 4) [101].

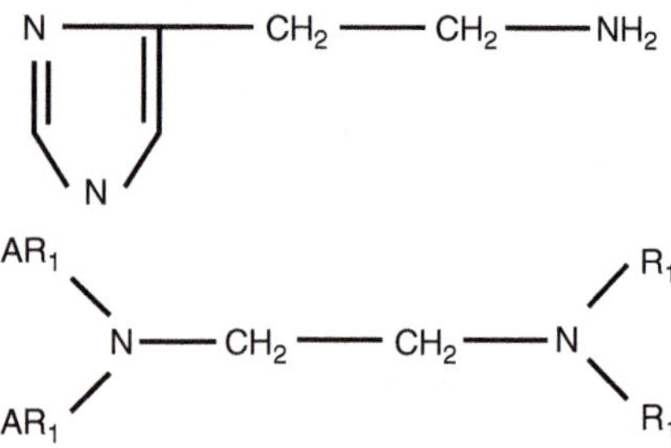

Fig. 5.13 Histamine (above) and antihistamine

Table 5.3 Histamine receptors

Receptor type	Expression	Effects
H_1	Mast cells, basophils, neutrophils, eosinophils, monocytes, myocytes, endothelium, exocrine gland epithelium, macrophages	Involvement in Th2-mediated inflammation; itching; systemic vasodilatation; smooth muscle constriction (e.g., bronchospasm); ileum contraction; mucus overproduction; stimulation of neutrophils and eosinophils chemotaxis; increase in cGMP
H_2	Exocrine gland epithelium, neutrophils, eosinophils, mast cells, basophils	Involvement in Th1-mediated inflammation; regulation of gastric HCl secretion; smooth muscle relaxation; inhibition of adaptive immune responses and cytokine production; sinus tachycardia; inhibition of neutrophils and eosinophils chemotaxis; increase in cAMP
H_3	Neurons, mast cells, basophils	The functioning of the blood-brain barrier; decrease in acetylcholine, serotonin, and norepinephrine presynaptic autoreceptors
H_4	Mast cells, basophils, leukocytes, enterocytes, colonocytes, hepatocytes, splenocytes, thymocytes, exocrine gland epithelium	Involvement in Th2-mediated inflammation; regulation of neutrophils and mast cells migration; promotion of eosinophil function

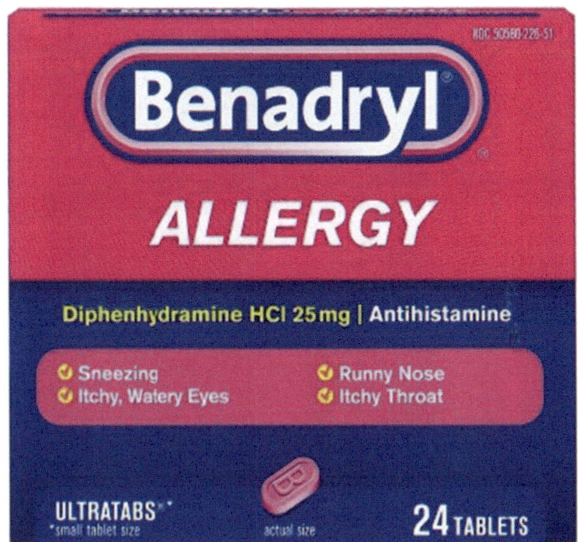

Fig. 5.14 Benadryl®

Antihistamines, H_1 blockers, compete with histamine for H_1 receptors and, as a result, diminish histamine's effects. They work best when taken before exposure to the allergen and may be used at the systemic and topical levels.

First-generation antihistamines, the oldest and nonselective, are used less often to treat allergies because they cause significant sedation and an anticholinergic side effect. They include:

Diphenhydramine (Benadryl® (see Fig. 5.14), Dimedrol®)
Clemastine (Tavegil® (see Fig. 5.15), Tavist®)
Chloropyramine (Suprastin®)
Cyproheptadine (Peritol®, Periactin®)

However, only some are manufactured in ampoule form (see Fig. 5.15) and may be used in urgent allergy cases. First-generation antihistamines are usually prescribed for a short term, no longer than 10 days.

Second-generation antihistamines, newer and much more selective for peripheral H_1 receptors, are currently used for allergy treatment. They do not cross the blood-brain barrier and act mainly in the periphery. However, analogous to the first-generation antihistamines, they are all "pro-medications" from which, in the course of biotransformation, active metabolites must be constituted. Second-generation antihistamines include:

Azelastine (Allergodil®)
Olopatadine (Opatanol®)
Loratadine (Claritin® (see Fig. 5.16), Alavert®)
Dimetindene (Fenistil®)
Cetirizine (Zyrtec®) (see Fig. 5.17)

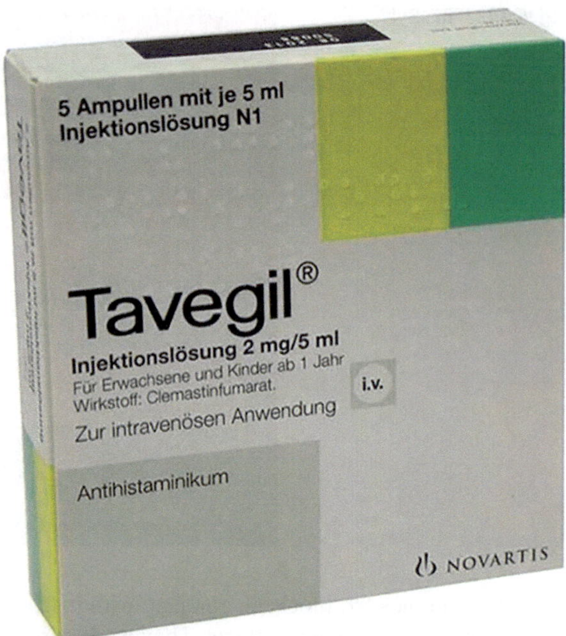

Fig. 5.15 Tavegil®

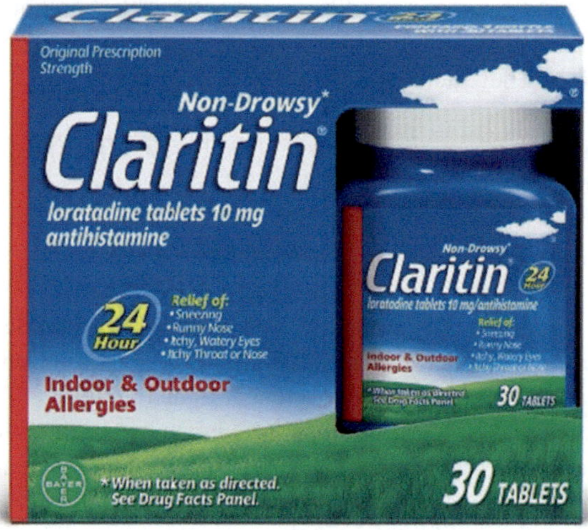

Fig. 5.16 Claritin®

Third-generation antihistamines, active metabolite derivatives of the second-generation drugs, do not pass the blood-brain barrier and have increased efficacy practically without side effects. They include:

Fexofenadine (Telfast®, Allegra®)
Desloratadine (Aerius® (see Fig. 5.18), Clarinex®)
Levocetirizine (Xyzal®)

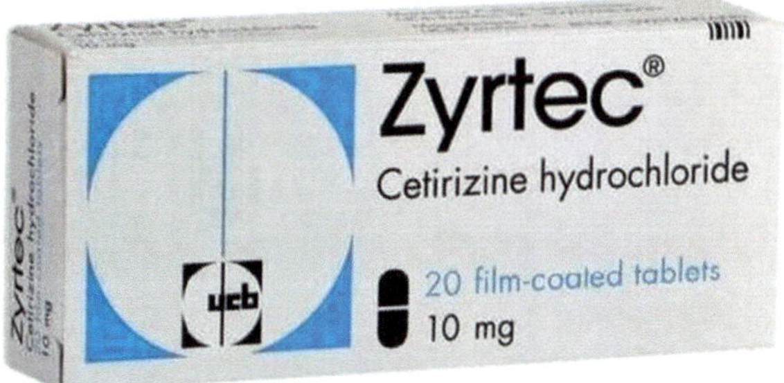

Fig. 5.17 Zyrtec®

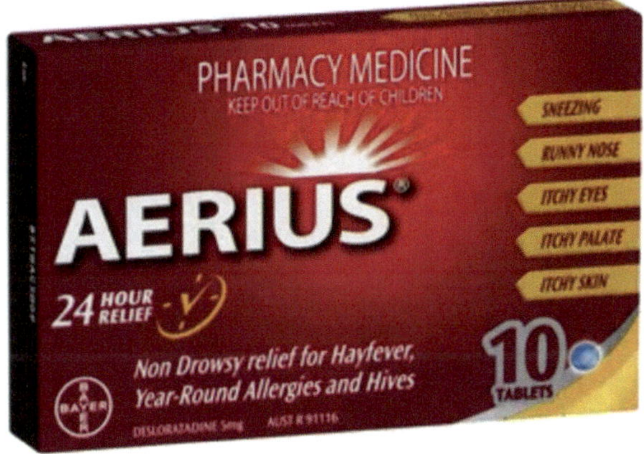

Fig. 5.18 Aerius®

Table 5.4 Prescription of antihistamines depending on age

Age	Antihistamine
From 1 month	Chloropyramine (Suprastin®), dimetindene (Fenistil®)
From 6 months	Cetirizine (Zyrtec®)
From 12 months	Clemastine (Tavegil®, Tavist®), desloratadine (Aerius®, Clarinex®)
From 24 months	Levocetirizine (Xysal®), loratadine (Claritin®, Alavert®)
From 6 years	Fexofenadine (Telfast®, Allegra®)

Second- and third-generation antihistamines are commonly prescribed for up to 3 weeks.

Antihistamines are prescribed depending on age (see Table 5.4).

Prescription of Antihistamines in Pregnant Women

If a daily antihistamine is required during pregnancy, second- and third-generation drugs are preferred because they are less sedating and have a better side effect profile. Loratadine and cetirizine are preferred second-generation antihistamines for pregnant women because they are the safest and most effective. They are generally considered to be safe at recommended doses for the treatment of allergic rhinitis during pregnancy.

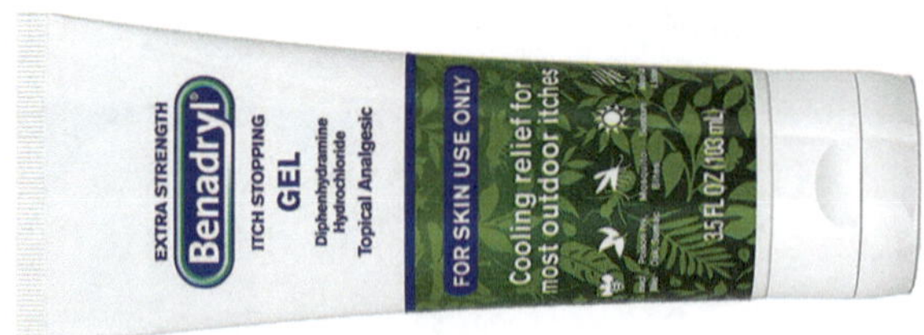

Fig. 5.19 Benadryl® gel

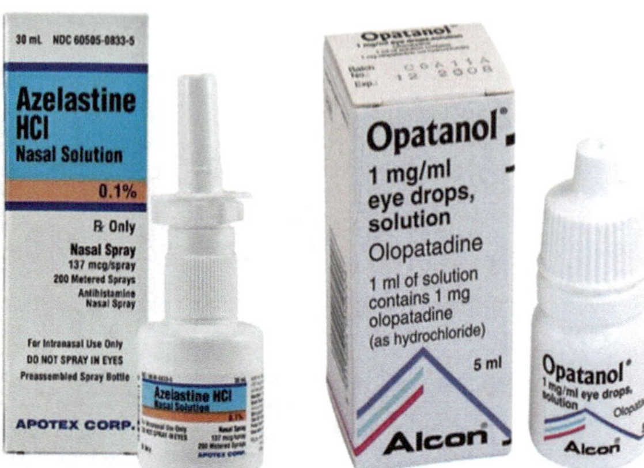

Fig. 5.20 Azelastine® nasal spray and opatanol® eye drops

There are now antihistamines in skin gel (see Fig. 5.19), nasal spray, and eye drops (see Fig. 5.20).

5.7.2 Membrane Stabilizers

Membrane stabilizers, ketotifen, and cromones (sodium cromoglycate and nedocromil), act by blocking histamine release from mast cells and basophils at the *early phase* of atopic allergic inflammation. They can be a helpful alternative to antihistamines in preventing allergic reactions. Their indications are prophylaxis and treatment for allergic asthma, rhinitis, allergic rhinoconjunctivitis, and manifestations of food allergy, as a part of the complex intervention. However, it takes some weeks for the therapeutic effects to be seen.

5.7.3 Topical Corticosteroids

Corticosteroids are almost identical to the natural hormone cortisol, produced by the body's adrenal glands. Corticosteroids, unlike antihistamines, can reduce reactions of three phases of atopic allergic inflammation, the *early phase*, *late phase*, and *chronic inflammation phase*. They suppress the B cell-mediated Th2-dependent response to allergens, inhibit the formation of new IgE molecules, downregulate both cellular forms of the allergic inflammation, with predomination of eosinophils and neutrophils, and prevent ongoing chronic allergic inflammation.

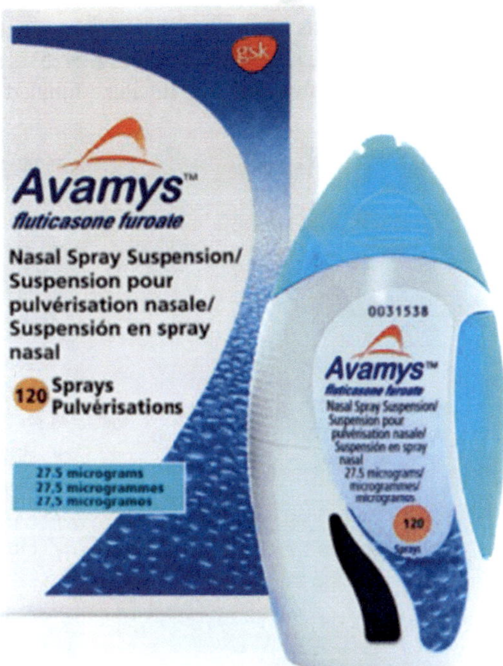

Fig. 5.21 Avamys® nasal spray

Nowadays, corticosteroids are used directly in the particular area of the body where the allergy symptoms are being noticed. It targets the symptoms and minimizes any possible side effects from the treatment, allowing the physician to keep the dose of medication to a minimum. Topical corticosteroids are used in the form of inhalers, nasal sprays, eye drops, gels, creams, and ointments.

Avamys® (fluticasone furoate) (see Fig. 5.21) and Nasonex® (mometasone furoate) (see Fig. 5.22) are used in the treatment of allergic rhinitis and conjunctivitis [53] in patients over 2 years of age. However, nose and throat dryness or irritation, blood-tinged mucus/phlegm, and nosebleeds may occur as side effects during treatment.

Inhaled corticosteroids are an established therapy for bronchial asthma [25]. Their success is based on their ability to improve control of asthma, avoid oral corticosteroids, and probably limit the risk of long-term disorder in lung function. There are three basic types of devices delivering inhaled medications, including corticosteroids in asthma:

1. A metered-dose inhaler (MDI) uses a chemical propellant to push the medication out of the inhaler.
2. A dry powder inhaler (DPI) delivers the medicine through fast and strong inhalation.
3. A nebulizer delivers fine liquid mists of the medication through a tube or a "mask" under pressure.

For example, Pulmicort® (budesonide) is prescribed to children over 6 months of age and adult patients through a nebulizer (see Figs. 5.23 and 5.24), whereas Flixotide® (fluticasone propionate) (see Fig. 5.25) is used in children over 12 months of age and adults through an inhaler. Inhaled corticosteroids are excellent

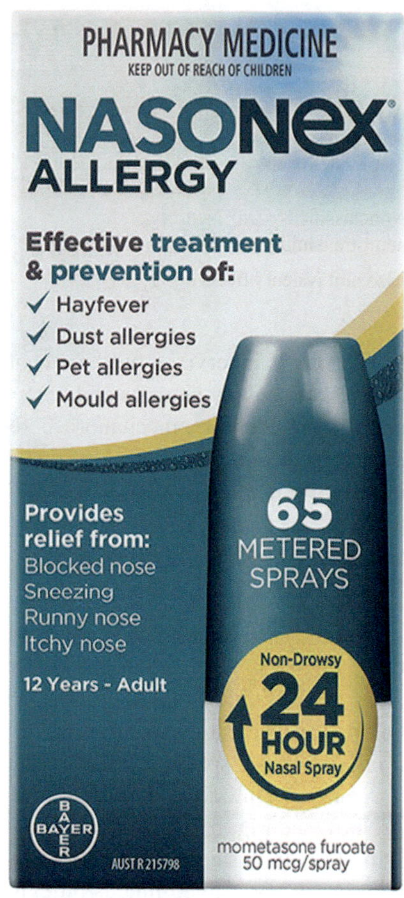

Fig. 5.22 Nasonex® nasal spray

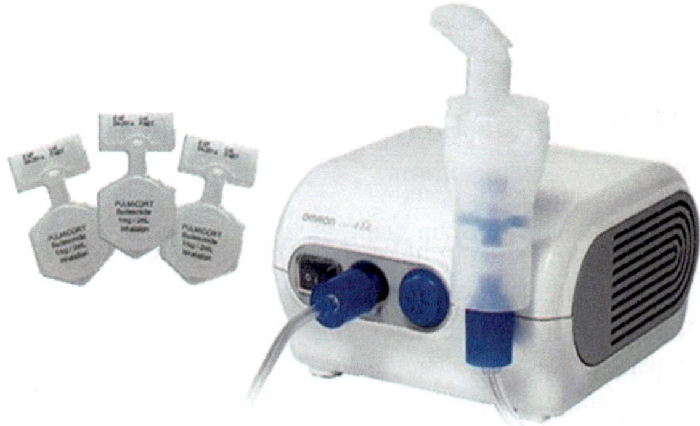

Fig. 5.23 Pulmicort® for inhalation

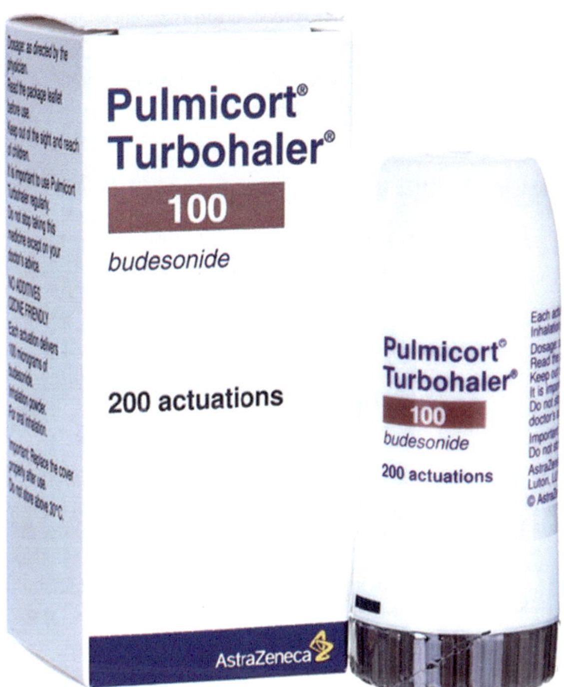

Fig. 5.24 Pulmicort® Turbohaler®

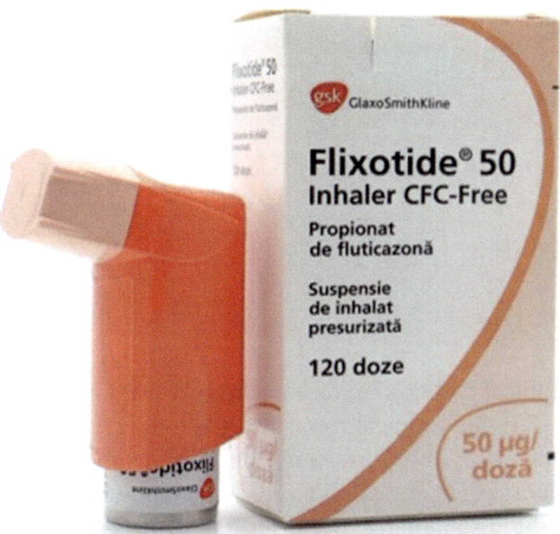

Fig. 5.25 Flixotide® Inhaler

medications for the treatment of asthma [25]. However, inhaled corticosteroids have common side effects: sore mouth or throat, hoarseness, fungus infection in the mouth and lungs, coughing, a decrease in bone thickness, and fluid buildup in the eye.

Table 5.5 Topical corticosteroid skin forms potency classes

Potency class	Generic name	Brand name	Concentration
Low	Hydrocortisone butyrate	Cortate®	0.1%, 0.5%, 1%, 2.5%
		Unicort®	
		Locoid®	
Medium	Betamethasone valerate	Celestoderm®	0.05%, 0.1%
		Betnovate®	
	Mometasone furoate	Elica® (see Fig. 5.26)	0.1%
	Triamcinolone acetonide	Ftorocort®	0.025%, 0.05%, 0.1%
		Aristocort D®	
		Aristocort R®	
		Vioderm-KC®	
		Kenacomb®	
	Fluocinolone acetonide	Flucinar®	0.01%, 0.025%, 0.01%
		Synalar®	
		Synamol®	
		Derma-smooth®	
High	Betamethasone dipropionate	Propaderm diprosone®	0.025%, 0.05%
		Diprolene glycol®	
		Akriderm®	
	Triamcinolone acetonide	Aristocort C®	0.5%
Highest	Clobetasol propionate	Dermovate® (see Fig. 5.27)	0.05%

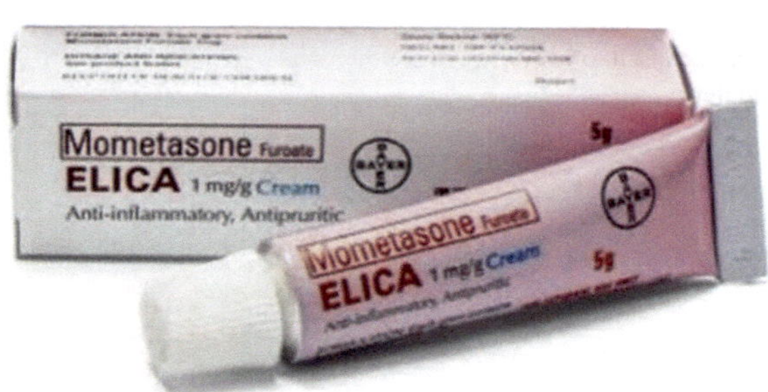

Fig. 5.26 Elica® (Mometasone furoate)

Topical corticosteroids are currently the mainstay of treatment for atopic dermatitis [85]. Skin topical forms include lotions, gels, creams, and ointments. In association with moisturization, the therapeutic effect may be suitable. Topical corticosteroids are categorized by action potency (see Table 5.5). Steroid therapy may be discontinued when lesions disappear and resumed when new rash elements occur.

The most common side effects of corticosteroids for skin use are observed mainly with long-term courses of treatment and include skin atrophy, striae, rosacea, perioral dermatitis, acne, and purpura. Side effects are unlikely to occur with short-term therapy.

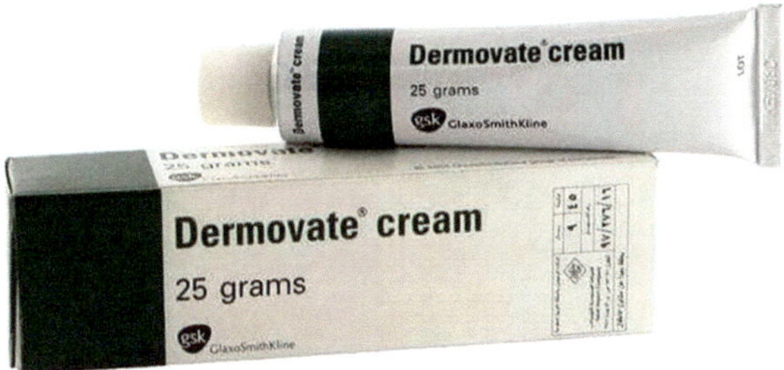

Fig. 5.27 Dermovate®

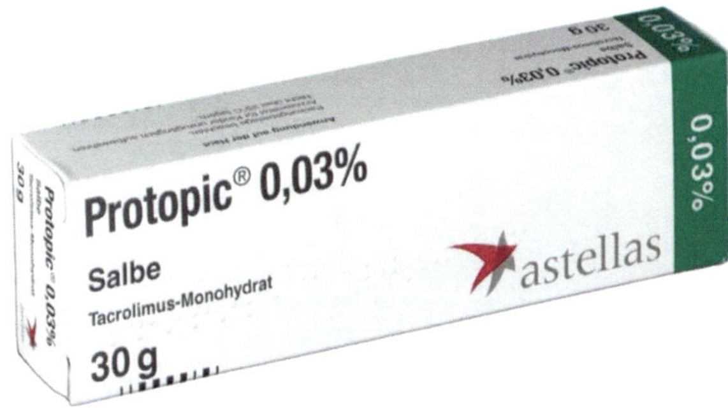

Fig. 5.28 Protopic®

5.7.4 Calcineurin Inhibitors

Calcineurin inhibitors downregulate the *IL-2 gene* transcription through the inactivation of the transcription factor NFAT. It eventually leads to reduced T cell proliferation in T cell clonal expansion and, correspondingly, the involvement of new lymphocytes in inflammation. Topical calcineurin inhibitors, such as pimecrolimus (cream Elidel®) and tacrolimus (ointment Protopic®) (see Fig. 5.28), are used in the short-term treatment for atopic dermatitis [85]. Side effects of these medications may include the development of immunocompromised skin conditions.

5.7.5 Leukotriene Receptor Antagonists

Leukotriene receptor antagonists reduce the *late phase* of atopic allergic inflammation and mucus production and work similar to corticosteroids but with fewer side effects. They include montelukast (Singular®) and zafirlukast (Accolate®) (see Fig. 5.29).

5.7.6 Biologics

In the past 15–20 years, monoclonal antibodies are rapidly growing biological medications becoming a dominant category of recombinant proteins currently presented

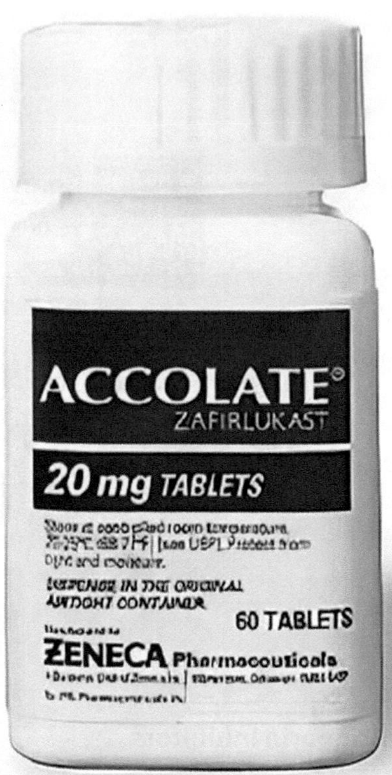

Fig. 5.29 Accolate®

in use. Like many other clinical disciplines, allergology is experiencing the early days of the development of new biologics that have entered the clinic [6]. See Table 5.6.

Omalizumab is the first, most studied biologic, which represents a humanized anti-IgE monoclonal antibody. FDA approved Xolair® in 2003. Anti-IgE therapy by omalizumab is used in severe allergic asthma [102] and chronic spontaneous urticaria [103, 104]. In addition, omalizumab efficacy has been studied in IgE-independent forms of urticaria [104]. Nowadays, omalizumab is on a clinical trial as an adjunct therapy to AIT in multiple food allergies [106–108]. This biologic downregulates the expression of FcεRI on mast cells (slowly), basophils (rapidly), and dendritic cells [107], blocks the interaction of free IgE with FcεRI on appropriate cells, and indirectly influence the production of Th2-associated cytokines [102]. As a result, the likelihood of allergen-IgE cross-linking is reduced, and anergy of IgE-bearing B cells occurs [103, 104]. The clinical efficacy of omalizumab has been shown in systematic reviews of published evidence [102, 104, 105].

Ligelizumab is a novel high-affinity anti-IgE antibody, currently in a clinical trial, particularly, in patients with chronic spontaneius urticaria [109]. The recent findings suggest ligelizumab has the potential to be more effective than Xolair® in treating chronic spontaneous urticaria. In addition, ligelizumab is actually in

Table 5.6 Biologics in therapy for allergic diseases

Generic name (brand name)	Monoclonal antibody	Indications	Current status
Omalizumab (Xolair®) (Fig. 5.30)	Anti-IgE	Moderate-to-severe persistent asthma, chronic spontaneous urticaria, nasal polyps	In use [102–105]
		Food allergies, AIT	On a trial [106–108]
Ligelizumab	Anti-IgE	Allergic asthma, chronic spontaneous urticaria, cholinergic urticaria, cold urticaria, atopic dermatitis, eosinophilic esophagitis, indolent systemic mastocytosis	On a trial [107, 109]
Mepolizumab (Nucala®) (Fig. 5.31)	Anti-IL-5	Severe eosinophilic asthma, late onset asthma, chronic rhinosinusitis with nasal polyps, eosinophilic granulomatosis with polyangiitis, hypereosinophilic syndrome	In use [102, 105, 108]
Reslizumab (Cinqair®)	Anti-IL-5	Severe eosinophilic asthma	In use [102, 105, 108]
Benralizumab (Fasenra®) (Fig. 5.32)	Anti-IL-5Rα	Severe eosinophilc asthma, late onset asthma	In use [102, 105, 108]
Dupilumab (Dupixent®) (Fig. 5.33)	Anti-IL-4Rα/IL-13Rα	Moderate-to-severe atopic dermatitis, severe eosinophil asthma, chronic rhinosinusitis with nasal polyposis	In use [82, 85, 102, 105]
		Eosinophilic asthma, aspirin-exacerbated respiratory disease, allergic rhinitis (with or without nasal polyps), severe eosinophilic chronic sinusitis, allergic bronchopulmonary aspergillosis, eosinophilic esophagitis, food allergies, AIT, chronic spontaneous urticaria, cholinergic urticaria	On a trial [102, 107, 108, 110]
Tralokinumab (Adtralza®)	Anti-IL-13	Moderate-to-severe atopic dermatitis	In use (EU only) [111]
Lebrikizumab	Anti-IL-13	Uncontrolled asthma, moderate-to-severe atopic dermatitis	On a trial [112, 113]
Etokimab	Anti-IL-33	Atopic dermatitis, eosinophilic asthma, chronic rhinosinusitis, food allergies, eosinophilic esophagitis	On a trial [107, 108, 114]
Itepekimab	Anti-IL-33	Moderate-to-severe asthma	On a trial [115]
Tezepelumab	Anti-TSLP	Severe asthma, moderate-to-severe atopic dermatitis, cat allergy, AIT	On a trial [107, 116]
Lirentelimab	Anti-SIGLEC8	Chronic spontaneous urticaria, indolent systemic mastocytosis, eosinophilic esophagitis, eosinophilic gastroenteritis, atopic keratoconjunctivitis	On a trial [107]

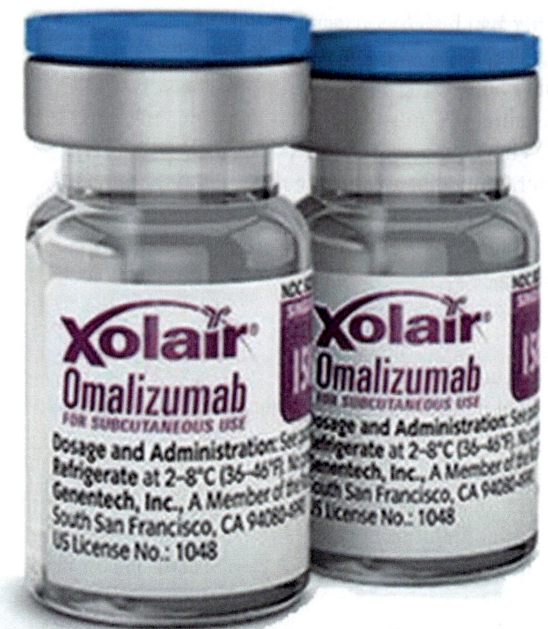

Fig. 5.30 Xolair®

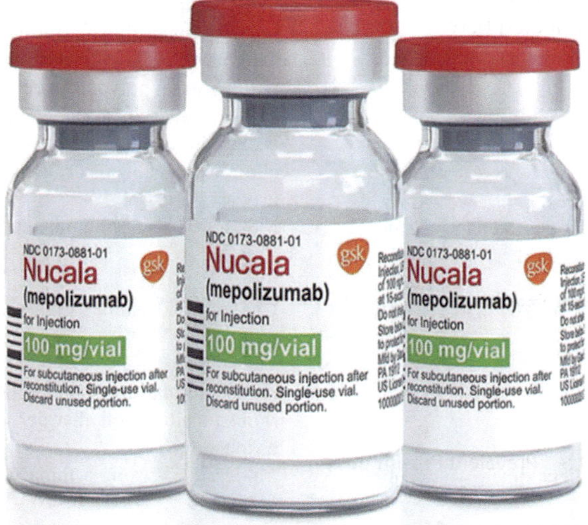

Fig. 5.31 Nucala®

clinical trials in patients with cholinergic urticaria, cold urticaria, indolent systemic mastocytosis, allergic asthma, atopic dermatitis, and eosinophilic esophagitis [107].

Mepolizumab (Nucala®) and *reslizumab* (Cinqair®), humanized monoclonal anti-IL-5 antibodies, were approved by the FDA in 2015 and 2016. According to published reports and a systematic review, these biologics significantly reduce the annual rate of exacerbations and improve asthma control and lung function [102].

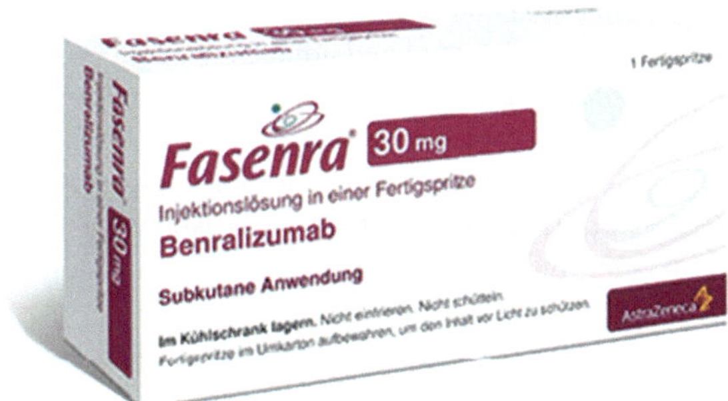

Fig. 5.32 Fasenra®

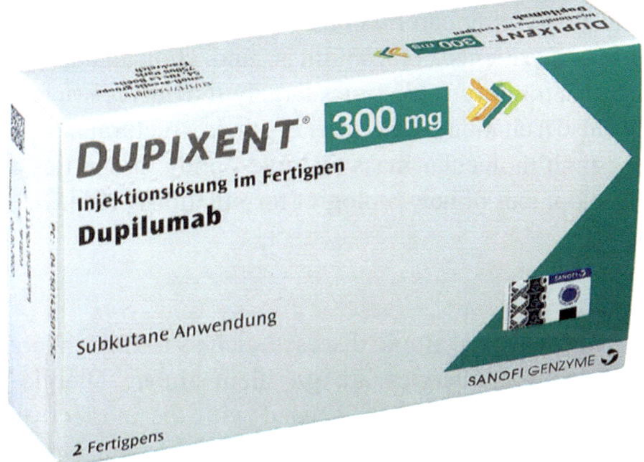

Fig. 5.33 Dupixent®

Benralizumab (Fasenra®), humanized monoclonal anti-IL-5Rα antibody, was approved by FDA in 2017. The clinical studies summarized in a systematic review have shown that benralizumab is efficient in significantly reducing the rate of recurrences and the symptoms of severe eosinophilic asthma and diminishing the required dose of oral corticosteroids [102].

Dupilumab (Dupixent®), the humanized monoclonal anti-IL-4Rα/IL-13Rα antibody, approved in 2017, is currently used for the treatment of moderate-to-severe atopic dermatitis, eosinophil asthma, and chronic rhinosinusitis with nasal polyposis. Dupilumab blocks IL-4 and IL-13 binding to the Rα chain, shared by both cytokines, and decreases allergic inflammation [110]. Dupilumab is reported capable of reducing the severity of asthma and the rate of exacerbations [102] and improving severe atopic dermatitis symptoms, as well as health-related quality of life [85]. So far, dupilumab is in clinical trials in patients with many allergic diseases [107], including combination therapy with AIT in persons with polysensitized food allergies [108].

Tralokinumab (Adtralza®), the fully human monoclonal anti-IL-13 antibody, was approved in the EU in 2021 for the treatment of persons with moderate-to-severe atopic dermatitis. Tralokinumab with concomitant topical corticosteroids improves the eczema area and severity index, reduces skin itch, and *Staphylococcus aureus* colonization on lesional and nonlesional skin [107].

Etokimab, the monoclonal anti-IL-33 antibody, is currently in clinical trials in patients with atopic dermatitis, Th2-high/eosinophilic asthma, chronic rhinosinusitis, food allergies, and eosinophilic esophagitis [108, 114]. In a phase 2 trial, *itepekimab* (anti-IL-33 antibody) displays a lower incidence of uncontrolled events and improvement of lung function as monotherapy for moderate-to-severe asthma [115].

Tezepelumab, the fully human monoclonal anti-TSLP antibody, is on a trial in patients with severe asthma [116], moderate-to-severe atopic dermatitis, and as an adjunct therapy to AIT in persons with cat allergy [107].

The number of biologics options increases. Therefore, the choice of them can be made only after careful consideration of the particular endotype and biomarkers of disease, patients comorbidities, and clinical data [102]. However, the route of administration for biologics largely remains restricted to injection, and side effects are also a challenge. Maintaining their structural integrity and activity and diminishing high molecular mass and hydrophilic properties are crucial for the successful development of new biologics formulations [105].

Key Points

1. Conventional atopic diseases such as asthma, allergic rhinitis, atopic dermatitis, and food allergies are prevalent among allergic conditions. If a recurrence occurs, it may be associated with the ineffectiveness of the therapy and the imbalance of pro-inflammatory and anti-inflammatory factors when pro-inflammatory factors are predominant.
2. International position papers define the basic medication therapy, including biologics, and allergen-specific immunotherapy (AIT) for allergies.
3. The component of “neurogenic inflammation” may contribute to the severity of the occurred exacerbation.
4. Syndromes identical to urticaria, angioedema, and anaphylaxis can be caused by IgE or IgG sensitization and be atopic, autoimmune, or toxico-allergic.

Take-Home Messages

1. Write a questionnaire on family history of a patient who has asthma.
2. Write a questionnaire on a social patient’s history who suffers from asthma.
3. Write a questionnaire on patients’ complaints in allergic rhinitis.
4. Write an essay about celebrities who suffered from seasonal allergies.
5. Make a flyer about allergic insects.
6. List separation of indoor and outdoor allergens in urticaria and angioedema.
7. Make a slide presentation on allergic skin diseases.

8. List causes of urticaria, angioedema, and anaphylaxis.
9. Write a paragraph about the classification of allergic asthma.
10. Write a paragraph about the classification of allergic rhinitis.
11. Make a flyer about basic medication therapy for allergies.
12. Write a paragraph about ScorAD.
13. List neuro molecules predominantly operate in the skin.
14. Write a paragraph about biologics.

Quiz B

Reading a question, please choose only one right answer.

Question 1

An endotype of asthma is characterized by a more severe course:

1. Th1/Th17/neutrophilic asthma's endotype.
2. Th2/eosinophilic asthma's endotype.
3. Asthma induced by physical exercise.
4. Asthma with allergic rhinitis.

Question 2

The order of a subsequent change of allergic target organs in "atopic march":

1. The bronchi, skin, nose/conjunctive.
2. The skin, nose/conjunctive, bronchi.
3. The nose/conjunctive, bronchi, skin.
4. The skin, bronchi, nose/conjunctive.

Question 3

Cells that provide the repeated episodes of allergic disease caused by the same allergen:

1. Dendritic cells.
2. Macrophages.
3. Memory cells.
4. Eosinophils.

Question 4

Allergological method taking into account the cytophilic property of IgE:

1. Component resolved diagnosis (CRD).
2. Allergic skin testing.
3. Video rhinoscopy.
4. Basophil activation test.

Question 5
Position paper related to asthma is:

1. GINA.
2. The skin prick test—European standards.
3. International consensus statement on allergy and rhinology.
4. ETFAD/EADV position paper.

Question 6
The perennial rhinitis commonly starts at the age of:

1. 1 year.
2. 12–15 years.
3. 10–12 years.
4. 3–5 years.

Question 7
Allergen tolerance breakdown does not resemble initial IgE-dependent response:

1. It resembles.
2. Does not resemble.
3. It resembles the adaptive CD4+ T cell response.
4. It resembles the adaptive CD8+ T cell response.

Question 8
ILC2 cells secrete:

1. IL-4, IL-6, IL10, and IL-13.
2. IFN-γ, IL-2, and TNF-β.
3. IL-5, IL-9, and IL-13.
4. IFN-α, IFN-β, and IL-18.

Question 9
ILC2 cells are activated by:

1. Alarmins: IL-25, IL-33, and TSLP.
2. Norepinephrine.
3. CGRP.
4. Histamine.

Question 10
Skin itch in atopic dermatitis is linked with:

1. Serotonin and GABA.
2. Histamine, TSLP, IL-31, IL-33, and NGF.

3. IL-4, IL-5, and IL-13.
4. IL-10, TGF-β, and IL-35.

Question 11
Alarmins activate:

1. Th1, Th17, and Th22.
2. Allergen-specific memory B cells.
3. Th2, ILC2, and DCs.
4. Mast cells and basophils.

Question 12
Follicular helper T cells (Tfh) originate from:

1. Memory T cells.
2. Th1 cells.
3. Peripheral Treg (pTreg) cells.
4. Naïve T cells.

Question 13
Endoscopic imaging in allergic rhinitis includes:

1. Mucosal edema.
2. Benign tumor.
3. Septal deviation.
4. Epistaxis.

Question 14
In the Northern hemisphere, there are ______ waves of allergen plant pollination:

1. Five.
2. Three.
3. One.
4. Six.

Question 15
The main symptom of urticaria is:

1. Papules.
2. Wheals.
3. Lichenification.
4. Crusts.

Question 16

The biologic based on anti-TSLP antibodies is:

1. Omalizumab.
2. Pascolizumab.
3. Mepolizumab.
4. Tezepelumab.

References

1. Holguin F. The atopic march: IgE is not the only road. Lancet. 2014;2(2):88–90. https://doi.org/10.1016/S2213-2600(13)70243-1.
2. Tham EH, Leung DYM. Mechanisms by which atopic dermatitis predisposes to food allergy and the atopic march. Allergy Asthma Immunol Res. 2019;11(1):4–15. https://doi.org/10.4168/aair.2019.11.1.4.
3. Banks TA, Gada SM. Filaggrin mutations as an archetype for understanding the pathophysiology of atopic dermatitis. J Am Acad Dermatol. 2014;71(3):592–3. https://doi.org/10.1016/j.jaad.2014.04.075.
4. Bantz SK, Zhu Z, Zheng T. The atopic march: progression from atopic dermatitis to allergic rhinitis and asthma. J Clin Cell Immunol. 2014;5(2):1–8. https://doi.org/10.4172/2155-9899.1000202.
5. Yamauchi K, Ogasawara M. The role of histamine in the pathophysiology of asthma and the clinical efficacy of antihistamines in asthma therapy. Int J Mol Sci. 2019;20:1733. https://doi.org/10.3390/ijms20071733.
6. Breiteneder H, Diamant Z, Eiwegger T, Fokkens WJ, Traidl-Hoffmann C, Nadeau K, et al. Future research trends in understanding the mechanisms underlying allergic diseases for improved patient care. Allergy. 2019;74:2293–311. https://doi.org/10.1111/all.13851.
7. Matricardi PM, Dramburg S, Potapova E, Skevaki C, Renz H. Molecular diagnosis for allergen immunotherapy. J Allergy Clin Immunol. 2019;143(3):831–43. https://doi.org/10.1016/j.jaci.2018.12.1021.
8. Van Hage M, Hamsten C, Valenta R. ImmunoCAP assays: pros and cons in allergology. J Allergy Clin Immunol. 2017;140(4):974–7. https://doi.org/10.1016/j.jaci.2017.05.008.
9. Di Fraia M, Arasi S, Castelli S, Dramburg S, Potapova E, Villalta D, Tripodi S, Sfika I, Zicari AM, Villella V, Perna S, Travaglini A, Verardo PL, Martricardi PM. A new molecular multiplex IgE assay for the diagnosis of pollen allergy in Mediterranean countries: a validation study. Clin Exp Allergy. 2019;49:341–9. https://doi.org/10.1111/cea.13264.
10. Brusca I, Barrale M, Onida R, La Chiusa SM, Gjomarkaj M, Uasuf CG. The extract, the molecular allergen or both for the in vitro diagnosis of peach and peanut sensitization? Clin Chim Acta. 2019;493:25–30. https://doi.org/10.1016/j.cca.2019.01.016.
11. Heinzerling L, Mari A, Bergmann KC, Bresciani M, Burbach G, Darsow U, et al. The skin prick test - European standards. Clin Transl Allergy. 2013;3(3):1–10. https://doi.org/10.1186/2045-7022-3-3.
12. Ebruster H. The prick test, a recent cutaneous test for the diagnosis of allergic disorders. Wien Klin Wochenschr. 1959;71:551–4.
13. Larenas-Linnemann D, Luna-Pech JA, Mësges R. Debates in allergy medicine: allergy skin testing cannot be replaced by molecular diagnosis in the near future. World Allergy Organ J. 2017;10(32):1–7. https://doi.org/10.1186/s40413-017-0164-1.
14. Klimov VV. Allergen-specific immunotherapy (ASIT). In: From basic to clinical immunology. Cham: Springer; 2019. https://doi.org/10.1007/978-3-030-0332301_11.

15. Agaché I, Bilò M, Braunstahl GJ, Delgado L, Demoly P, Eigenmann P, Gomes E, Hellings P, Horak F, Muraro A, Werfel T, Jutel M. *In vivo* diagnosis of allergic diseases - allergen provocation tests. Allergy. 2015;70(4):355–65. https://doi.org/10.1111/all.12586.
16. Wise SK, Lin SY, Toskala E, Orlandi RR, Akdis AA, Alt JA, et al. International consensus statement on allergy and rhinology: allergic rhinitis. Int Forum Allergy Rhinol. 2018;8(2):108–352. https://doi.org/10.1002/alr.22073.
17. Patel G, Saltoun C. Skin testing in allergy. Allergy Asthma Proc. 2019;40(6):366–8. https://doi.org/10.2500/aap.2019.40.4248.
18. Campo P, Eguiluz-Gracia I, Bogas G, Salas M, Plaza Seron C, Perez N, et al. Local allergic rhinitis: implications for management. Clin Exp Allergy. 2019;49(1):6–16. https://doi.org/10.1111/cea.13192.
19. Jensen-Jarolim E, Jensen AN, Canonica GW. Debates in allergy medicine: molecular allergy diagnosis with ISAC will replace screenings by skin prick test in the future. World Allergy Organ J. 2017;10(1):33. https://doi.org/10.1186/s40413-017-0162-3.
20. Mansouri M, Rafiee E, Darougar S, Mesdaghi M, Chavoshzadeh Z. Is the atopy patch test reliable in the evaluation of food allergy-related atopic dermatitis? Int Arch Allergy Immunol. 2018;175(1–2):85–90. https://doi.org/10.1159/000485126.
21. Gao W, Gong J, Mu M, Zhu Y, Wang W, Chen W, et al. The pathogenesis of eosinophilic asthma: a positive feedback mechanism that promotes Th2 immune response via filaggrin deficiency. Front Immunol. 2021;12:672312. https://doi.org/10.3389/fimmu.2021.672312.
22. Hough KP, Curtiss ML, Blain TJ, Liu R-M, Trevor J, Deshane JS, Thannickal VJ. Airway remodeling in asthma. Front Med. 2020;7:191. https://doi.org/10.3389/fmed.2020.00191.
23. Hirose K, Iwata A, Tamachi T, Nakajima H. Allergic airway inflammation: key players beyond the Th2 cell pathway. Immunol Rev. 2017;278(1):145–61. https://doi.org/10.1111/imr.12540.
24. Lin T-Y, Poon AH, Hamid Q. Asthma phenotypes and endotypes. Curr Opin Pulm Med. 2013;19:18–23. https://doi.org/10.1097/MCP.0b013e32835b10ec.
25. Global Initiative for Asthma. Global strategy for asthma management and prevention. 2021. www.ginasthma.org.
26. Bellanti JA. Phenotypic classification of asthma based on a new type 2-high and type 2-low endotypic classification: it all began with Rackemann. J Prec Respir Med. 2020;3(1):9–20. https://doi.org/10.2500/jprm.2020.3.200001.
27. Pembrey L, Barreto ML, Douwes J, Cooper P, Henderson J, Mpairwe H, et al. Understanding asthma phenotypes: the World Asthma Phenotypes (WASP) international collaboration. ERJ Open Res. 2018;4:00013–2018. https://doi.org/10.1183/23120541.00013-2018.
28. Radermecker C, Louis R, Bureau F, Marichal T. Role of neutrophils in allergic asthma. Curr Opin Immunol. 2018;54:28–34. https://doi.org/10.1016/j.coi.2018.05.006.
29. Barnes PJ, Burney PGJ, Silverman EK, Celli BR, Vestbo J, Wedzicha JA, Wounters FM. Chronic obstructive pulmonary disease. Nat Rev Dis Primers. 2015;1:15076. https://doi.org/10.1038/nrdp.2015.76.
30. Guida G, Antonelli A. Eosinophilic phenotype: the lesson from research models to severe asthma. In: Fucs O, Athari SS, editors. Cells of the immune system. London: IntechOpen; 2020. p. 1-22. https://doi.org/10.5772/intechopen.92123.
31. Moldaver DM, Lanché M, Rudulier CD. An update on lymphocyte subtypes in asthma and airway disease. Chest. 2017;151(5):1122–30. https://doi.org/10.1016/j.chest.2016.10.038.
32. Bush A. Cytokines and chemokines as biomarkers of future asthma. Front Pediatr. 2019;7:72. https://doi.org/10.3389/fped.2019.00072.
33. Murrison LB, Brandt EB, Meyers JB, Hershey GKK. Environmental exposures and mechanisms in allergy and asthma development. J Clin Invest. 2019;124(4):1504–15. https://doi.org/10.1172/JCI124612.
34. Chan A, Yu JE. Food allergy and asthma. J Food Allergy. 2020;2(1):44–7. https://doi.org/10.2500/jfa.2020.2.200003.

35. Wang Y-H, Lue K-H. Association between sensitized to food allergens and childhood allergic respiratory diseases in Taiwan. J Microbiol Immunol Infect. 2020;53(5):812–20. https://doi.org/10.1016/j.jmii.2019.01.005.
36. Emons JAM, van Wijk GR. Food allergy and asthma: is there a link? Curr Treat Options Allergy. 2018;5:436–44. https://doi.org/10.1007/s40521-018-0185-1.
37. Foong R-X, Swan K, Fox AT. Asthma and food allergies. EMJ Allergy Immunol. 2018;3(1):82–8.
38. Campo P, Eguiluz-Gracia I, Plaza-Seron M, Salas M, Rodriguez MJ, Perez-Sanchez N, Gonzalez M, Molina A, Mayorga C, Torres MJ, Rondón C. Bronchial asthma triggered by house dust mites in patients with local allergic rhinitis. Allergy. 2019;74(8):1502–10. https://doi.org/10.1111/all.13775.
39. Yamana Y, Fukuda K, Ko R, Uchio E. Local allergic conjunctivitis: a phenotype of allergic conjunctivitis. Int Ophthalmol. 2019;39:2539–44. https://doi.org/10.1007/s10792-019-01101-z.
40. Voisin T, Bouvier A, Chiu IV. Neuro-immune interactions in allergic diseases: novel targets for therapeutics. Int Immunol. 2017;29(6):247–61. https://doi.org/10.1093/intimm/dxx040.
41. Licari A, Castagnoli R, Brambilla I, Marseglia A, Tosca MA, Marseglia GL, Ciprandi G. Asthma endotyping and biomarkers in childhood asthma. Pediatr Allergy Immunol Pulmonol. 2018;31(2):44–58. https://doi.org/10.1089/ped.2018.0886.
42. Nekoee H, Graulich E, Schleich F, Guissard F, Paulus V, Henket M, et al. Are type-2 biomarkers of any help in asthma diagnosis? ERJ Open Res. 2020;6:00169–2020. https://doi.org/10.1183/23120541.00169-2020.
43. Kunc P, Fabry J, Lucanska M, Pecova R. Biomarkers of bronchial asthma. Physiol Res. 2020;69(Suppl 1):29–34. https://doi.org/10.33549/physiolres.934398.
44. Lugogo NL, Akuthota P. Type 2 biomarkers in asthma: yet another reflection of heterogeneity. J Allergy Clin Immunol Pract. 2021;9(3):1276–7. https://doi.org/10.1016/j.jaip.2020.12.032.
45. Popović-Grle S, Stajduhar A, Lampalo M, Rnjak D. Biomarkers in different asthma phenotypes. Genes. 2021;12:801. https://doi.org/10.3390/genes12060801.
46. Diamant Z, Vijverberg S, Alvig K, Bakirtas A, Bjermer L, Custovic A, et al. Toward clinically applicable biomarkers for asthma: an EAACI position paper. Allergy. 2019;74(10):1835–51. https://doi.org/10.1111/all.13806.
47. Su J. A brief history of Charcot-Leyden crystal protein/galectin-10 research. Molecules. 2018;23(11):2931. https://doi.org/10.3390/molecules23112931.
48. Kuruvilla ME, Lee FE-H, Lee GB. Understanding asthma phenotypes, endotypes, and mechanisms of disease. Clin Rev Allergy Immunol. 2019;56:219–33. https://doi.org/10.1007/s12016-018-8712-1.
49. Heaney LG, Busby J, Hanratty CE, Djukanovic R, Woodcock A, Walker SM, et al. Composite type-2 biomarker strategy versus a symptom–risk-based algorithm to adjust corticosteroid dose in patients with severe asthma: a multicentre, single-blind, parallel group, randomised controlled trial. Lancet. 2021;9(1):57–68. https://doi.org/10.1016/S2213-2600(20)30397-0.
50. Lee Y, Quoc QL, Park H-S. Biomarkers for severe asthma: lessons from longitudinal cohort studies. Allergy Asthma Immunol Res. 2021;13(3):375–89. https://doi.org/10.4168/aair.2021.13.3.375.
51. Tashiro H, Takahashi K, Sadamatsu H, Kurihara Y, Haraguchi T, Tajiri A, et al. Biomarkers for overweight in adult-onset asthma. J Asthma Allergy. 2020;13:409–14. https://doi.org/10.2147/JAA.S276371.
52. Hue L, Salimi M, Panse I, Mjosberg JM, McKenzie ANJ, Spits H, et al. Prostaglandin D2 activates group 2 innate lymphoid cells through chemoattractant receptor-homologous molecule expressed on TH2 cells. J Allergy Clin Immunol. 2014;133(4):1184–94.e7. https://doi.org/10.1016/j.jaci.2013.10.056.
53. Bousquet J, Schunemann HJ, Togias A, Bachert C, Erhola M, Hellings PW, et al. Next-generation Allergic Rhinitis and its Impact on Asthma (ARIA) guidelines for allergic rhinitis based on Grading of Recommendations Assessment, Development and Evaluation

(GRADE) and real-world evidence. J Allergy Clin Immunol. 2020;145(1):70–80.e3. https://doi.org/10.1016/j.jaci.2019.06.049.
54. Passali D, Cingi C, Staffa P, Passali F, Muluk NB, Bellussi ML. The international study of the allergic rhinitis survey: outcomes from 4 geographical regions. Asia Pac Allergy. 2018;8(1):e7. https://doi.org/10.5415/apallergy.2018.8.e7.
55. Romano MR, James S, Farrington E, Perry R, Elliott L. The impact of perennial allergic rhinitis with/without allergic asthma on sleep, work and activity level. Allergy Asthma Clin Immunol. 2020;16:12. https://doi.org/10.1186/s13223-020-0408-4.
56. Okubo K, Kurono Y, Ichimura K, Enomoto T, Okamoto Y, Kawauchi H, et al. Japanese guidelines for allergic rhinitis 2017. Allergol Int. 2017;66(2):205–19. https://doi.org/10.1016/j.alit.2016.11.001.
57. Jung C-G, Lee J-H, Ban G-Y, et al. Prevalence and clinical characteristics of local allergic rhinitis to house dust mites. Yonsei Med J. 2017;58(5):1047–50. https://doi.org/10.3349/ymj.2017.58.5.1047.
58. Bousquet J, Anto JM, Bachert C, Baiardini I, Bosnic-Anticevich S, Canonica GW, et al. Allergic rhinitis. Nat Rev Dis Primers. 2020;6:95. https://doi.org/10.1038/s41572-020-00227-0.
59. Watts AM, Cripps AW, West NP, Cox AJ. Modulation of allergic inflammation in the nasal mucosa of allergic rhinitis sufferers with topical pharmaceutical agents. Front Pharmacol. 2019;10:294. https://doi.org/10.3389/fphar.2019.00294.
60. Nozad CH, Michael LM, Lew DB, Michael CF. Non-allergic rhinitis: a case report and review. Clin Mol Allergy. 2010;8(1):1–9. https://doi.org/10.1186/1476-7961-8-1.
61. Scadding GK, Kariyawasam HH, Scadding G, Mirakan R, Buckley RJ, Dixon T, et al. BSACI guideline for the diagnosis and management of allergic and non-allergic rhinitis (revised edition 2017; first edition 2007). Clin Exp Allergy. 2017;47:856–89. https://doi.org/10.1111/cea.12953.
62. Galimberti M, Passalacqua G, Incorvaia C, Castella V, Costantino MT, Cucchi B, et al. Catching allergy by a simple questionnaire. World Allergy Organ J. 2015;8:1–7. https://doi.org/10.1186/s40413-015-0067-y.
63. Eifan AO, Durham SR. Pathogenesis of rhinitis. Clin Exp Allergy. 2016;46(9):1139–51. https://doi.org/spiral.imperial.ac.uk:8443/handle/10044/1/37061.
64. Caimmi D, Baiz N, Sanyal S, Banerjee S, Demoly P, Annesi-Maesano I. Discriminating severe seasonal allergic rhinitis. Results from a large nation-wide database. PLoS One. 2018;13(11):e0207290. https://doi.org/10.1371/journal.pone.020729.
65. Leung AK, Hon KL. Seasonal allergic rhinitis. Recent Pat Inflamm Allergy Drug Discov. 2013;7(3):187–201. https://doi.org/10.2174/1872213x113079990022.
66. Tomazic PV, Darnhofer B, Birner-Gruenberger R. Nasal mucus proteome and its involvement in allergic rhinitis. Expert Rev Proteomics. 2020;17(2):191–9. https://doi.org/10.1080/14789450.2020.1748502.
67. Maoz-Segal R, Machnes-Maayan D, Veksler-Offengenden I, Frizinsky S, Hajyahia S, Agmon-Levin N. Local allergic rhinitis: an old story but a new entity. In: Gendeh BS, Turkalj M, editors. Rhinosinusitis. London: IntechOpen; 2019. p. 1–9. https://doi.org/10.5772/intechopen.86212.
68. Papadopoulos NG, Bernstein JA, Demoly P, Dykewicz M, Fokkiens W, Hellings PW, et al. Phenotypes and endotypes of rhinitis and their impact on management: a PRACTALL report. Allergy. 2015;70:474–94. https://doi.org/10.1111/all.12573.
69. De Greve G, Hellings PW, Fokkens WJ, Pugin B, Steelant B, Seys SF. Endotype-driven treatment in chronic upper airway diseases. Clin Transl Allergy. 2017;7(22):1–14. https://doi.org/10.1186/s13601-017-0157-8.
70. Klimov AV, Isaev PY, Klimov VV, Sviridova VS. Endotypes of allergic rhinitis and asthma accompanying food allergy. Bull Sib Med. 2019;18(2):287–9. https://doi.org/10.20538/1682-0363-2019-2-287-289.
71. Wen HC, Czarnowicki T, Noda S, Malik K, Pavel AB, Nakajima S, et al. Serum from Asian patients with atopic dermatitis is characterized by TH2/TH22 activation, which is highly

correlated with nonlesional skin measures. J Allergy Clin Immunol. 2018;142:324–8.e11. https://doi.org/10.1016/j.jaci.2018.02.047.
72. Ständer S. Atopic dermatitis. N Engl J Med. 2021;384:1136–43. https://doi.org/10.1056/NEJMra2023911.
73. Banzon T, Leung DYM, Schneider LC. Food allergy and atopic dermatitis. J Food Allergy. 2020;2(1):35–8. https://doi.org/10.2500/jfa.2020.2.200018.
74. Oranje AP. Practical issues on interpretation of scoring atopic dermatitis: SCORAD Index, objective SCORAD, patient-oriented SCORAD and three-item severity score. In: Shiohara T, editor. Pathogenesis and management of atopic dermatitis. Curr Probl Dermatol, vol. 41. Basel: Karger; 2011. p. 149–55. https://doi.org/10.1159/000323308.
75. Avena-Woods C. Overview of atopic dermatitis. Am J Manag Care. 2017;23(8):S115–23.
76. Carlton SM. Nociceptive primary afferents: they have a mind of their own. J Physiol. 2014;592(16):3403–11. https://doi.org/10.1113/jphysiol.2013.269654.
77. Pondeljak N, Lugović-Mihić L. Stress-induced interaction of skin immune cells, hormones, and neurotransmitters. Clin Ther. 2020;42(5):757–70. https://doi.org/10.1016/j.clinthera.2020.03.008.
78. Thijs JL, de Bruin-Weller MS, Hijnen D. Current and future biomarkers in atopic dermatitis. Immunol Allergy Clin N Am. 2017;37:51–61. https://doi.org/10.1016/j.iac.2016.08.008.
79. Renert-Yuval Y, Thyssen JP, Bissonnette R, Bieber T, Kabashima K, Hijnen D, Guttman-Yassky E. Biomarkers in atopic dermatitis-a review on behalf of the International Eczema Council. J Allergy Clin Immunol. 2021;147(4):1174–90.e1. https://doi.org/10.1016/j.jaci.2021.01.013.
80. Ungar B, Garcet SD, Gonzalez J, Dhingra N, da Rosa JC, Shemer A, et al. An integrated model of atopic dermatitis biomarkers highlights the systemic nature of the disease. J Invest Dermatol. 2017;137:603–13. https://doi.org/10.1016/j.jid.2016.09.037.
81. Kaplan MH, Engle S, Chang C-Y, Satterwhite A, Ulrich B, Hayes T, et al. Biomarker prediction of pediatric atopic dermatitis severity. J Immunol. 2020;204(Suppl 1):147.20.
82. He H, Olesen CM, Pavel AB, Clausen M-L, Wu J, Estrada Y, et al. Tape-strip proteomic profiling of atopic dermatitis on dupilumab identifies minimally invasive biomarkers. Front Immunol. 2020;11:1768. https://doi.org/10.3389/fimmu.2020.01768.
83. Pavel AB, Zhou L, Diaz A, Ungar B, Dan J, He H, et al. The proteomic skin profile of moderate-to-severe atopic dermatitis patients shows an inflammatory signature. J Am Acad Dermatol. 2020;82:690–9. https://doi.org/10.1016/j.jaad.2019.10.039.
84. Hernández-Rodríguez RT, Amezcua-Guerra LM. The potential role of microRNAs as biomarkers in atopic dermatitis: a systematic review. Eur Rev Med Pharmacol Sci. 2020;24(22):11804–9. https://doi.org/10.26355/eurrev_202011_23837.
85. Wollenberg A, Christen-Zach S, Taieb A, Paul C, Thyssen JP, de Bruin-Weller M, et al. ETFAD/EADV Eczema task force 2020 position paper on diagnosis and treatment of atopic dermatitis in adults and children. J Eur Acad Dermatol Venereol. 2020;34(12):2717–44. https://doi.org/10.1111/jdv.16892.
86. Azmy V, Brooks JP, Hsu FI. Clinical presentation of hereditary angioedema. Allergy Asthma Proc. 2021;41(Suppl 1):S18–21. https://doi.org/10.2500/aap.2020.41.200065.
87. Forjaz MJ, Ayala A, Caminoa M, Prior N, Pérez-Fernández E, Caballero T, et al. HAE-AS: a specific disease activity scale for hereditary angioedema with C1-inhibitor deficiency. J Investig Allergol Clin Immunol. 2021;31(3):246–52. https://doi.org/10.18176/jiaci.0479.
88. Kurowski K, Boxer RW. Food allergies: detection and management. Am Fam Physician. 2008;77(12):1678–86.
89. Pali-Schöll I, Blank S, Verhoeckx K, Mueller RS, Janda J, Marti E, Seida AA, Rhynar C, DeBoer DJ, Jensen-Jarolim E. EAACI position paper: comparing insect hypersensitivity induced by bite, sting, inhalation or ingestion in human beings and animals. Allergy. 2019;74:874–87. https://doi.org/10.1111/all.13722.
90. Gonzalez-Estrada A, Silvers SK, Klein A, Zell K, Wang X-F, Lang DM. Epidemiology of anaphylaxis at a tertiary care center: a report of 730 cases. Ann Allergy Asthma Immunol. 2017;118(1):80–5. https://doi.org/10.1016/j.anai.2016.10.025.

91. Vidal C, Armisén M, Monsalve R, González-Vidal T, Lojo S, López-Freire S, et al. Anaphylaxis to Vespa velutina nigrithorax: pattern of sensitization for an emerging problem in Western countries. J Investig Allergol Clin Immunol. 2021;31(3):228–35. https://doi.org/10.18176/jiaci.0474.
92. Brockow K. Drug allergy: definitions and phenotypes. In: Khan DA, Ji AB, editors. Drug allergy testing, Chapter 3. St. Louis, Missouri: Elsevier; 2018. p. 19–26. https://doi.org/10.1016/B978-0-323-48551-7.00003-1.
93. Radonjic-Hoesli S, Hofmeier KS, Micaletto S, Schmid-Grendelmeier P, Bitcher A, Simon D. Urticaria and angioedema: an update on classification and pathogenesis. Clin Rev Allergy Immunol. 2018;54(1):88–101. https://doi.org/10.1007/s12016-017-8628-1.
94. Hon KL, Leung AKC, Ng WGG, Loo SK. Chronic urticaria: an overview of treatment and recent patents. Recent Pat Inflamm Allergy Drug Discov. 2019;13(1):27–37. https://doi.org/10.2174/1872213X13666190328164931.
95. Kasumagic-Halilovic E, Beslic N, Ovcina-Kurtovic N. Thyroid autoimmunity in patients with chronic urticaria. Med Arch. 2017;71(1):29–31. https://doi.org/10.5455/medarh.2017.71.29-31.
96. Porebski G, Kwiecien K, Pawica M, Kwitniewski M. Mas-related G protein-coupled receptor-X2 (MRGPRX2) in drug hypersensitivity reactions. Front Immunol. 2018;9:3027. https://doi.org/10.3389/fimmu.2018.03027.
97. Maurer M, Eyerich K, Eyerich S, Ferrer M, Gutermuth J, Hartmann K, et al. Urticaria: Collegium Internationale Allergologicum (CIA) update 2020. Int Arch Allergy Immunol. 2020;181:321–33. https://doi.org/10.1159/000507218.
98. Simons FER, Ebisawa M, Sanchez-Borges M, Thong BY, Worm M, Tanno LK, Lockey RF, El-Gamal YM, SGA B, Park H-S, Sheikh A. 2015 update of the evidence base: World Allergy Organization anaphylaxis guidelines. World Allergy Organ J. 2015;8:32. https://doi.org/10.1186/s40413-015-0080-1.
99. Fromar L. Prevention of anaphylaxis: the role of the epinephrine auto-injector. Am J Med. 2016;129(12):1244–50. https://doi.org/10.1016/j.amjmed.2016.07.018.
100. Reber LL, Hernandez JD, Galli SJ. The pathophysiology of anaphylaxis. J Allergy Clin Immunol. 2017;140(2):335–48. https://doi.org/10.1016/j.jaci.2017.06.003.
101. Thangam EB, Jemima EA, Singh H, Baig MS, Khan M, Mathias CB, et al. The role of histamine and histamine receptors in mast cell-mediated allergy and inflammation: the hunt for new therapeutic targets. Front Immunol. 2018;9:1873. https://doi.org/10.3389/fimmu.2018.01873.
102. Menzella F, Ruggiero P, Ghidoni G, Fontana M, Bagnasco D, Livrieri F, et al. Anti-IL5 therapies for severe eosinophilic asthma: literature review and practical insights. J Asthma Allergy. 2020;13:301–13.
103. Curto-Barredo L, Spertino J, Figueras-Nart I, Expósito-Serrano V, Guilabert A, Melé-Ninot G, et al. Omalizumab updosing allows disease activity control in patients with refractory chronic spontaneous urticaria. Br J Dermatol. 2018;179(1):210–2. https://doi.org/10.1111/bjd.16379.
104. Maurer M, Metz M, Brehler R, Hillen U, Jakob T, Mahler V, et al. Omalizumab treatment in patients with chronic inducible urticaria: a systematic review of published evidence. J Allergy Clin Immunol. 2018;141(2):638–49. https://doi.org/10.1016/j.jaci.2017.06.032.
105. Liang W, Pan HW, Vilasaliu D, Lam JKW. Pulmonary delivery of biological drugs. Pharmaceutics. 2020;12:1025. https://doi.org/10.3390/pharmaceutics12111025.
106. Brandström J, Vetander M, Sundqvist A-C, Lilija G, Johansson SGO, Melén E, et al. Individually dosed omalizumab facilitates peanut oral immunotherapy in peanut allergic adolescents. Clin Exp Allergy. 2019;49(10):1328–41. https://doi.org/10.1111/cea.13469.
107. Tontini C, Bulfone-Paus S. Novel approaches in the inhibition of IgE-induced mast cell reactivity in food allergy. Front Immunol. 2021;12:613461. https://doi.org/10.3389/fimmu.2021.613461.

108. Chen M, Zhang W, Lee L, Saxena J, Sindher S, Chinthrajah RS, Dant C, Nadeau K. Biologic therapy for food allergy. J Food Allergy. 2020;2(1):86–90. https://doi.org/10.2500/jfa.2020.2.200004.
109. Maurer M, Giménez-Arnau AM, Sussman G, Metz M, Baker DR, Bauer A, et al. Ligelizumab for chronic spontaneous urticaria. N Engl J Med. 2019;381:1321–32. https://doi.org/10.1056/NEJMoa1900408.
110. Bagnasco D, Ferrando M, Varricchi G, Passalacqua G, Canonica GW. A critical evaluation of anti-IL-13 and anti-IL-4 strategies in severe asthma. Int Arch Allergy Immunol. 2016;170:122–31. https://doi.org/10.1159/000447692.
111. Silverberg JI, Futtman-Yassky E, Gooderham M, Worm M, Rippon S, O'Quinn S, et al. Health-related quality of life with tralokinumab in moderate-to-severe atopic dermatitis. A phase 2b randomized study. Ann Allergy Asthma Immunol. 2021;126:576–83. https://doi.org/10.1016/j.anai.2020.12.004.
112. Austin CD, Gonzalez Edick M, Ferrando RE, Solon M, Baca M, Mesh K, et al. A randomized, placebo-controlled trial evaluating effects of lebrikizumab on airway eosinophilic inflammation and remodelling in uncontrolled asthma (CLAVIER). Clin Exp Allergy. 2020;50:1342–51. https://doi.org/10.1111/cea.13731.
113. Guttman-Yassky E, Blauvelt A, Eichenfield LF, Paller AS, Armstrong AW, Drew J, et al. Efficacy and safety of lebrikizumab, a high-affinity interleukin 13 inhibitor, in adults with moderate to severe atopic dermatitis. A phase 2b randomized clinical trial. JAMA Dermatol. 2020;156(4):411–20. https://doi.org/10.1001/jamadermatol.2020.0079.
114. Chen Y-L, Gutowska-Owsiak D, Hardman CS, Westmoreland M, MacKenzie T, Cifuentes L, et al. Proof-of-concept clinical trial of etokimab shows a key role for IL-33 in atopic dermatitis pathogenesis. Sci Transl Med. 2019;11(515):eaax2945. https://doi.org/10.1126/scitranslmed.aax2945.
115. Wechsler M, Ruddy MK, Pavord ID, Israel E, Rabe KF, Ford LB, et al. Efficacy and safety of itepekimab in patients with moderate-to-severe asthma. N Engl J Med. 2021;385:1656–68. https://doi.org/10.1056/NEJMoa2024257.
116. Menzies-Cow A, Corren J, Bourdin A, Chupp G, Israel E, Wechsler ME, et al. Tezepelumab in adults and adolescents with severe, uncontrolled asthma. N Engl J Med. 2021;384:1800–9. https://doi.org/10.1056/NEJMoa2034975.

Local Atopic Disorders in the Unified Airway

6

Contents

Didactics

Knowledge. Upon successful completion of this chapter, students should be able to:

1. List the groups of local atopic diseases.
2. Be familiar with the interpretation of patient's history, clinical, component resolved data for diagnosis, and results of skin prick testing (SPT) concerning patients with local allergic rhinitis.
3. Differentiate roles of various allergology methods of investigation.
4. Draw clinical symptoms of local atopic disorders.
5. Define allergen tolerance maintenance and breakdown of local atopic conditions. Distinguish between conventional and local allergic rhinitis.
6. Describe the pathology and clinical symptoms of "dual" allergic rhinitis.

Supplementary Information The online version contains supplementary material available at [https://doi.org/10.1007/978-3-031-04309-3_6].

V. V. Klimov, *Textbook of Allergen Tolerance*,
https://doi.org/10.1007/978-3-031-04309-3_6

Acquired Skills. Upon successful completion of this chapter, students should demonstrate the following skills:

1. Interpret the knowledge related to routine allergology.
2. Critically evaluate the clinical literature about conventional and local atopic diseases.
3. Discuss the scientific articles from the current research literature to criticize experimental and clinical data and formulate new hypotheses in allergy.
4. Obtain a patient's history, including a history of present illness, past medical history, social, family, and occupational history, and review of systems of a patient with local atopic disorder.
5. Perform a patient's physical examination thoroughly.
6. Explain the rationale for the choice of diagnosis of a patient with a local allergy.
7. Have a clear perception of the presented allergology definitions expressed orally and in written form.
8. Formulate the presented immunology and allergy terms.
9. Correctly answer the quiz questions.

Attitude and Professional Behaviors. Students should be able to:

1. Have the readiness to be hard-working.
2. Behave professionally at all times.
3. Recognize the importance of studying and demonstrate a commitment.
4. Demonstrate the consideration of the patient's feelings, ethnic, religious, cultural, and social background, and display empathy.

6.1 Introduction

▶ **Definition** Local allergen tolerance breakdown is a specific type of allergen tolerance breakdown different from a breakdown at the organism level. Local atopic disorders are specific atopic conditions pathogenically based on a breakdown at the regional level.

Thanks to multinational, randomized placebo-controlled studies, the atopic clinical manifestation pattern has been confirmed as being linked with sensitization patterns in people with atopic heredity [1–4]. However, the number of people with atopic heredity and clinical allergic symptoms does not coincide with the number of practically healthy people with atopic heredity but without symptoms due to the phenomenon of allergen tolerance [5–8]. Nearly healthy though allergen-sensitized people always make up more than patients who suffer from clinical allergic diseases.

The unified airway is a specific anatomical site that undergoes aeroallergen attacks, mainly by European house dust mite, *Dermatophagoides pteronissinus*, and American house dust mite, *Dermatophagoides farinae* [9, 10]. Conventional atopic entities of the unified airway, allergic asthma, and allergic rhinitis

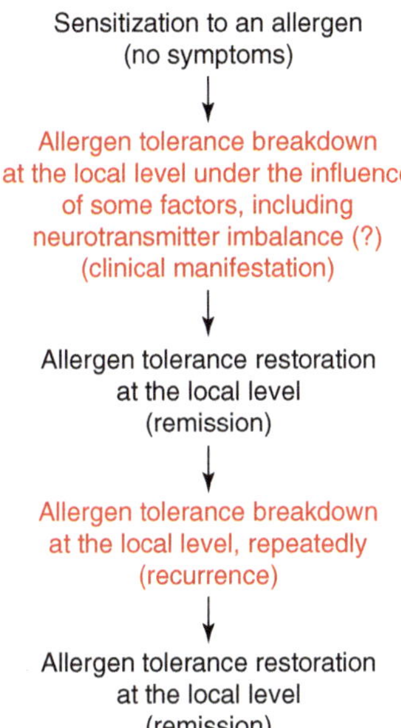

Fig. 6.1 Cycling local atopic disorders in the unified airway

(rhinoconjunctivitis) have been already studied and, long ago, included in the consensus position papers on diagnostics and therapy [11–13]. In the last decade, Rondón et al. [14] described a new atopic disorder, local allergic rhinitis (LAR), which has to date been studied in detail. However, local allergic asthma and local allergic conjunctivitis have recently been identified too [15, 16], and "local respiratory allergy" [17] became the whole spectrum of pathology. Unfortunately, it remains almost unknown to most allergist communities worldwide. Compared to the conventional atopic endotype, the local atopic endotype is mainly recognized by the absence of systemic allergen tolerance breakdown. The patients have the typical allergic symptoms from the unified airway but not from the other organs (e.g., the skin and gastrointestinal tract). They did not show positive allergic skin tests, high serum total IgE, and component-specific IgE assays [14].

Local atopic disorders in the unified airway proceed in a cyclic manner (see Fig. 6.1).

6.2 Local Allergic Asthma

► **Definition** Local asthma is a recently discovered endotype of allergic bronchial asthma, whose pathogenesis is yet imprecisely known.

Local allergic asthma [15, 18–20] is a novel area for pathogenic and clinical perception, the development of diagnostics and therapy, and fertile for research and debate.

Recently, Campo et al. [15] proposed the appearance of a new endotype/phenotype after complex functional and immunological investigation. At the initial stage, 245 patients aged 14–65 years with perennial rhinitis and asthma were invited to participate in the study. All the rhinitis persons also had clinical asthmatic episodes for at least 3 years. As a result of the exclusion protocol based on GINA criteria [12], only 65 patients with significantly confirmed sensitization to house dust mites remained in the study. The cohort included 28 persons with local allergic rhinitis (LAR), 18 with conventional allergic rhinitis (AR), and 19 with nonallergic rhinitis. They had no differences in the severity of asthma. The induced sputum was not proved to be the suitable material for the determination of special IgE. Conversely, the bronchial allergen provocation test was positive in some patients, particularly with LAR when systemic atopy was absent.

The peculiarity of both conventional and local endotypes of allergic rhinitis and asthma is very similar due to the unified airway's linked counterparts from the histological and immunological viewpoint. The mucosa of the upper and lower airways is almost identical, containing ciliated columnar epithelium and particular cells such as M cells, goblet cells, γδT cells, and pulmonary neuroendocrine cells (PNEC). PNECs or Kulchitsky cells recognize different aerosols, pollutants, allergens, and pathogens in inhaled air, detect hypoxia, secrete many bioactive molecules, and impact tissue regeneration. PNECs regulate many lung functions at the systemic and regional levels, including the production of neurotransmitters (GABA, serotonin, acetylcholine, etc.) and neuropeptides (CGRP) [21–23]. The overactivation of PNECs has been described in allergic asthma and other pulmonary diseases; it leads to the amplification of allergic inflammation and bronchial remodeling. Besides, small cell lung cancer originates from the PNECs [21]. Recent single-cell RNA sequencing analyses revealed that PNECs account for 0.01% of all lung cells [24].

In the submucosa, there are eosinophils, neutrophils, macrophages, ILC2, mast cells, etc. [11, 25]. The main difference in submucosal components is the absence of smooth muscles in the upper airways compared to the lower airways and the lack of extensive subepithelial capillary and arterial systems and cavernous venous sinusoids in the lower airways in comparison with the upper airways. The complex of cells and biomolecules (see Fig. 6.2) orchestrate the various events in the lung on which either the balance or imbalance, or allergen tolerance, or allergic inflammation depend.

The ciliated epithelium with in-built mucus-secreting goblet cells is the primary barrier against the entry of aeroallergens, including substances from house dust mites. The submucosal macrophages serve as a second barrier against allergens if they overcame the epithelium and passed through M cells and DCs. Submucosal DCs are represented by type 1 (myeloid, mDC) and type 2 (plasmacytoid, pDC) cells. They are allergen-presenting cells required for type 2 helper T (Th2) cell activation and adaptive B cell response with IgE end-production [25, 26].

On the one hand, these immature DCs involve endocytosis and processing allergens. During maturation, the DCs acquire characteristic long outgrowths called dendrites, which are used for allergen presentation. On the other hand, if respiratory infection at that time occurs in the lung, pathogen-associated molecular patterns (PAMP) are recognized by pattern recognition receptors (PRR), including Toll-like

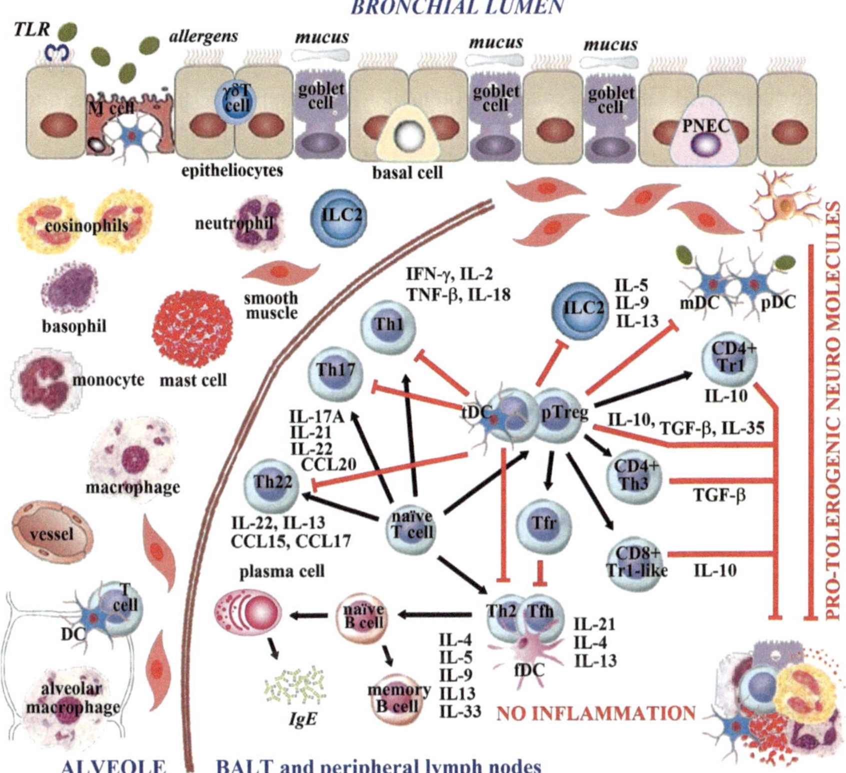

Fig. 6.2 Allergen tolerance maintenance in endotypes of allergic asthma. In physiological conditions, tolerance implies inhibiting all pathways of allergen-specific responses, including those controlled by type 2 helper T cells. Tolerogenic dendritic (tDCs) cells and allergen-specific CD4+CD25+FoxP3 Treg cells can stop activation and clonal expansion of sensitized Th2 cells and B cells and proliferation of IgE-producing plasma cells. The inhibition of follicular DC (fDC) cells leads to a decrease in a pool of allergen-specific memory T cells and B cells, and upregulation of T follicular regulatory (Tfr) cells results in suppression of follicular helper T (Tfh) cells. Pro-tolerogenic neuro molecules, specifically for the lung-relevant serotonin, calcitonin-gene-related peptide (CGRP), and nitric oxide, participate in the process. Hence, there are no IgE production and pathological effects associated with mast cells, eosinophils, neutrophils, vessels, smooth muscles, and hypersecretion. ILC2 group 2 innate lymphoid cell, mDC myeloid dendritic cell, pDC plasmacytoid DC, tDC tolerogenic DC, Tfh follicular helper T cell, Tfr T follicular regulatory cell, fDC follicular DC, pTreg peripheral Treg cell, Tr1 type 1 regulatory T cell, Th3 type 3 helper T cell, Tr1-like type 1 regulatory T cell-like, PNEC pulmonary neuroendocrine cell

receptors (TLR) and C-type lectins [27]. Upon activation of PRR, epithelial cells, ILC2 [28–30], and macrophages produce cytokines, chemokines, and other mediators that recruit a series of immune system cells to contribute to inflammation and downregulation of allergen tolerance.

The mechanisms of tolerance induction to allergens in the unified airway associated with systemic immunosuppressor networks in the periphery develop in bronchus-associated lymphoid tissue (BALT) and regional draining lymph nodes, i.e., in the local compartment of the neuroimmune system. Atopic allergic responses originate in the context of the failure of tolerance toward specific allergens and lead to the production of allergen-specific IgE under the control of Th2 cells [6]. Naïve regulatory T (nTreg) cells possess a low diversity of TCR and hence have weak allergen-specific potency. Allergen-specific pTreg cells have a wide variety of TCR and play a central role in the induction and maintenance of allergen tolerance [7]. They originate from naïve T cells by the influence of IL-27, IL-2, IL-10, TGF-β [31, 32], and promote some new subsets: type 1 regulatory T (Tr1) cells, type 3 helper T (Th3) cells, etc. (see Chap. 3). The progression of allergen-specific Treg cells can limit the manifestation of allergic disorders. It has been proven that tolerance to allergens is critically dependent on the generation of allergen-specific Treg cells, which upregulate a state of sustained unresponsiveness to constantly invading allergens in healthy individuals. Also, some DCs' subsets because of their extensive functional plasticity and, in a particular extracellular microenvironment, including cytokines and neurotransmitters, enable the differentiation into the tDCs, which matter very much in allergen tolerance maintenance [33].

The immunosuppressive hormones and neurotransmitters, such as glucocorticoids, GABA, and serotonin, appear to have a significant but not quite specialized meaning in allergen tolerance [23, 34]. It has been known for decades that glucocorticoids show their pro-tolerogenic and anti-inflammatory effects due to the inhibition of stimulatory biomolecules expression at the transcriptional level and inactivation of all types of adaptive immune responses.

Apart from regulating gastrointestinal peristalsis, vasoconstriction, blood clotting, and feeling pleasure, serotonin is also involved in the immune responses and allergen tolerance by controlling the release of various biomolecules [35]. Mainly, serotonin being a pro-tolerogenic neurotransmitter, inhibits CXCL10 (IP-10) production, differentiation of inflammatory DCs, Th1 and Th17 cells pathways, and promotes IL-10 synthesis [33].

Various causes can trigger allergen tolerance breakdown and reactivation of a Th2 cell-dependent B cell-mediated adaptive immune response with IgE end-production. Commonly, genetics and epigenetics belong to one essential group of this subject [36]. Environmental factors, including excessive exposure to allergens by inhalation, ingestion, injection or direct contact, infection, stress, depression, anxiety, endocrine imbalance, occupational factors, etc., constitute the other group [5, 26]. Besides, the individual non-tolerogenic lung's microbiota [37] and excess of allergen-associated molecular patterns (AAMP) in the bronchial secretion [38] can contribute to the local allergen tolerance breakdown.

In contrast to the skin and gastrointestinal tract, innervation of the unified airway is characterized by a distinctive peculiarity. The unified airway is provided with the somatosensory neurons and the vegetative nervous system (VNS), which function locally and mediate different local processes [39]. The VNS that innervates the unified airway is composed of parasympathetic neurons whose cell bodies reside in the petrosal ganglion and brainstem, and sympathetic neurons whose cell bodies reside in the paravertebral ganglia [39, 40].

The predominant neuro molecules originating from neurons, which innervate the lung, and nonneuronal sources are acetylcholine, serotonin, CGRP, nitric oxide, and substance P. There is no prevalence of either pro-tolerogenic or pro-immunogenic neurotransmitters and neuropeptides in the respiratory tract neuroimmune unit [40]. Hence, an inequality of neuro molecules may appear quickly. Hypothetically, when systemic allergen tolerance maintenance is still available, but regional imbalance happens to activate pro-immunogenic cells and neuro molecules in the unified airway, the VNS may become responsible for the autonomous allergen tolerance breakdown and atopic exacerbation only in this area. Probably, it is not such a frequent event compared to conventional respiratory allergies.

Conversely, the gastrointestinal tract has its own autonomic, self-contained nervous system called the enteric nervous system (ENS) that consists of interneurons and intrinsic neurons of the myenteric and submucosal plexuses, while extrinsic neurons of the VNS associated with the ENS participate in the innervation of the gut [39]. This system, rich in pro-tolerogenic neuro molecules, appears to maintain allergen tolerance in the gut.

6.3 Local Allergic Rhinitis

▶ **Definition** Local allergic rhinitis is an atopic inflammation in the nose, which is the particular endotype having specific pathogenesis of allergen tolerance breakdown at the regional level.

6.3.1 Previous Studies in Local Allergic Rhinitis and Their Discussion

For the last decade, both researchers in allergy and otorhinolaryngology have focused on the various aspects of LAR [41]. One group of researchers [42] just supposed that LAR did not fit into the classical systemic allergic (atopic) rhinitis (AR) vs. nonallergic rhinitis, and LAR was hence a new rhinitis's phenotype. However, another group of researchers [43–45] substantiated that LAR is an endotype of allergic rhinitis as it does not display all atopic biomarkers at the systemic level but exhibits them in the nasal mucosa.

Patients with LAR have the same classic symptoms as those with conventional allergic rhinitis, such as nasal obstruction, sneezing, itching, and rhinorrhea. A study comparing patients with allergic rhinitis and LAR also confirmed that both share a similar clinical phenotype. They are caused by sensitization to *Dermatophagoides* house dust mites, occur preferentially in nonsmokers, display a severe persistent clinical picture, often with conjunctival and asthma symptoms, and develop in children and adults [44].

A retrospective, follow-up study for longer than 7 years displayed the conversion of LAR into conventional systemic airway allergic reactions in almost half of the observed patients ($n = 42$) [46]. Another 10-year follow-up study of a cohort of 176 patients with LAR [47] demonstrated a low rate of development of systemic atopy, including allergic asthma.

In the experiment, the mice were intranasally sensitized with 400 or 25 μg ovalbumin for 5 or 14 days, respectively. As a result, researchers found that mice treated with 25 μg ovalbumin sensitized for 14 days could manifest the major features of human LAR such as allergic nasal symptoms and localized but not systemic specific IgE. LAR was likely to occur if the allergen was exposed repeatedly at a low dose [48].

Due to their high cost and complexity, nasal provocation tests with house dust mite allergens and detection of specific IgE in nasal secretions are not yet recommended in everyday clinical practice. Therefore, some patients with LAR, including elderly persons [49], are still being classified into the nonallergic rhinitis group in most clinics [50], which negatively affects the treatment efficacy.

From a theoretical viewpoint, allergic rhinitis and local allergic rhinitis pathogenesis share almost all features of the allergic inflammation in the nose but differ in terms of mechanisms and level of the allergen tolerance breakdown. At the systemic level, allergen tolerance maintenance seems to be associated with a network of pro-tolerogenic cells and biomolecules such as pTreg cells, tDC cells, IL-10, IL-35, and TGF-β [5, 25]. At the local (nasal) level, allergen tolerance appears to depend on peculiarities of nose's innervation and local set of neurotransmitters and neuropeptides.

Rhinitis linked with autonomic nervous system dysfunction has been described, but there is no information on the type of this rhinitis: conventional allergic, local allergic, or nonallergic [51].

6.3.2 Neurotransmitter Immunoregulation in Allergic Rhinitis

It has been shown that allergic rhinitis induced anxiety-like behavior in humans and altered social interaction in rodents, along with the increased expression of Th2 cells [52]. Higher levels of tryptophan, a precursor of serotonin, were preferentially found in nonresponders to AIT in allergic rhinitis [53].

The concentration of L-glutamate, a precursor of GABA, in the nasal mucosa in patients with allergic rhinitis was significantly higher, whereas GABA corresponded to the control level [54]. The well-studied GABAergic system exists not only in the brain but also in airway epithelial cells playing a pro-tolerogenic role. In experiments, GABA inhibits the overproduction of mucus and synthesis of IL-13 in mice with allergic reactions induced by ovalbumin [55].

In a pilot study [56], patients with allergic rhinitis were exposed to a standardized trier social stress test (TSST), followed by allergic skin tests. Stress responders were estimated based on the salivary cortisol concentrations, anxiety scale and serum norepinephrine, and oxytocin levels. The baseline concentrations, independent of TSST, norepinephrine, and oxytocin, were significantly higher in allergic persons. So, patients with allergic rhinitis are more stressed unresisting. Furthermore, mast cells and macrophages in the mucosa express oxytocin receptors under elevated oxytocin concentrations, which may interfere with local allergic responses, linking neuronal emotions and inflammation [57]. Unfortunately, similar clinical studies in selected groups of conventional allergic rhinitis and local allergic rhinitis in humans and experiments in rodents have not yet been carried out.

6.3.3 Preliminary Clinical Diagnostic Markers of Local Allergic Rhinitis

In the beginning, any suspected allergic rhinitis patients should be studied according to the rhinology/allergy position papers [11, 13]. This algorithm includes:

1. A patient's history
2. Clinical examination
3. Nasal endoscopy (video rhinoscopy),
4. Rhinomanometry and acoustic rhinometry
5. Sinonasal radiographic imaging (radiology)
6. Nasal cytology or histology
7. Allergic skin tests
8. Serum total IgE content

Routine ENT examination mainly includes nasal endoscopy and radiology. The endoscopy does not demonstrate an essential difference in patients with AR and LAR. However, video rhinoscopy is the main method to identify the allergic nature of rhinitis compared to nonallergic forms of rhinitis. Commonly, it reveals mucosal edema, mucosal cyanosis, nasal obstruction, and, in some patients, septal deviation, rhinosinusitis, and polyps. Radiology specifies the anatomical and inflammatory comorbidities like septal deviation, nasal crest, rhinosinusitis, sinus cyst, polyps, turbinate hypertrophy, central compartment atopy, etc. [58, 59].

Information about allergic skin tests was published in 1959. They are divided into skin prick testing (SPT) [60] and intradermal tests. According to several prospective studies and systematic reviews, SPT is a safe method of allergy testing [61]. Besides, SPT executes in any age group [11].

Intradermal testing is rarely used as a primary testing modality, and it is often a secondary method following SPT. Interestingly, the skin intradermal testing appears to be more sensitive when indoor allergens are being tested. It is unclear on what this higher sensitivity depends [11].

The performance and reliability of serum total IgE measuring are affected by several factors, including the choice of reagents and modernization of equipment.

Some authors demonstrated an insufficient diagnostic accuracy of this marker to define allergic conditions regardless of its value [62, 63].

According to the ongoing scientific discussion [64], new techniques of IgE detection like allergic skin tests cannot be replaced by such new methods of specific IgE detection like component resolved diagnosis [65]. It seems to be connected with the fact that IgE is the only cytophilic antibody among other immunoglobulin isotypes. The high-affinity FcεRI is expressed on basophils and mast cells and binds to IgE/allergen complex triggering atopic inflammation [66].

6.3.4 Corroborative Clinical Diagnostic Markers of Local Allergic Rhinitis

The confirmatory identification of LAR is based on the following algorithm [15, 67]:

1. Absence of systemic atopic disorders such as food, insect allergies, or atopic dermatitis if they are not independent comorbidities
2. Negative allergic skin tests
3. Absence of the elevated level of serum total IgE if it is not associated with an alternative sensitization
4. Evidence of IgE sensitization at the local level

Lack of systemic atopic diseases and enhanced serum total IgE, and negative allergic skin tests confirm allergen tolerance maintenance at the systemic level in those patients. However, local atopic disorders in the unified airway, including local allergic rhinitis, may be manifested in some of the patients. Hence, the evidence of IgE presence in the nose is an essential subject for the proper diagnosing and missing diagnostic errors.

There are three methods of nasal-specific IgE detection:

(a) Nasal allergen provocation test (NAPT), or allergen challenge test [11, 68–71] using the visual analog scale (VAS) (a, i) or rhinomanometry (a, ii)
(b) Nasal allergen-specific IgE determination [11, 72–74] in the secretion of the nose (b, i) or using nasal mucosal brush biopsy (MBB) (b, ii)
(c) Basophil activation test (BAT) [11, 41, 75, 76].

To learn more about methods and their different specificity and sensitivity see Table 6.1.

The allergen for the NAPT procedure may be administered by various devices, including syringes, nasal sprays, nose droppers, micropipettes, etc. The result of a NAPT can be evaluated 20 min after allergen application by several methods such as VAS, rhinomanometry, acoustic rhinometry, inflammatory markers in the nasal secretion, and nasal NO^- concentration. A NAPT procedure is conducted separately for the allergens *D. pteronyssinus* and *D. farinae* at a dose of 5000 standardized biological units (SBU)/mL each, administered at 0.2 mL via a calibrated tool into both nostrils at room temperature [70].

Table 6.1 Specificity and sensitivity of the detection IgE sensitization to house dust mite allergens in local allergic rhinitis

Tests	Specificity	Sensitivity
(a, i) Nasal provocation test (NAPT) by VAS assessment	77.4% [68]	90.6% [68]
(a, ii) Nasal provocation test (NAPT) by rhinomanometry assessment	100% [71]	83.7% [71]
(b, i) Nasal-specific IgE by detection in secretion of the nose	>90% [76]	22–40% [76]
(b, ii) Nasal-specific IgE using MBB	100% [77]	–
(c) Basophil activation test (BAT)	93% [78]	50% [78]
	>90% [76]	50% [76]

As a result of a NAPT, VAS allows for assessing the change of nasal symptom patterns such as rhinorrhea, itching, sneezing, and obstruction, and achieving a significant difference in LAR compared to nonallergic rhinitis [68]. Nowadays, the VAS incorporated applications have been developed for smartphones to assess disease control with a high efficacy [69, 79].

NAPT's rhinomanometric examination serves to analyze nasal airway resistance for the flow rates measured in the right and left nasal passage separately during normal breathing [70]. So, the NAPT has a high specificity and sensitivity (see Table 6.1) to be the "gold standard" for the diagnosis of LAR [41, 45]. However, the NAPT requires technical resources and skilled personnel, and can lead to eosinophil infiltrations in the nose.

Evidence of nasal-specific IgE in the nasal secretions for LAR's clinical diagnosis is important but hard to access [11]. Using the immunoCAP technique [72] the content of IgE is positive if its concentration >0.35 kU/L [72]. Nasal secretions are collected via absorptive filter paper applied to the inferior turbinates for 5 min [80], and allergen-specific IgE to house dust mites is then assayed via the immunoCAP technique. Different methods have been described concerning identifying the best nasal sIgE, including nasal lavage, mucosal biopsy, and MBB [11, 73, 77]. However, in clinical practice, noninvasive methods might be preferable [41]. Thus, nasal allergen-specific IgE has a high specificity and medium-grade sensitivity for the diagnosis of LAR.

The BAT is a flow cytometry-based assay performed on the patient's peripheral blood, where the expression of some activation markers like CD63 is measured following stimulation with house dust mite or other allergens [41]. BAT may be a proper additional method when the diagnosis of LAR is in doubt, the allergen responsible for clinical symptoms is unknown, and it requires assessing the response to allergen-specific immunotherapy (AIT) [11, 75]. As seen in Table 6.1, BAT has a high specificity and medium-grade sensitivity.

From a clinical viewpoint, eosinophil cationic protein, tryptase, cytokines, and chemokines are additional, specifying markers for both LAR and AR [43, 81].

According to the peculiarity of allergen tolerance breakdown, a psychosomatic marker is probably more inherent in LAR than AR. For this reason, the questionnaire by Spitzer et al. [82] can be a valuable tool for the differential diagnosis between these endotypes of allergic rhinitis.

Thus, LAR and AR share similar clinical and endoscopic symptoms. However, the diagnosis of LAR is based on the demonstration of a positive response to NAPT or the detection of nasal-specific IgE or a positive BAT in the absence of systemic

IgE sensitization [11, 83]. The NAPT is the "gold standard" for LAR identification, as it displays the optimal specificity and sensitivity [45]. Unfortunately, LAR often remains underdiagnosed and refers to nonallergic rhinitis. Currently, there are only licensed pharmacological treatments available for LAR [70]. However, some investigations show encouraging results with using AIT in LAR [84].

6.4 "Dual" Allergic Rhinitis

There is the endotype of allergic rhinitis in which SPT with different allergens may coexist in the same patient [85]. For example, a patient suffers from perennial and seasonal rhinitis, but his/her SPT displays sensitivity only to seasonal allergens, whereas his/her NAPT is positive to perennial and seasonal allergens [41]. "Dual" allergic rhinitis has not been described yet among elderly populations [17]. Similar to AR and LAR, patients with "dual" allergic rhinitis show IgE sensitizations and nasal eosinophilic infiltrate if NAPT executes.

6.5 Local Allergic Conjunctivitis

▶ **Definition** Local allergic conjunctivitis is a particular, recently described endotype of atopic inflammation in the eyes.

The conjunctiva via the *canalis nasolacrimalis* connects with the unified airway. Respectively, Campo et al. [15] postulate that one local atopic disorder (e.g., LAR) rapidly evolves toward clinical worsening and association with others (e.g., asthma and conjunctivitis).

Yamana et al. [16] studied 83 patients with allergic conjunctivitis, who were positive for total IgA in tear fluids. Diagnosis of allergic conjunctivitis was based on Japanese guidelines for allergic conjunctival diseases [86]. Among these people, 69 (83.1%) persons were positive for some allergens, including *Dermatophagoides pteronissinus*, and 14 (about 16.9%) persons had no detectable serum-specific IgE. Researchers suggested the existence of local allergic conjunctivitis as a new endotype/phenotype of allergic conjunctivitis.

Key Points

1. Local atopic diseases occurring only in the unified airway have been recently identified but remain a still not decrypted group of allergies. The novel respiratory pathology includes local asthma, local allergic rhinitis, "dual" allergic rhinitis, and local allergic conjunctivitis.
2. It is clear that these endotypes stay the underdiagnosed pathology and, by error, are classified as nonallergic diseases. Therefore, this research is highly required as it is cutting edge.
3. The prevalent neuro molecules originating from neurons and nonneuronal sources, which innervate the lung, are acetylcholine, serotonin, CGRP, nitric

oxide, and substance P. Hypothetically, the local unit of the neuroimmune system upon an imbalance of neuro molecules may matter much for the pathogenesis of local respiratory allergy.

Take-Home Messages

1. Write a flyer about local atopic disorders in the unified airway.
2. Write a paragraph about the diagnosis of local allergic rhinitis.
3. Write an essay about local asthma.
4. Write an essay about local allergic rhinitis.
5. Write a paragraph about local seasonal rhinitis.
6. Write a flyer about "dual" allergic rhinitis.
7. List allergens that cause local atopic disorders in the unified airway.
8. Draw the waves of pollination seasons in local seasonal allergies.
9. Write a paragraph about the differential diagnosis of conventional and local allergic rhinitis.
10. Make a slide presentation about the diagnosis of local atopic disorders in the unified airway.

Quiz

Reading a question, please choose only one right answer.

Question 1

Pro-tolerogenic neuro molecules are relevant for the lung:

1. GABA and glycine.
2. Serotonin, CGLP, and nitric oxide.
3. Norepinephrine and oxytocin.
4. CGRP and VIP.

Question 2

Pro-immunogenic neuro molecules are relevant for the lung:

1. Neuromedin U and dopamine.
2. L-glutamate and histamine.
3. Acetylcholine and substance P.
4. Substance P and L-glutamate.

Question 3

This disease is not related to the atopic entities:

1. Local allergic rhinitis.
2. Atopic dermatitis.
3. Local allergic asthma.
4. "Dual" allergic rhinitis.

Question 4
The local atopic pathology develops in a target organ:

1. The unified airway.
2. The skin.
3. The gastrointestinal tract.
4. The genitourinary tract.

Question 5
This biomarker is relevant for local atopic entities:

1. Eosinophilia.
2. Decreased serum total IgE.
3. Elevated serum total IgE.
4. Positive SPT.

Question 6
This biomarker is relevant for local allergic rhinitis:

1. Negative SPT.
2. Video rhinoscopy: mucosal edema, cyanosis.
3. Eosinophilia.
4. Lymphocytosis.

Question 7
This biomarker is relevant for local allergic rhinitis:

1. Eosinophilia.
2. Positive SPT.
3. Elevated serum total IgE.
4. Positive nasal allergen provocation test.

Question 8
The following test has the highest sensitivity in local allergic rhinitis:

1. Nasal allergen provocation test.
2. Nasal-specific IgE.
3. Basophil activation test.
4. Serum-specific IgE.

Question 9
This disease is related to the local atopic entities:

1. Conventional asthma.
2. Localized infection.

3. Local allergic asthma.
4. Atopic dermatitis.

Question 10
Allergy scarification tests include:

1. Allergic application test.
2. Skin prick testing (SPT).
3. Nasal allergen provocation test.
4. Basophil activation test.

Question 11
Systemic atopic disorders are:

1. Food allergies.
2. Local allergic rhinitis.
3. Local allergic asthma.
4. Local allergic conjunctivitis.

Question 12
"Dual" allergic rhinitis has not yet been described among:

1. Young patients.
2. Females.
3. Elderly patients.
4. Patients with local perennial rhinitis.

Question 13
Patients with conventional seasonal rhinitis can also suffer from local perennial rhinitis:

1. No.
2. Yes.
3. Never.
4. No way.

Question 14
Pathogenesis of local atopic entities is thoroughly studied:

1. No.
2. Yes.
3. Unknown data.
4. Researches are classified.

Question 15
Local allergic rhinitis is mainly caused by:

1. Food allergens.
2. HDMs' allergens.
3. Pets' allergens.
4. Unknown.

Question 16
Conventional allergic rhinitis is mainly caused by:

1. Pets' allergens.
2. HDMs' allergens.
3. Food allergens.
4. Insect allergens.

References

1. Chen Q, Zhong X, Acosta L, et al. Allergic sensitization patterns identified through latent class analysis among NYC asthmatic and non-asthmatic children. Ann Allergy Asthma Immunol. 2016;116(3):212–8. https://doi.org/10.1016/j.anai.2016.01.006.
2. Hose AJ, Depner M, Illi S, Ege MJ. Latent class analysis reveals clinically relevant atopy phenotypes in 2 birth cohorts. J Allergy Clin Immunol. 2017;139(6):1935–45. https://doi.org/10.1016/j.jaci.2016.08.046.
3. Passali D, Cingi C, Staffa P, et al. The international study of the allergic rhinitis survey: outcomes from 4 geographical regions. Asia Pac Allergy. 2018;8(1):e7. https://doi.org/10.5415/apallergy.2018.8.e7.
4. Simon D. Recent advances in clinical allergy and immunology 2019. Int Arch Allergy Immunol. 2019;180(4):291–305. https://doi.org/10.1159/000504364.
5. Wisniewski J, Agrawal R, Woodfolk JA. Mechanisms of tolerance induction in allergic disease: integrating current and emerging concepts. Clin Exp Allergy. 2013;43(2):164–76. https://doi.org/10.1111/cea.12016.
6. Abdel-Gadir A, Massoud AH, Chatila TA. Antigen-specific Treg cells in immunological tolerance: implications for allergic diseases. F1000Res. 2018;7:1–13. https://doi.org/10.12688/f1000research.12650.
7. Calzada D, Baos S, Cremades-Jimeno L, Cárdaba B. Immunological mechanisms in allergic diseases and allergen tolerance: the role of Treg cells. J Immunol Res. 2018;2018:6012053. https://doi.org/10.1155/2018/6012053.
8. Calderón MA, Linneberg A, Kleine-Tebbe J, De Bay F, de Rojas DHF, Virchow JC. Respiratory allergy caused by house dust mites: what do we really know? J Allergy Clin Immunol. 2015;136(1):38–47. https://doi.org/10.1016/j.jaci.2014.10.012.
9. Thomas WR. Hierarchy and molecular properties of house dust mite allergens. Allergol Int. 2015;64:304–11. https://doi.org/10.1016/j.alit.2015.05.004.
10. Huang F-L, Liao E-C, Yu SJ. House dust mite allergy: its innate immune response and immunotherapy. Immunobiology. 2018;223(3):300–2. https://doi.org/10.1016/j.imbio.2017.10.035.
11. Wise SK, Lin SY, Toskala E, Orlandi RR, Akdis CA, Alt JA, et al. International consensus statement on allergy and rhinology: allergic rhinitis. Int Forum Allergy Rhinol. 2018;8(2):108–352. https://doi.org/10.1002/alr.22073.

12. Global Initiative for Asthma. Global strategy for asthma management and prevention. 2021. www.ginasthma.org.
13. Bousquet J, Schunemann HJ, Togias A, Bachert C, Erhola M, Hellings PW, et al. Next-generation Allergic Rhinitis and its Impact on Asthma (ARIA) guidelines for allergic rhinitis based on Grading of Recommendations Assessment, Development and Evaluation (GRADE) and real-world evidence. J Allergy Clin Immunol. 2020;145(1):70–80.e3. https://doi.org/10.1016/j.jaci.2019.06.049.
14. Rondón C, Canto G, Blanca M. Local allergic rhinitis: a new entity, characterization and further studies. Curr Opin Allergy Clin Immunol. 2010;10(1):1–7. https://doi.org/10.1097/ACI.0b013e328334f5fb.
15. Campo P, Eguiluz-Gracia I, Salas M, Rodriguez MJ, Perez-Sanchez N, Gonzalez M, Molina A, Mayorga C, Torres MJ, Rondón C, et al. Bronchial asthma triggered by house dust mites in patients with local allergic rhinitis. Allergy. 2019;74(8):1502–10. https://doi.org/10.1111/all.13775.
16. Yamana Y, Fukuda K, Ko R, Uchio E. Local allergic conjunctivitis: a phenotype of allergic conjunctivitis. Int Ophthalmol. 2019;39:2539–44. https://doi.org/10.1007/s10792-019-01101-z.
17. Testera-Montes A, Salas M, Palomares F, Ariza A, Torres MJ, Rondón C, Eguiluz-Gracia I. Local respiratory allergy: from rhinitis phenotype to disease spectrum. Front Immunol. 2021;12:691964. https://doi.org/10.3389/fimmu.2021.691964.
18. Froidure A, Mouthuy J, Durham SR. Asthma phenotypes and IgE responses. Eur Respir J. 2015;12:1–16. https://doi.org/10.1183/13993003.01824-2014.
19. Kılıç E, Kutlu A, Hastalıkları G, Hastanesi KD, Servisi AI, et al. Does local allergy (entopy) exists in asthma? J Clin Anal Med. 2016. Letters to Editors from 01.02.2016; https://doi.org/10.4328/JCAM.3272.
20. Klimov AV, Isaev PY, Klimov VV, Sviridova VS. Endotypes of allergic rhinitis and asthma accompanying food allergy. Bull Sib Med. 2019;18(2):287–9. https://doi.org/10.20538/1682-0363-2019-2-287-289.
21. Noguchi M, Furukawa KT, Morimoto M. Pulmonary neuroendocrine cells: physiology, tissue homeostasis and disease. Dis Model Mech. 2020;13(12):dmm046920. https://doi.org/10.1242/dmm.046920.
22. Sui P, Wiesner DL, Xu J, Zhang Y, Lee J, van Dyken S, et al. Pulmonary neuroendocrine cells amplify allergic asthma responses. Science. 2018;360:6393. https://doi.org/10.1126/science.aan8546.
23. Kabata H, Artis D. Neuro-immune crosstalk and allergic inflammation. J Clin Invest. 2019;129(4):1475–82. https://doi.org/10.1172/JCI124609.
24. Travaglini KJ, Nabhan AN, Penland L, Sinha R, Gillich A, Sit RV, et al. A molecular cell atlas of the human lung from single cell RNA sequencing. Nature. 2020;587(7835):619–25. https://doi.org/10.1038/s41586-020-2922-4.
25. Klimov VV. Skin and mucosal immune system. In: From basic to clinical immunology. 1st ed. Cham: Springer Nature; 2019. p. 101–25. https://doi.org/10.1007/978-3-030-03323-1_2.
26. Tang MLK. The physiological induction of tolerance to allergens. Mechanisms of airway tolerance. In: Wahn U, Sampson HA, editors. Allergy, immunity and tolerance in early childhood. Paris: Academic Press; 2016. p. 153–70. https://doi.org/10.1016/B978-0-12-420226-9.00010-3.
27. Scheurer S, Toda M, Vieths S. What makes an allergen? Clin Exp Allergy. 2015;45(7):1150–61. https://doi.org/10.1111/cea.12571.
28. Zheng H, Zhang Y, Pan J, Liu N, Qin L, Liu M, Wang T. The role of type 2 innate lymphoid cells in allergic diseases. Front Immunol. 2021;12:586078. https://doi.org/10.3389/fimmu.2021.586078.
29. Pasha MA, Patel G, Hopp R, Yang Q. Role of innate lymphoid cells in allergic diseases. Allergy Asthma Proc. 2019;40(3):138–45. https://doi.org/10.2500/aap.2019.40.4217.
30. Gurram RK, Zhu J. Orchestration between ILC2s and Th2 cells in shaping type 2 immune responses. Cell Mol Immunol. 2019;16:225–35. https://doi.org/10.1038/s41423-019-0210-8.

31. Yoshida H, Hunter CA. The immunobiology of interleukin-27. Annu Rev Immunol. 2015;33:417–43. https://doi.org/10.1146/annurev-immunol-032414-112134.
32. Hall BM, Tran GT, Robinson CM, Hodgkinson SJ. Induction of antigen specific CD4+CD25+Foxp3+T regulatory cells from naïve natural thymic derived T regulatory cells. Int Immunopharmacol. 2015;28(2):975–86. https://doi.org/10.1016/j.intimp.2015.03.049.
33. Švajger U, Rožman P. Induction of tolerogenic dendritic cells by endogenous biomolecules: an update. Front Immunol. 2018;9:2482. https://doi.org/10.3389/fimmu.2018.02482.
34. Kerage D, Sloan EK, Mattarollo SR, McCombe PA. Interaction of neurotransmitters and neurochemicals with lymphocytes. J Neuroimmunol. 2019;332:99–111. https://doi.org/10.1016/j.jneuroim.2019.04.006.
35. Szabo A, Gogolak P, Koncz G, Foldvari Z, Pazmandi K, Miltner M, Poliska S, Bacsi A, Djurovic S, Rajnavolgyi E. Immunomodulatory capacity of the serotonin receptor 5-HT2B in a subset of human dendritic cells. Sci Rep. 2018;8:1765. https://doi.org/10.1038/s41598-018-20173-y.
36. Bellanti JA, Settipane RA. Genetics, epigenetics, and allergic disease: a gun loaded by genetics and a trigger pulled by epigenetics. Allergy Asthma Proc. 2019;40(2):73–5. https://doi.org/10.2500/aap.2019.40.4206.
37. Huffnagle GB. The microbiota and allergies/asthma. PLoS Pathog. 2010;6(5):e1000549. https://doi.org/10.1371/journal.ppat.1000549.
38. Pali-Schöll I, Jensen-Jarolim E. The concept of allergen-associated molecular patterns (AAMP). Curr Opin Immunol. 2016;42:113–8. https://doi.org/10.1016/j.coi.2016.08.004.
39. Voisin T, Bouvier A, Chiu IV. Neuro-immune interactions in allergic diseases: novel targets for therapeutics. Int Immunol. 2017;29(6):247–61. https://doi.org/10.1093/intimm/dxx040.
40. De Virgillis F, Di Giovanni S. Lung innervation in the eye of a cytokine storm: neuroimmune interactions and COVID-19. Nat Rev Neurol. 2020;16:645–52. https://doi.org/10.1038/s41582-020-0402-y.
41. Maoz-Segal R, Machnes-Maayan D, Veksler-Offengenden I, Frizinsky S, Hajyahia S, Agmon-Levin N. Local allergic rhinitis: an old story but a new entity. In: Gendeh BS, Turkalj M, editors. Rhinosinusitis. London: IntechOpen; 2019. p. 1–9. https://doi.org/10.5772/intechopen.86212.
42. Forester JP, Calabria CW. Local production of IgE in the respiratory mucosa and the concept of entopy: does allergy exist in nonallergic rhinitis? Ann Allergy Asthma Immunol. 2010;105(4):249–55. https://doi.org/10.1016/j.anai.2010.02.001.
43. Incorvaia C, Fuiano N, Martignago I, Gritti BL, Ridolo E. Local allergic rhinitis: evolution of concepts. Clin Transl Allergy. 2017;7(38):1–4. https://doi.org/10.1186/s13601-017-0174-7.
44. De Mello JF. Local allergic rhinitis. Braz J Otorhinolaryngol. 2016;82(6):621–2. https://doi.org/10.1016/j.bjorl.2016.09.001.
45. Eguiluz-Gracia I, Pérez-Sánchez N, Bogas G, Campo P, Rondón C. How to diagnose and treat local allergic rhinitis: a challenge for clinicians. J Clin Med. 2019;8(7):1062–74. https://doi.org/10.3390/jcm8071062.
46. Sennekamp J, Joest I, Filipiak-Pittroff B, et al. Local allergic nasal reactions convert to classic systemic allergic reactions: a long-term follow-up. Int Arch Allergy Immunol. 2015;166:154–60. https://doi.org/10.1159/000380852.
47. Rondón C, Campo P, Togias A, Powe DG, Mullol J, Blanca M. Local allergic rhinitis: concept, pathophysiology, and management. J Allergy Clin Immunol. 2012;129:1460–7. https://doi.org/10.1111/all.12002.
48. Liang M-J, Xu R. Local allergic rhinitis and its relation to allergic rhinitis. Otolaryngology (Sunnyvale). 2016;6(4):249–50. https://doi.org/10.4172/2161-119X.1000249.
49. Bozek A, Ignasiak B, Kasperska-Zajac A, Scierski W, Crzanka A, Karzab J. Local allergic rhinitis in elderly patients. Ann Allergy Asthma Immunol. 2015;114(3):199–202. https://doi.org/10.1016/j.anai.2014.12.013.
50. Hellings PW, Klimek L, Cingi C, Agache I, Akdis C, Bachet C, et al. Non-allergic rhinitis: position paper of the European Academy of Allergy and Clinical Immunology. Allergy. 2017;72:1657–65. https://doi.org/10.1111/all.13200.
51. Yao A, Wilson JA, Ball SL. Autonomic nervous system dysfunction and sinonasal symptoms. Allergy Rhinol (Providence). 2018;9:1–9. https://doi.org/10.1177/2152656718764233.

52. Tonelli LH, Katz M, Kovacsics CE, Gould TD, Joppy B, Hoshino A, Hoffman G, Komarow H, Postolache TT. Allergic rhinitis induces anxiety-like behavior and altered social interaction in rodents. Brain Behav Immun. 2009;23(6):784–93. https://doi.org/10.1016/j.bbi.2009.02.017.
53. Gostner JM, Becker K, Kofler H, Strasser B, Fuchs D. Tryptophan metabolism in allergic disorders. Int Arch Allergy Immunol. 2016;169:203–15. https://doi.org/10.1159/000445500.
54. Lee H-S, Goh E-K, Wang S-G, Chon K-M, Kim H-K, Roh H-J. Detection of amino acids in human nasal mucosa using microdialysis technique: increased glutamate in allergic rhinitis. Asian Pac J Allergy Immunol. 2006;23(4):213–9. https://www.researchgate.net/publication/7206172.
55. Xiang Y-Y, Wang S, Liu M, Hirota JA, Li J, Ju W, et al. A GABAergic system in airway epithelium is essential for mucus overproduction in asthma. Nat Med. 2007;3(7):862–7. https://doi.org/10.1038/nm1604.
56. Gotovina J, Pranger CL, Jensen AN, Wagner S, Kothgassner OD, Mothes-Luksch N, et al. Elevated oxytocin and noradrenaline indicate higher stress levels in allergic rhinitis patients: implications for the skin prick diagnosis in a pilot study. PLoS One. 2018;13(5):e0196879. https://doi.org/10.1371/journal.pone.0196879.
57. Szeto A, Nation DA, Mendez AJ, Dominguez-Bendala J, Brooks LG, Schneiderman N, Philip M, McCabe PM. Oxytocin attenuates NADPH-dependent superoxide activity and IL-6 secretion in macrophages and vascular cells. Am J Physiol Endocrinol Metab. 2008;295(6):E1495–501. https://doi.org/10.1152/ajpendo.90718.2008.
58. DelGaudio JM, Loftus PA, Hamizan AW, Harvey RJ, Wise SK. Central compartment atopic disease. Am J Rhinol Allergy. 2017;31:228–34. https://doi.org/10.2500/ajra.2017.31.4443.
59. Marcus S, Schertzer J, Roland LT, Wise SK, Levy JM, DelGaudio JM. Central compartment atopic disease: prevalence of allergy and asthma compared with other subtypes of chronic rhinosinusitis with nasal polyps. Int Forum Allergy Rhinol. 2020;10(2):183–9. https://doi.org/10.1002/alr.22454.
60. Heinzerling L, Mari A, Bergmann KC, Bresciani M, Burbach G, Darsow U, et al. The skin prick test - European standards. Clin Transl Allergy. 2013;3(3):1–10. https://doi.org/10.1186/2045-7022-3-3.
61. Bernstein IL, Li JT, Bernstein DI, Hamiltin R, Spector SL, Tan R, Sicherer S, et al. Allergy diagnostic testing: an updated practice parameter. Ann Allergy Asthma Immunol. 2008;100(3):S1–148. https://doi.org/10.1016/s1081-1206(10)60305-5.
62. Satwani H, Rehman A, Ashraf S, Hassan A. Is serum total IgE levels a good predictor of allergies in children? J Pak Med Assoc. 2009;59(10):698–702.
63. Tu YL, Chang SW, Tsai HJ, Chen L-C, Lee W-I, Hua M-C, et al. Total serum IgE in a population-based study of Asian children in Taiwan: reference value and significance in the diagnosis of allergy. PLoS One. 2013;8:e80996. https://doi.org/10.1371/journal.pone.0080996.
64. Larenas-Linnemann D, Luna-Pech JA, Mösges R. Debates in allergy medicine: allergy skin testing cannot be replaced by molecular diagnosis in the near future. World Allergy Organ J. 2017;10(32):1–7. https://doi.org/10.1186/s40413-017-0164-1.
65. Sastre J, Sastre-Ibanez M. Molecular diagnosis and immunotherapy. Curr Opin Allergy Clin Immunol. 2016;16:565–70. https://doi.org/10.1097/ACI.0000000000000318.
66. Sutton BJ, Davies AM. Structure and dynamics of IgE-receptor interactions: FcεRI and CD23/FcεRII. Immunol Rev. 2015;268(1):222–35. https://doi.org/10.1111/imr.12340.
67. Krzych-Fałta E, Namysłowski A, Samoliński B. Dilemmas associated with local allergic rhinitis. Adv Dermatol Allergol. 2018;35(3):243–5. https://doi.org/10.5114/ada.2018.76215.
68. Jung C-G, Lee J-H, Ban G-Y, Park H-S, Shin YS. Prevalence and clinical characteristics of local allergic rhinitis to house dust mites. Yonsei Med J. 2017;58(5):1047–450. https://doi.org/10.3349/ymj.2017.58.5.1047.
69. Klimek L, Bergmann K-C, Biedermann T, Bousqut J, Hellings P, Jung K, et al. Visual analogue scales (VAS): measuring instruments for the documentation of symptoms and therapy monitoring in cases of allergic rhinitis in everyday health care. Allergo J Int. 2017;26(1):16–24. https://doi.org/10.1007/s40629-016-0006-7.

70. Wojas O, Samoliński B, Krzych-Fałta E. Local allergic rhinitis: nasal allergen provocation testing as a good tool in the differential diagnosis. Int J Occup Med Environ Health. 2020;33(2):241–6. https://doi.org/10.13075/ijomeh.1896.01503.
71. De Blay F, Doyen V, Lutz C, Godet J, Barnig C, Qi S, Braun J-J. A new, faster, and safe nasal provocation test method for diagnosing mite allergic rhinitis. Ann Allergy Asthma Immunol. 2015;115:385–90.e1. https://doi.org/10.1016/j.anai.2015.07.014.
72. Meng Y, Lou H, Wang Y, Wang C, Zhang L. The use of specific immunoglobulin E in nasal secretions for the diagnosis of allergic rhinitis. Laryngoscope. 2018;128:E311–5. https://doi.org/10.1002/lary.27120.
73. Hamizan A, Alvarado R, Rimmer J, Sewell WA, Barham HP, Kalish L, Harvey R. Nasal mucosal brushing as a diagnostic method for allergic rhinitis. Allergy Asthma Proc. 2019;40(3):167–72. https://doi.org/10.2500/aap.2019.40.4209.
74. De Schryver E, Devuyst L, Derycke L, Dullaers M, Van Zele T, Bachert C, Gevaert P. Local immunoglobulin E in the nasal mucosa: clinical implications. Allergy Asthma Immunol Res. 2015;7(4):321–31. https://doi.org/10.4168/aair.2015.7.4.321.
75. Hemmings O, Kwok M, McKendry R, Santos AF. Basophil activation test: old and new applications in allergy. Curr Allergy Asthma Rep. 2019;19(12):58. https://doi.org/10.1007/s11882-019-0889-8.
76. Campo P, Eguiluz-Gracia I, Bogas G, Salas M, Plaza Serón C, Perez N, Mayorga C, Torres MJ, Shamji MH, Rondón C. Local allergic rhinitis: implications for management. Clin Exp Allergy. 2019;49(1):6–16. https://doi.org/10.1111/cea.13192.
77. Reisacher WR. Detecting local immunoglobulin E from mucosal brush biopsy of the inferior turbinates using microarray analysis. Int Forum Allergy Rhinol. 2013;3:399–403. https://doi.org/10.1002/alr.21111.
78. Gomez E, Campo P, Rondón C, Barrionuevo E, Blanca-Lopez N, Torres MJ, et al. Role of the basophil activation test in the diagnosis of local allergic rhinitis. J Allergy Clin Immunol. 2013;132(4):975–6. https://doi.org/10.1016/j.jaci.2013.07.016.
79. Courbis A-L, Murray RB, Arnavielhe S, Caimmi D, Bedbrook A, Van Eerd M, et al. Electronic clinical decision support system for allergic rhinitis management: MASK e-CDSS. Clin Exp Allergy. 2018;48(12):1640–53. https://doi.org/10.1111/cea.13230.
80. Hamed A, Palacios T, Khokhar D, Aj S, Steinke JW, Platts-Mills AE, Lawrence MG, Borish L. Local IgE production in allergic (AR) and non-allergic rhinitis (NAR). J Allergy Clin Immunol. 2017;139(2, suppl):AB155. https://doi.org/10.1016/j.jaci.2016.12.510.
81. Hoyte FCL, Nelson HS. Recent advances in allergic rhinitis. F1000Res. 2018;7:1333. https://doi.org/10.12688/f1000research.15367.1.
82. Spitzer RL, Kroenke K, Williams JBW, Lowe B. A brief measure for assessing generalized anxiety disorder. The GAD-7. Arch Intern Med. 2006;166:1092–7. https://doi.org/10.1001/archinte.166.10.1092.
83. Bousquet J, Anto JM, Bachert C, Baiardini I, Bosnic-Anticevich S, Canonica GW, et al. Allergic rhinitis. Nat Rev Dis Primers. 2020;6:95. https://doi.org/10.1038/s41572-020-00227-0.
84. Rondón C, Campo P, Salas M, Aranda A, Molina A, González M, et al. Efficacy and safety of *D. pteronyssinus* immunotherapy in local allergic rhinitis: a double-blind placebo-controlled clinical trial. Allergy. 2016;71:1057–61. https://doi.org/10.1111/all.12889.
85. Eguiluz-Gracia I, Fernandez-Santamaria R, Almudena Testera-Montes A, Ariza A, Campo P, et al. Coexistence of nasal reactivity to allergens with and without IgE sensitization in patients with allergic rhinitis. Allergy. 2020;1:1689–98. https://doi.org/10.1111/all.14206.
86. Takamura E, Uchio E, Ebihara N, Ohno S, Ohashi Y, Okamoto S, et al. Japanese guideline for allergic conjunctival diseases. Allergol Int. 2017;66(2):220–9. https://doi.org/10.1016/j.alit.2016.12.004.

Food Allergies and Oral Tolerance

7

Contents

Didactics

Knowledge. Upon successful completion of this chapter, students should be able to:

1. List the groups of conventional atopic diseases.
2. Be familiar with the definitions of oral tolerance, food allergies, and food intolerance.
3. List "The Big Eight" food allergens.
4. Describe the autonomous enteric nervous system (ENS).
5. Draw clinical symptoms of food allergies.
6. List the prevalent forms of food allergies in children and adults in Canada.
7. Explain, why anaphylaxis happens to some, but not to all atopic individuals.
8. List clinical forms of allergic disorders in the gut.

Supplementary Information The online version contains supplementary material available at [https://doi.org/10.1007/978-3-031-04309-3_7].

V. V. Klimov, *Textbook of Allergen Tolerance*,
https://doi.org/10.1007/978-3-031-04309-3_7

Acquired Skills. Upon successful completion of this chapter, students should demonstrate the following skills:

1. Interpret the knowledge related to the autonomous enteric nervous system (ENS).
2. Critically evaluate the clinical literature about food allergies.
3. Discuss the scientific articles from the current research literature to criticize clinical data concerning food anaphylaxis.
4. Obtain a patient's history, including the history of present illness, past medical history, social, family, and occupational history, and review of systems of patients with food allergy.
5. Perform a patient's physical examination thoroughly.
6. Describe the management of food allergies.
7. Have a clear perception of the presented allergology definitions expressed orally and in written form.
8. Formulate the presented immunology and allergy terms.
9. Correctly answer the quiz questions.

Attitude and Professional Behaviors. Students should be able to:

1. Have the readiness to be hard-working.
2. Behave professionally at all times.
3. Recognize the importance of studying and demonstrate a commitment.
4. Demonstrate the consideration of the patient's feelings, ethnic, religious, cultural, and social background, and display empathy.

7.1 Introduction

► **Definition** Food allergies represent an allergic syndrome based on different pathogenic mechanisms, with or without the immune system's involvement. Food intolerance is a pathologic response of the gastrointestinal tract to food due to enzymatic insufficiency.

Food eating is a daily physiologic process, and nutrients encounter distinct factors such as digestive enzymes, microbiota, individual gastrointestinal tract's peculiarities, immune cells and molecules, neurotransmitters, genes, and epigenetic impact. This co-influence is multiple, ambiguous, may be beneficial or harmful, and is characterized by different terms related to food adverse reactions [1].

Food allergy and *food intolerance* are two distinct conditions but are commonly confused because they occasionally share similar symptoms. A food allergy is caused by the immune system reacting to harmless food, while inadequate digestive enzymes cause food intolerance to breaking down food. Food intolerance does not involve the immune system and does not result in severe allergic reactions known as anaphylaxis. Moreover, food intolerance shows negative allergic skin testing.

Milk remains one of the most common food problems, which leads to the immune system's response to one or more of its proteins (food allergy) [2]. Besides, milk may fail the digestive system, which cannot produce enough lactase enzyme to cleave the milk's lactose sugar (food intolerance). Ultimately, food allergies occur in 3–4% of adult persons, whereas food intolerance affects more than half the world's population.

Food allergies may develop in different phenotypes such as Th2-high (IgE-dependent), Th2-low, IgE-independent, and immune system-independent phenotypes. Atopic sensitization due to IgE overproduction is prevalent [3]. According to a survey [4], >26 million US adults suffer from food allergies in various clinical forms. Sometimes, food allergies may be extremely tough, and their diagnostics be complex [5]. Nowadays, knowledge of the pathways underpinning the development of atopic food allergy has increased but current evidence does not fully explain why life-threatening anaphylaxis occurs in only some individuals among those allergic to food allergens. Genetics and epigenetics are likely involved in some of these differences.

7.2 Autonomous Enteric Neuroimmune System

▶ **Definition** The enteric nervous system (ENS) is an autonomous compartment of the body's nervous system present in the gut and different from the vegetative nervous system.

The gastrointestinal tract is innervated by three types of peripheral nervous system counterparts under the supreme control of the central nervous system [6]. They are structured in the (1) somatosensory nervous system, (2) vegetative nervous system (VNS), and (3) autonomous enteric nervous system (ENS). Among the target organs, the gastrointestinal tract possesses its own unique self-contained nervous system, called the enteric nervous system, metaphorically speaking, "the second brain" (see Fig. 7.1) [7]. The ENS can be found from the beginning of the esophagus to the anus embedded in the gut lining, being in direct contact with the central nervous system through innervation by the VNS [6, 8]. The ENS consists of several hundred million neurons with cell bodies located in the intestinal wall, structured in two plexuses, submucosal (disposed between the circular muscle layer and epithelium) and myenteric (located between the longitudinal and circular muscle layers) containing intrinsic neurons and interneurons. Submucosal neurons regulate gut secretions, nutrient absorption, and local blood flow, whereas myenteric neurons coordinate smooth muscle contractions [9, 10]. The cell bodies of extrinsic vegetative neurons functionally associated with the ENS are outside the gastrointestinal tract in the paravertebral ganglia (sympathetic) and the nodose/jugular ganglia and brainstem (parasympathetic) [6]. The cell bodies of extrinsic sensory neurons reside in the dorsal root ganglia, and sensory fibers are mainly carried by the vagus nerve.

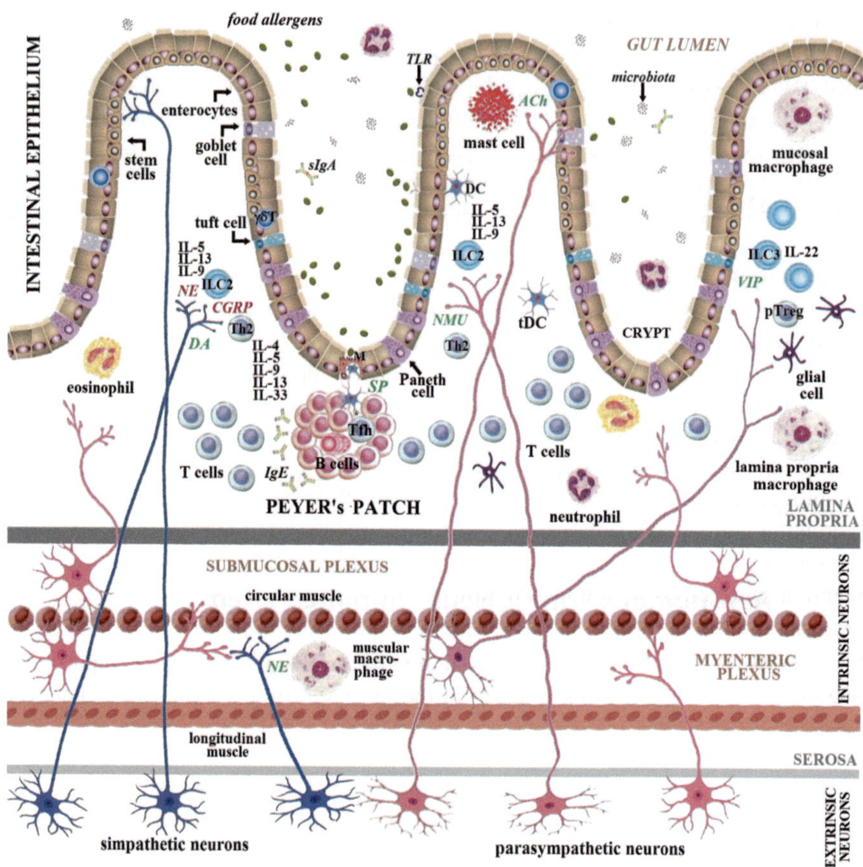

Fig. 7.1 Enteric nervous system. The cell bodies of the ENS intrinsic neurons are located in submucosal and myenteric plexuses but via neuro molecules contribute to the functioning of the gut epithelium, lamina propria, and plexuses immune cells. Neuropeptide neuromedin U activates ILC2 cells, which produce IL-5, IL-9, and IL-13. In contrast, adrenergic neurotransmitter norepinephrine and neuropeptide CGRP inhibit ILC2 cells. Dopamine upregulates Th2/Tfh-dependent IgE-response. Enteric glial cell-derived neurotrophic factors and cholinergic neuron-originated neuropeptide VIP stimulate ILC3 cells to secrete IL-22, a cytokine promoting gut barrier integrity. Cholinergic neurotransmitter acetylcholine amplifies the degranulation of mast cells and promotes goblet cells to secrete mucus. Besides, neuropeptide substance P stimulates the migration of allergen-presenting DCs required for initiation of Th2-dependent responses. In the myenteric plexus, norepinephrine induces anti-inflammatory, tissue-protective M2-phenotype of muscular macrophages. Th2 type 2 helper T cell, Tfh follicular helper T cell, ILC2 group 2 innate lymphoid cell, ILC3 group 3 innate lymphoid cell, DC dendritic cell, M cell "microfold" cell, NMU neuromedin U, NE norepinephrine, DA dopamine, VIP vasoactive intestinal peptide, CGRP calcitonin-gene-related peptide, Ach acetylcholine, SP substance P

The ENS operates with motor (excitatory, inhibitory, and secretomotor), sensory neurons (90% of all extrinsic), and interneurons. Other essential players in the ENS are enteric glial cells and glial cells/neurons/microbiota-derived neurotransmitters and neuropeptides [9]. The intrinsic neurons respond to nutrient changes in the gut lumen, gut microbes, and mechanical distortion and then send reflex signals through enteric interneurons [8]. Extrinsic neurons of the VNS are either cholinergic functioning through α7ACh-receptors or adrenergic using β_2-adrenoreceptors.

The ENS is rich in pro-tolerogenic neuro molecules controlling gut tolerance. The potent pro-tolerogenic neurotransmitter serotonin is synthesized both in the brain and enterochromaffin cells and in enteric neurons. Adenosine triphosphate (ATP), a pro-tolerogenic atypical neurotransmitter, acts through the purinergic receptors, P1, P2X, and P2Y, found in the myenteric plexus. The essential pro-tolerogenic neurotransmitter GABA, synthesized in the brain and various cells, contributes via $GABA_A$ receptor to regulating the ENS and inhibiting T cell-mediated responses in the gut. In contrast to the brain, GABA is engaged in neuronal excitability within the ENS [8]. Pro-tolerogenic neuropeptides, calcitonin-gene-related peptide (CGRP) and vasoactive intestinal peptide (VIP), are found in intrinsic primary afferent neurons of myenteric and submucosal plexuses. They participate in upregulating the gut's symbiotic microbiota against enteric bacterial pathogens [11]. These neuro molecules synthesized in both enteric neurons and gut microbiota allow the ENS to interact with the central nervous system [7].

The predominant neuro molecules originating from ENS and operating in the gut are serotonin, GABA, CGRP, norepinephrine, and dopamine [8, 12, 13].

The researchers used single-cell RNA sequencing (RAISIN RNA-seq and MIRACL-seq) to profile lots of transcriptomes from the ENS of mice and human samples and came to the following results:

- Neuron subsets are characterized by heterogeneity depending on the source.
- There is a circadian control of ENS function, nutrient absorption, and metabolism.
- ENS is enriched for the expression of several cytokines and cytokine receptors, which signal to cells of the immune system to shape mucosal immunity.
- Dysfunction in the ENS may exacerbate central nervous system diseases, including neurodegeneration [14].

Parasympathetic and sympathetic nerves also send efferent information from the central nervous system to the gut by signaling to the ENS to mediate nutrient sensation, mucus production, and gut motility. Recently, many two-way interactions between neurons and immune cells have been discovered due to the proximity between nerve fibers and immune cells in mucosal and barrier tissues. Releasing neuropeptides and neurotransmitters act, on the one hand, as immunosuppressors, and on the other hand, as pro-inflammatory factors producing vasodilatation, plasma extravasation, edema. It has been shown that allergic inflammation is linked with abdominal pain [15]. This observation reflects the concept that neuronal signaling can produce a "neurogenic inflammation" when neurons damage the tissue they innervate [16]. Mast cells, essential for allergic responses, are in close contact with nerves in the gut. DCs are also found closely opposed to the peripheral nerve terminals of vagal sensory neurons. Eosinophils, a critical innate effector cell type in allergic reactions, have been revealed to localize close to cholinergic nerves in the gut.

As an important defensive organ, the gastrointestinal tract is covered by simple columnar epithelium with microvilli and associated with a layer of glycocalyx on their luminal surface to protect epitheliocytes from the acid pH. Among epitheliocytes, there are many cell types, but enterocytes and colonocytes are the dominant types. The epithelium sits on the underlying connective tissue called lamina propria, constituting villi and crypts, while neutrophil-like Paneth cells are located on the crypt's bottom. The Paneth cells release many antibacterial factors providing the crypts with a sterile condition. Almost every week, a new epitheliocyte regenerates from stem cells in-built in the epithelial monolayer. The other cell types are goblet cells, M cells, CD8αα+ γδT cells (IELs), tuft cells, and enteroendocrine cells (EEC).

The goblet cells secrete 30 mm-one-layer mucus in the small intestine and 480 mm-two-layer mucus in the large intestine, and the mucus may serve as a "trap" for microbes to inhibit their colonization [17]. Tuft cells are chemosensory cells able to communicate with neurons and release acetylcholine, an alarmin IL-25, cysteinyl leukotrienes, enzymes, etc. There are minimal data on their role in food allergies. FcεRII (CD23) constitutively expressed by epitheliocytes provides the transcytosis of IgE linked with food allergen that contributes to food allergy due to promoting by intraepithelial lymphocytes CD8αα+ γδT cells and stimulating by CCL20 (MIP-3α) [18]. There are other food allergen transcytosis routes, including impaired epithelium integrity, M cells, goblet cell-associated passage (GAP), and uptake by long outgrowths of DC [18].

Enteroendocrine (EEC) cells, similar to the neuroendocrine (NEC) cells [19], secrete over 30 gastrointestinal regulatory peptides, neurotransmitters (histamine and serotonin), and neuropeptides (CGRP, VIP, and substance P), which promote appropriate effects in the gastrointestinal tract, ENS, VNS, and central nervous system [20, 21]. EECs have been studied by single-cell RNA sequencing combined with a real-time fluorescence analysis and displayed hormonal plasticity in the course of their maturation and phenotypic heterogeneity [22].

Mucosal macrophages (M2) located close to epithelium are responsible for the survival and differentiation of enterocytes, intestinal stem cells, M cells, goblet cells, and Paneth cells, epithelial barrier integrity and repair in its disruption, and surveillance for tolerogenic as well as potentially inflammatory gut microbiota [8, 23].

Peyer's patches, solitary (isolated) follicles, and the appendix are lymphoid aggregates of the gut. The scattered lymphoid elements in the esophagus and stomach do not organize similar aggregates. In the aggregated lymphoid follicles, there are B cell areas where fDCs and Tfh take part in controlling the advanced B cell-mediated immune response. Formed plasma cells secrete sIgA, IgG, and IgE, transported into the lumen employing secretory component for sIgA (sIgA > IgG). Some antigen-specific dendritic cells may migrate via draining lymphatics to mesenteric lymph nodes, where they can also trigger an advanced B cell-mediated immune response [17].

The structure of the lamina propria is very compressible and elastic, which allows it to support the nourishment of the epithelium and its functioning. Cell types of lymphoid aggregates such as Peyer's patches and of lamina propria are myeloid (conventional) dendritic (mDC-1 and mDC-2) cells and plasmacytoid dendritic (pDC) cells, CD103+ tolerogenic dendritic (CD103+tDC) cells, enteric glial cells, fibroblasts, lamina propria's macrophages (M2), neutrophils, mast cells, and eosinophils. CD103+tDCs are present only in the gut and express integrin α_E (CD103+), complexed with molecule β_7 to shape $\alpha_E\beta_7$ receptor for E-cadherin and essential for homing of new T cells in the gastrointestinal tract [24]. A subset of tDCs expressing CD103+ is also responsible for delivering allergens to the draining lymph node and inducing pTregs. Besides, these tDC cells promote the recently primed pTregs to home back to the lamina propria where they operate, supporting oral tolerance [25]. Enteric glial cells modulate the interactions between neurons and maintain the epithelial barrier integrity [9, 10]. Lamina propria's macrophages (M2) are self-maintaining, long-lived, ENS-associated, and display different transcriptional profiles specific to their microanatomic location [23]. Muscular macrophages (M2) in the myenteric plexus via β_2 adrenergic receptors and norepinephrine suppress both innate and adaptive immunity [8].

Thus, ENS is a source of different stimuli, anti-inflammatory and pro-inflammatory, with the prevalence of anti-inflammatory (pro-tolerogenic), and a container for immune cells, molecules, microbiota, and digestive enzymes. Due to ENS, the gastrointestinal tract is the uncommon target organ different from the skin and unified airway. It does not develop typical chronic atopic diseases like atopic dermatitis, asthma, and allergic rhinitis as the gut is a zone of allergen tolerance provided with ENS, normal microbiota, pro-tolerogenic neuro molecules, M2 macrophages, tDCs, pTreg cells, and other components of the allergen tolerance maintenance system instead. The predominance of food allergies is approximately 10-fold lower than respiratory allergies [1, 26]. The *dual-allergen exposure hypothesis* postulates that early oral exposure to food allergens induces tolerance, whereas exposure at non-gastrointestinal sites, such as the skin or respiratory tract, results in food sensitization and allergy development [27, 28]. Therefore, a food allergy (series of allergic episodes) does not look like a typical atopic disease and represents a known exception to the rule conceived by evolution.

The prevalence of food allergies is continuously growing, including severe cases, and it is a paradoxical problem in the face of evolution. However, this challenge is inherent to our civilization and will be resolved on the basis of new knowledge and technologies.

7.3 Allergenicity of Food Proteins and Sensitization to Them

Not all food proteins are allergens; therefore, the subject of food allergens *allergenicity* is very important. There are some families and three classes of food allergens. *Class 1 food allergens* (cow's milk, peanut, hen's egg, etc.) are oral allergens that cause sensitization via the gastrointestinal tract and display severe clinical symptoms. *Class 2 food allergens* (e.g., apple, celery, carrot, melon, and kiwi) are cross-reactive with aeroallergens that evoke sensitization via the respiratory tract and exert not severe cross-reactions termed "oral allergy syndrome" [1, 29, 30]. *Class 3 food allergens* (e.g., small food proteins <10 kDa, additives, colorants like tartrazine, and contaminants) do not have the capacity of cross-reactivity, which sensitizes via the unified airway or skin and frequently cause occupational allergies [31]. Some researchers have developed classifications within plant and animal food allergens.

Regarding food allergies, the allergenicity of food nutrients, which are proteins and glycoproteins, including novel and genetically modified food ingredients, is evaluated by many methods such as bioinformatics analysis, serological assays, mass spectrometry, cell experiments, and animal models [32–34]. Food protein allergenicity depends on many factors: antigenic structure (multiple epitopes capable of linear IgE binding), molecular weight lower than 70 kDa, stability, solubility in water, interaction with lipids, abundance in food, biochemical characteristics of proteins (that allow them to survive the extremes of food processing and denaturation and proteolysis by digestive enzymes), combination with adjuvants in food, ability to promote the production of high levels of allergen-specific IgE and high-affinity allergen-specific IgE, pathologic deviations in the gut microbiota, damaged mucosal barriers, decreased enzyme secretion, deficiency in sIgA, atopic predisposition of a person, etc. [35–37]. Besides, food allergens can generally be divided into heat-stable and heat-labile molecules. Heat-stable allergens are resistant to heat and acid and can cause systemic reactions. In contrast, heat-labile allergens are highly sensitive to heat and acid and may lead to cross-reactivity if they get into the body as pollen particles [38].

A food allergen enters the body via the gastrointestinal tract, respiratory tract, skin [1, 39], or genitourinary tract (see Chap. 9). If it does not degrade by digestive enzymes in the gut, this allergen occurs before the epithelial barrier (see Fig. 7.2). SIgA and mucus may neutralize it. One more obstacle is the allergen tolerance system, which possesses uncommon power in the gastrointestinal tract. Penetrating through the epithelium using GAP, M cells, long outgrowths of DC, and epithelium defects [18] food allergen turns on Th2-controlled B cell-mediated immune response that then leads to allergen-specific IgE production and memory B and T cells establishment. Before the beginning of the immune response, ILC2, APC, and Th2 cells were activated by epithelium-derived alarmins, IL-25, IL-33, TSLP, and ILC2 were on separation upregulated by neuromedin U [40–42]. Th2 cells produce type 2 cytokines such as IL-4, IL-5, IL-9, IL-13, and IL-33 and function as regulatory cells that drive allergic inflammation. Cytokine IL-33 is important for mast cell maturation and readiness for degranulation [39]. At this time, Tregs acquire Th2 phenotype and lose the ability to suppress the mast cell activation [43, 44]. Tfh secrete IL-21, IL-4, and IL-13, which are essential for promoting IgE class switch recombination in B cells, maturing plasma cells, and growing allergen-specific IgE affinity [17].

At this time, the allergen-specific Treg occurs due to tDCs [45]. In contrast, if tolerance is constituted, the clinical symptoms do not manifest. This allergen may break the tolerance during the second entry, activate IgE production, and involve inflammatory cells and biomolecules that develop food allergy symptoms in the gut and other target organs. Inflammation may become long-lasting and life-threatening if allergenic complexes in a large amount get into circulation. But it is more frequently only an episode as allergen tolerance is restored. One of the mechanisms

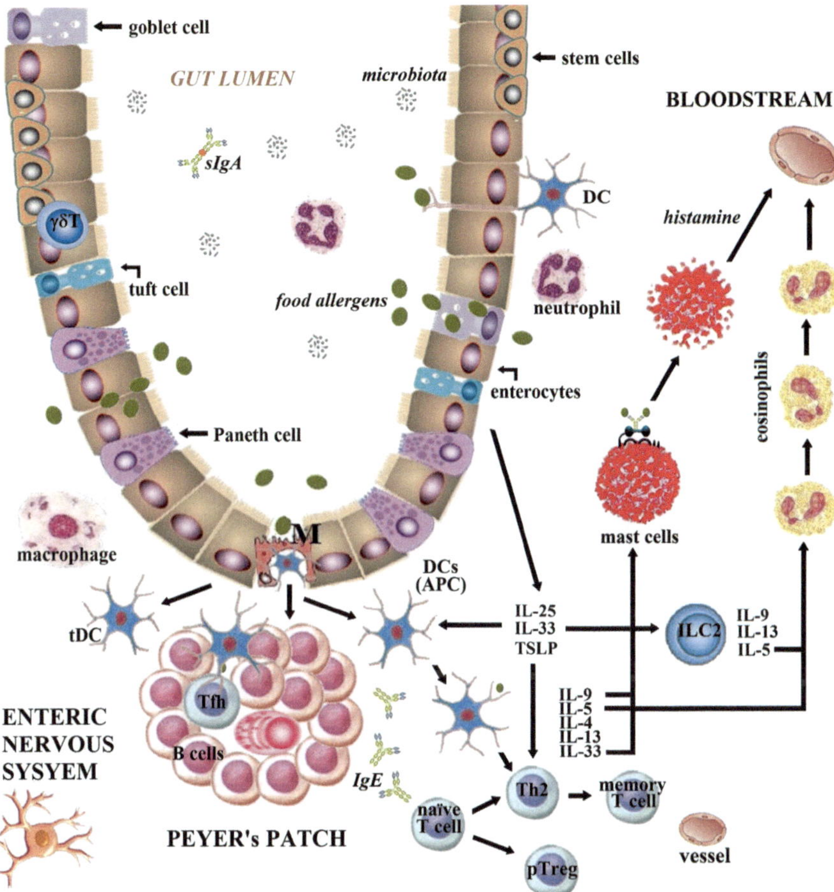

Fig. 7.2 Sensitization and allergen tolerance breakdown in food allergy. Penetrating through the epithelium using GAP, M cells, DC, and epithelium defects, a food allergen appears in the submucosa filled in various cells. The epithelium generates alarmins, IL-25, IL-33, and TSLP, upregulating ILC2, APC, and Th2 cells. Activated ILC2 secretes IL-5, IL-9, and IL-13 affecting eosinophils and mast cells. Food allergen is engulfed by submucosal DCs, processed, and presented to Th2 cells that trigger B cell Th2-controlled B cell response with IgE end-production promotion and memory B and memory T cells establishment. This process proceeds in Peyer's patches. Th2 cells produce type 2 cytokines such as IL-4, IL-5, IL-9, IL-13, and IL-33 and function as regulatory cells that drive allergic inflammation. IL-33 is essential for the maturation of mast cells. Tfh secrete IL-21, IL-4, and IL-13, important for upregulating IgE class switch recombination in B cells, maturing plasma cells, and growing allergen-specific IgE affinity. Since ENS fills in pro-tolerogenic neurotransmitters, food allergen cannot easily overcome the system of allergen tolerance maintenance. However, if it happens, allergic inflammation develops, and food allergies manifest. APC allergen-presenting cell, ILC2 group 2 innate lymphoid cell, TSLP thymic stromal lymphopoietin, tDC tolerogenic dendritic cell, pTreg peripheral regulatory T cell, Tfh follicular helper T cell

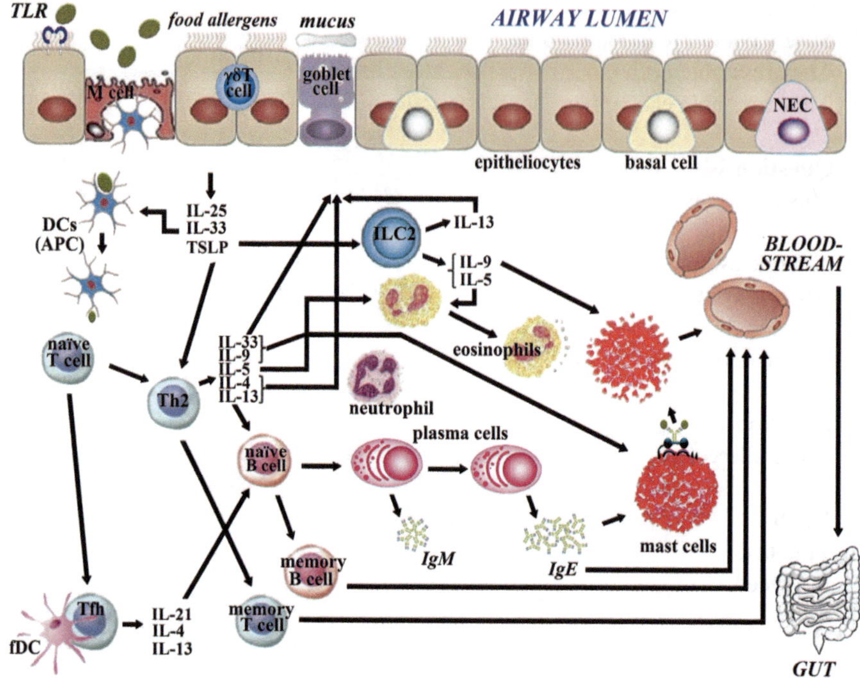

Fig. 7.3 The unified airway route of food sensitization. Food allergens enter the body via the unified airway route, get into the nasal and lung submucosae, and promote Th2-dependent IgE-response. When the immune response is completed, memory B cells, T cells, and IgE antibodies get into the bloodstream and then into the gastrointestinal tract. DCs dendritic cells, APC allergen-presenting cells, Th2 type 2 helper T cells, Tfh follicular helper T cells, fDC follicular dendritic cells, ILC2 group 2 innate lymphoid cells, NEC neuroendocrine cells, TLR toll-like receptors

presents the induction of synthesis of IgG antibodies competing with IgE antibodies. The other mechanisms of allergen tolerance maintenance, including neuro molecules, tDCs, and pTregs, are recruiting too. However, immunologic memory about the history of this food allergen is lifelong.

New sensitization to food allergens may occur if they come by inhalation promoting food allergies, and exacerbating the course of asthma, allergic rhinitis, and atopic dermatitis development. Exposure to food allergens may proceed at home, in schools, restaurants, grocery stores, commercial flights, and occupational environments [31, 46]. Food allergens penetrating the body via the unified airway route get into the nasal and lung submucosae, where the immune system responds to these allergens (see Fig. 7.3). Researchers have demonstrated that peanut allergens have triggered IL-33 and TSLP synthesis in primary human nasal or bronchial epitheliocytes and stimulated the maturation and migration of peanut-specific lung mDC-1 cells to draining lymph nodes. In addition, inhalational exposure to peanut and indoor dust has induced peanut-specific Th2 cell differentiation and accumulation of Tfh cells in draining lymph nodes, which were associated with increased B cells numbers and peanut-specific IgE and IgG_1 production [27].

The transcutaneous sensitization to food allergens plays a role in the pathogenesis of food allergies and atopic dermatitis, especially if *filaggrin gene* mutations are available [47–49].

Quiz A

Reading a question, please choose only one right answer.

Question 1

Innervation of the gastrointestinal tract is provided with:

1. Enteric nervous system.
2. Somatosensory neurons and enteric nervous system.
3. Somatosensory neurons, vegetative nervous system, and enteric nervous system.
4. Somatosensory neurons.

Question 2

Innervation of the gastrointestinal tract differs from innervation of the unified airway by:

1. Presence of self nervous system.
2. Absence of vegetative nervous system.
3. Involvement of nociceptive neurons.
4. Involvement of the vagus nerve.

Question 3

Sensitization and repeated immune response to the food allergen develop in:

1. Intestinal simple columnar epithelium.
2. Intestinal lumen.
3. Mouth only.
4. Submucosa and lymphoid aggregates of the gut.

Question 4

The enteric nervous system contains:

1. Nociceptive neurons.
2. Sympathetic neurons.
3. The myenteric plexus and submucosal plexus.
4. Parasympathetic and somatosensory fibers.

Question 5

Food intolerance is caused by:

1. Inadequate functioning of digestive enzymes.
2. Irritable bowel syndrome.
3. Ulcerative colitis.
4. Reactions of the immune system to harmless food.

Question 6

A type of gut macrophages involved in constant surveillance for tolerogenic microbiota is:

1. Mucosal macrophages.
2. Kupffer's cells.
3. Lamina propria's macrophages.
4. Muscular macrophages.

Question 7

The large intestine contains the following lymphoid aggregates:

1. Tonsils.
2. Solitary follicles.
3. Lymph nodes.
4. Scattered lymphoid elements.

Question 8

This MALT's compartment refers to the gastrointestinal tract:

1. NALT.
2. TALT.
3. GALT.
4. BALT.

Question 9

Serotonin is synthesized in:

1. Dopaminergic neurons.
2. Enteric neurons.
3. Thyroid.
4. Tonsils.

Question 10

Food protein allergenicity depends on:

1. Antigenic structure.
2. NALT.
3. BALT.
4. Lymphoid aggregates in the nasopharynx.

Question 11

Food protein allergenicity depends on:

1. BALT.
2. Resistance to denaturation and proteolysis by digestive enzymes.

3. Conditions of the thyroid.
4. Conditions of the adrenal gland.

Question 12
This neurotransmitter is not related to pro-tolerogenic:

1. GABA.
2. Serotonin.
3. Acetylcholine.
4. Norepinephrine.

Question 13
Allergic response to a food protein is controlled by:

1. Mast cells.
2. Th2 cells.
3. Eosinophils.
4. Neutrophils.

Question 14
Th2 cells secrete the following cytokines:

1. IFN-γ and IL-2.
2. IL-4, IL-5, IL-9, and IL-13.
3. IL-35, TGF-β, IL-27, and IL-10.
4. IL-1β and IL-6.

Question 15
The enteric nervous system produces more neuro molecules:

1. Pro-inflammatory cytokines and chemokines.
2. Pro-immunogenic neuro molecules.
3. Pro-tolerogenic neuro molecules.
4. Acetylcholine.

Question 16
Tfh cells produce the following cytokines:

1. IL-1β and IL-6.
2. IL-35, TGF-β, IL-27, and IL-10.
3. IFN-γ and IL-2.
4. IL-21, IL-4, and IL-13.

7.4 Oral Tolerance and Food Allergies

▶ **Definition** Oral tolerance, a form of allergen tolerance, is a physiologic process of nutrient absorption with no adverse reaction. A food allergy is a pathologic process associated with food eating when the immune system responds to nutrients as allergens develop allergic inflammation in the gut, unified airway, skin, and even genitourinary tract. Cross-reactions ("oral allergy syndrome") are the combination of food allergy and pollen allergy.

7.4.1 Role of Intestinal Microbiota in Oral Tolerance

Much of our current understanding of mechanisms responsible for oral tolerance and food allergies has been derived from animal models. Experimental data demonstrated that key factors in the regulation of oral tolerance versus food allergies are defects of the intestinal epithelium, imbalance in gut microbiota (*dysbiosis*), and involvement of innate immunity (ILC2 and inflammatory cells) [50].

In children, the gastrointestinal tract's immaturity may play a role in the increased prevalence of gastrointestinal microbiota and food allergies seen in the first 4 years of life. In general, in children and adults, the gastrointestinal tract's main function is to process ingested food into a form that can be absorbed and used for energy and growth, and simultaneously prevent the multiplication of undesirable microbiota in the body. Ingestion of food proteins normally results in local and systemic immune unresponsiveness in a process termed oral tolerance [51, 52].

The gut microbiota is a potent factor of oral tolerance at any age [53–56]. From the first minutes after birth, a baby's body is colonized with many microbes, collectively termed the microbiota or microbiome. The microbiome adds a magnitude of genes to the human genome, increasing it up to 200 times [57]. Unfavorable factors such as cesarean delivery, lack of breastfeeding, early-life-antibiotic exposure, and a low-fiber/high-fat diet induce gut microbiota dysbiosis, promoting allergen tolerance breakdown [58]. Adults develop dysbiosis due to diseases, unhealthy diet (a decrease in fibers, vital vitamins, trace elements, and increase in fat, sugar, salt, junk foods, etc.), tobacco and alcohol use, unhealthy lifestyle, lack of environmental sanitation, immobility, etc. The genetic and epigenetic background also play a role.

Bacteria of the microbiota are heterogeneous and divided into two groups, inflammatory and immunoregulatory [59]. Inflammatory microbes are prone to promote the maturation of Th1 and Th17, share features with both pathogens and symbionts, and cause pathological processes under specific conditions. The immunoregulatory commensals, certain bacterial strains (e.g., *Bifidobacterium longum 35624*, *Clostridia*, *Bacteroides fragilis*, *Lactobacillus rhamnosus JB-1*, etc.) regulate the host immune processes, including allergen tolerance [60]. Their metabolites, like eight short-chain fatty acids (butyrate, propionate, acetate, etc.), have an anti-inflammatory action and stimulate differentiation of pTregs from naïve T cells. pTregs, and pro-tolerogenic neurotransmitters and neuropeptides (serotonin, norepinephrine, GABA, etc.), maintain allergen tolerance in the gut and prevent food allergies. Besides, short-chain fatty acids promote functioning CD103+tDC and amplify IL-10 production [61]. The abundance of gut microbiota metabolites if dysbiosis is absent allows the modulation of tolerogenic systems in the unified airway and skin [62]. The presence or absence of specific immunologically important microbiota members can determine a person's susceptibility to disease and highlight the role of microbiota composition in human pathology [59]. In addition, normal immunoregulatory microbiota through short-chain fatty acids and pTregs influences the enterocytes and colonocytes regeneration inducing renewal of intestinal stem cells and inhibition of the Th1, Th2, and Th17 lymphocytes activity [63].

The communities of microbes comprising the gut microbiome are complex and dynamic, from infancy to adulthood. Factors affecting the diversity and development of the gut microbiome show that the microbiome can dramatically influence the outcome of immune responses in the gut, including those to food peptides (allergens). Furthermore, this circumstance appears to be the leading cause of IgE-dependent food allergies to start or not [18, 51, 64]. However, a ratio of constant tolerance versus food allergy episodes remains questionable, particularly why most individuals do not get sensitized during their lifespan at all [65].

The gut microbiota also synthesizes neuro molecules, serotonin, GABA, opioids, dopamine, etc., required for the immunoregulation in the gut and interaction with the enteric nervous system and central nervous system [7, 66]. It is one more essential role of the microbiota in the body.

In non-atopic adults, IgE-dependent food allergies must not occur, but IgG-mediated food allergies may appear at any age if gastrointestinal disorders are available. There are also food-allergic reactions previously called "*pseudo allergies*." IgE-mediated food-allergic reactions may present in different tissues such as skin, gastrointestinal, respiratory, and genitourinary tracts, and allergens penetrate the body in the same ways [1, 45, 51]. However, there is not yet a full explanation as to why food allergies occur in only some atopic persons but not in all.

From a clinical viewpoint, persons with a suspect "pseudo allergy" should be examined comprehensively, including gastrointestinal conditions.

In summary, the human microbiome is enriched by contact with natural environment that promotes immune homeostasis and protects from allergy and inflammatory disorders regarding the biodiversity hypothesis. The biosphere balance is lost, and there is an ecological necessity to protect, restore and return to the natural world [67].

7.4.2 Prerequisites of Oral Tolerance Breakdown

Oral tolerance depends on multiple factors, which can maintain or destabilize it under the everyday entry of food proteins, dynamic gut microbiota, changing signals from neuro molecules, and continuous trafficking of pro-inflammatory cells and molecules. In general, genetic predisposition, epigenetic modifications, and environmental exposures may be the risk factors [52, 68]. In detail, delivery route (cesarean delivery), home and farm animal exposure, parents smoking, air pollution, and daycare as environmental factors can matter for the development of food allergies in infants [68].

Damaged oral mucosal epithelial barrier integrity may predispose to food allergies, at least, profilin-mediated cases (with sensitization to peanut, kiwi, celery, melon, etc.). In patients, histologic features of progressive oral mucosal remodeling have been found, with increased acanthosis, angiogenesis, and a greater density of collagen fibers. These histologic features were comparable with those previously described in oral mucosa in patients with inflammatory pathologies such as gingivitis and periodontal disease [69].

A survey investigated whether native and foreign-born residents of the US have different risks of food sensitization, whether the risk of food sensitization differs by the immigration status of a child's parent, and whether the timing of immigration affects the risk of food and aeroallergen sensitization [70]. On the whole, oral tolerance to food and its loss results from a complicated interaction between the allergens in the food, the microbiome inhabiting the gut, immune and nonimmune cells in the gut-associated lymphoid tissue (GALT), and specialized neurotransmitters found in the autonomous enteric nervous system. The particular tDCs subset, intestinal CD103+tDCs, operates in the gut and mesenteric lymph nodes using heterodimeric integrin $\alpha_E\beta_7$ [24, 71] and also plays a role in oral tolerance.

See factors affecting food tolerance breakdown and oral tolerance in Table 7.1.

Thus, oral tolerance must meet the following main criteria:

1. Potent allergen tolerance maintenance system in the gut
2. Balance in intestinal microbiota with a significant amount of useful microbes
3. Integrity of the gastrointestinal barriers

The loss of oral tolerance promotes the development of food allergies.

Table. 7.1 Factors affecting the homeostasis in oral tolerance

Pro-tolerogenic (oral tolerance)	Pro-immunogenic (food allergies)
Activation of tDCs	Inactivation of tDCs
Activation of pTregs	Inactivation of pTregs
Expression of the immunosuppressive cytokines	Expression of the pro-inflammatory cytokines
Overexpression of coinhibitory molecules	Inhibition of coinhibitory molecules
Inactivation of pro-inflammatory cells, prevalence of lymphocytes somewhere in the gut	Prevalence of pro-inflammatory cells somewhere in the gut
Gastrointestinal barriers integrity	Damaged gastrointestinal barriers
Balance in gut microbiota	Inadequate change of the gut microbiota; hypothetically, constant excess of PAMP in the gut microbiota and AAMP in the food
Predominance of signals from pro-tolerogenic neuro molecules (serotonin, norepinephrine, CGRP, etc.)	Predominance of signals from pro-immunogenic neuro molecules (substance P, neuromedin U, etc.)

7.4.3 Polymorphisms of Food Allergies

The term "food allergy" is exploited to describe an adverse immunologic response to a food protein (allergen). Several hypotheses have been formulated to explain the pathogenesis of food allergies: the hygiene hypothesis and "old friends" hypothesis (exposure to a lack of infections in early childhood promotes an imbalance in favor of the Th2), dual-allergen exposure hypothesis (food allergen exposure via the skin is rather than oral route), allergen avoidance hypothesis (food allergen avoidance in early life would prevent sensitization), vitamin D hypothesis (cholecalciferol deficiency), microbiota hypothesis (the presence of specific bacterial strains in the gut), "false alarm hypothesis" (a high level of advanced glycation food products), and nutritional immunomodulation hypothesis (dietary factors with immunomodulatory properties might affect risks) [52, 72].

Food-related reactions are linked with a broad range of signs and symptoms such as skin itch, urticaria, red rash, angioedema, bronchospasms, difficulty swallowing, feeling sick or vomiting, abdominal pain, or diarrhea, and anaphylaxis. It may involve any body system, including target organs. It is important to distinguish food allergies from other nonimmune-mediated adverse reactions to foods [73, 74]. A recent survey of over 15,022 individuals estimated the prevalence of food allergies in Canada amounts to 7.5% (see Table 7.2).

Table 7.2 Prevalence for self-reported food allergy in Canada ([73], modified)

Food allergen			Prevalence (%)	
Name	Species	Major allergen	Children	Adults
Peanut [75]	*Arachis hypogaea*	*Ara h 2, Ara h 6*	2.2	0.6
Hazelnut [76]	*Corylus avellana*	*Cor a 9, Cor a 14*	1.5	1.0
Carp [77]	*Cyprinus carpio*	*Cyp c 1*	0.9	0.5
Shrimp [78]	*Penaeus aztecus*	*Pen a 1*	0.8	1.6
Milk [79]	*Bos domesticus*	*Bos d 5, Bos d 8*	0.2	0.2
Egg [80]	*Gallus domesticus*	*Gal d 1, Gal d 2*	1.0	0.5
Wheat [81]	*Triticum aestivum*	*Tri a 19*	0.2	0.2

It is estimated that 3–4% of adults and 5% of children under 4 years of age in industrialized/westernized countries have food allergies. Furthermore, extensive data suggest that food allergies are even up to 10% affected [52]. "The Big Eight" food allergens cause about 90% of all food-allergic reactions. They are cow's milk, eggs, peanut, tree nuts, soy, wheat, fish, and crustacean shellfish. Food allergies to cow's milk, egg, and wheat often are outgrown as persons acquire allergen tolerance, whereas allergies to peanut, tree nuts, fish, and shellfish commonly persist over a lifetime and have a high association with anaphylaxis [1, 73, 82].

Baker and Sampson [3] created a classification of phenotypes and endotypes of IgE-mediated food allergies based on clinical characteristics and known immunologic mechanisms. They proposed some phenotypes: classic (prevalent), intermittent (cross-reactive allergy), aerosolized sensitization, and α-Gal syndrome (mammalian meat allergy). The corresponding endotypes specified the phenotypes' peculiarities were described as follows: persistent, transient, local and systemic reactions, and drugs/exercise/alcohol-induced.

In other words, food allergies may develop in different phenotypes such as Th2-high (IgE-dependent), Th2-low, IgE-independent, and immune system-independent phenotypes. Atopic sensitization due to IgE overproduction is prevalent [3].

The cross-reaction based on food allergies is called "oral allergy syndrome" or "pollen food allergy syndrome" [1, 83]. The cross-reaction may be explained by the biochemical proximity of allergens, which are present in both pollens and food. The list of cross-reactions is extensive. A typical sample is sensitization to birch, alder, elm, associated with food allergy to apple, peach, cherry, kiwi, carrot, tomato, etc., and hypersensitivity to ragweed linked with food allergy to banana, watermelon, zucchini, cucumber, etc. Besides, allergy to grass is associated with hypersensitivity to orange, melon, honey, etc. [73]. Chitinases are a group of allergens often found in plant food (wheat, rice, tomato, raspberry, grape, banana, coffee, etc.), latex (hevein), arthropods (HDM), and insects (silkworm). Accordingly, chitinases develop cross-reactivity syndrome and may cause anaphylaxis [84]. Naturally, most people become tolerant of the cross-allergy if products containing heat-labile allergens have been baked, cooked, and roasted.

However, food-allergic reactions among several clinical atopic diseases remain controversial. The diagnosis of food allergy requires a detailed past medical history, physical examination, skin prick testing (SPT), serologic IgE analyses based on biotechnologically engineered allergens (component resolved assays) [74] (see Chap. 5), atopy patch tests [85], and referral to an allergist. In some cases, it may require the oral food challenge, which an allergist conducts in the allergist's office taking into account the risk of acute allergic reactions of unpredictable severity. However, the oral food challenge currently represents the "gold standard" test to diagnose food allergies [5]. Once the diagnosis of food allergy is confirmed, strict elimination of the offending food allergen from the diet is generally necessary.

Treatment management of food allergies [86] consists of educating the patient about allergen avoidance, prescribing biologics [87], and the method of oral AIT [88–91] (see Chap. 8). Epicutaneous AIT has been developing, whereas sublingual AIT is generally not as efficacious [73]. In severe cases, an epinephrine auto-injector (EAI) should prescribe. Prevention of food allergy by early introduction of food has been discussed. Some researchers suggest that the early introduction of six allergenic foods (peanut, cooked egg, cow's milk, sesame, whitefish, and wheat) in exclusively breastfed infants with a genetic risk of developing food allergy who were 3 months of age would reduce the prevalence of food allergy by the age of 3 [73, 92]. The idea of the early introduction of allergenic food matches the dual-allergen exposure hypothesis [68, 93]. However, this approach did not display efficacy concerning all main food allergens [72, 94].

Natural recovery from a food allergy episode is possible and sometimes appears. Reverting food allergy to allergen tolerance is characterized by a loss of Th2 cells and an increase in Th1 cells, the simultaneous induction of blocking IgG antibodies, and suppression of inflammation's effector cell functions [95].

Researchers have begun to describe the molecular structure of food allergens and have fulfilled chip-based assays for multiple allergens. A study of the structure of causative food allergens has allowed the engineering of synthetic and recombinant vaccines [1, 96].

7.5 Why Does Anaphylaxis Happen to Some, But Not to Others?

▶ **Definition** Food anaphylaxis, a life-threatening systemic syndrome, has particular features and occurs only in some atopic individuals who suffer from food allergies.

In some cases, the immune system releases a wide range of chemicals in greater quantity than usual, causing reactions in multiple body areas. Collectively, these reactions are known as anaphylaxis. There is currently no explanation for why life-threatening anaphylaxis occurs in only some individuals among those who are allergic to food allergens [39, 97]. Genetic and epigenetic factors in food anaphylaxis are of high interest and directly and indirectly involved in IgE-mediated food allergies pathogenesis [98]. Although genetics plays a vital role in the manifestation of most atopic diseases, epigenetics matters much through three epigenetic mechanisms: DNA methylation, covalent posttranslational histone modifications, and micro-RNA-mediated gene silencing. So, it may be essential for the interactions between various susceptibility genes, immunologic processes, and environmental factors [99].

Eighty children at age 1–18 years with diagnosed allergies to eggs, peanut, tree nuts, and 14 healthy children (no food allergy) were recruited to study the *TLR2*, *TLR4*, and *CD14 gene* expression. Patients with nut allergies had lower expression of *TLR genes* than those with egg allergies or without food allergies. Methylation in the promoter regions of *TLR2* was associated with a decrease in *TLR gene* expression in all children. The study showed that genetic alterations in two *PRR* and *CD14 genes* and epigenetic modifications changed the course of food allergies [98].

Monogenic disorders leading to atopic inflammation are distinct from immunodeficiency, autoimmune, or autoinflammatory phenotypes. The definition "primary atopic disorders" is proposed to categorize heritable genetic diseases, which present with deregulated pathogenic allergic effector responses irrespective of sensitization. The primary atopic diseases include genetic disorders leading to urticaria, anaphylaxis, and other consequences of abnormal mast cell degranulation, chronic polarization to type 2 helper T cells, eosinophil-mediated allergic inflammation, and excited IgE production [100, 101]. Monogenic mutations associated with only severe food allergy have not been found, but separate facts about some mutations causing metabolic disturbances have been accumulating. For example, mutations in the phosphoglucomutase 3 (*PGM3 gene*) gene (6q14.1) are linked with food allergy and food protein-induced enteropathy [100]. D816V mutations in the gene (*KIT gene*) (on 4q12) encoded the tyrosine kinase receptor KIT are found in some patients with clonal mast cell disorders, including mastocytosis, and some persons with recurrent anaphylaxis but without mastocytosis [102].

On the whole, there is a series of causes why life-threatening anaphylaxis occurs in only some individuals among those who are allergic to food allergens:

- The obligatory atopic predisposition of the body
- Individual selectiveness to separate allergens
- Dose and pathway of penetrating causative allergens
- Repeated entry of the same allergen, which already resulted in anaphylaxis
- Secondary genetic alterations and epigenetic modifications leading to the weakness of the allergen tolerance system

Reviewing data with impaired TCR signaling [100] in humans, most mutations in pathways critical for propagating TCR signals were first reported in the context of recessive severe combined immunodeficiencies. For example, mutations in tyrosine kinases like ZAP70 resulted in an extreme Th2 cell polarization weakening the allergen tolerance. In patients with the hyper-IgE syndrome caused by dominant mutations in the signal transducer and activator of transcription 3 ($STAT3^{DN}$), altered TGF-β signaling has been found. In persons with X-linked recessive mutations in FoxP3, there was immune dysregulation polyendocrinopathy enteropathy X-linked (IPEX) syndrome. Both nTregs and pTregs were absent, IL-10 was decreased, and, as a result, the allergen tolerance system was becoming weaker. In all reviewed episodes, food anaphylaxis occurred [100].

In atopic individuals, if an allergy to food allergens such as peanut, tree nuts, fish, and shellfish once occurred, it can repeat during the patient's lifetime. Furthermore, these food allergies are highly associated with anaphylaxis and are lifelong in approximately 80% of patients. In patients with food allergies, about ~200 allergen-specific B cells per million are detected among B cells, whereas allergen-specific CD4+ T cells account for 9 through 100 cells per million T cells [82]. Since specific IgE-expressing cells have a short lifespan, the crucial role in maintaining food allergies is played by memory B cells and T cells, among which memory B cells regularly replenish pools of IgE-secreting cells. Some researchers explain lifelong food allergies, which humans observe, as the manifestation of constant exposure to food allergens that recurrently activate memory cells and identify them as a target with disease-transforming potential [103].

An interesting study concerning the mechanism by which IgE reappears in repeated anaphylaxis has been carried out. A novel culture system and application of single-cell RNA sequencing displayed the transcriptomic signature of human peanut-reactive B cells and T cells and IL-4/IL-13 signal transduction as a signaling pathway essential for the IgE reactivation response. Certainly, interruption of this pathway not only prevented IgE production and anaphylaxis but also reprogrammed the response against peanut [104].

In everyday life, hidden allergens must not be forgotten. Much consumed food is prepared outside the home, and meals may be composed of different ingredients, including hidden allergens. In atopic sensitized individuals, anaphylaxis can occur to a composite food. The best way to evaluate the likelihood of a hidden allergen provoking an allergic reaction is a good knowledge of commonly used ingredients, presence of cofactors, and type of food and where it was consumed [105].

The problem of anaphylaxis is still unresolved. It is unlikely that lifelong food allergies depend only on gene mutations. Future in-depth studies of food anaphylaxis will promote the discovery of predictive biomarkers and therapeutic targets for diagnosing and treating severe food allergies.

From a clinical viewpoint, anaphylaxis remains a clinical diagnosis and biomarkers have no role in acute management. However, they are important to confirm the diagnosis and distinguish anaphylaxis from its mimics such as severe asthma, hypotensive crisis, somatoform disorders, vocal cord dysfunction, due to nonallergic causes. The measurement of serum total mast cell *tryptase* remains the "gold standard," which may help differentiate anaphylaxis from its mimics [106]. Higher levels of IL-4 and histamine have been reported in the serum of human patients with severe anaphylaxis contributing to the molecular mechanisms of food-induced anaphylaxis severity [107].

7.6 Allergic Inflammation in the Gastrointestinal Tract

The gut is a zone of powerful pro-tolerogenic influence due to the autonomous enteric nervous system (ENS) competing with vegetative neurons and pro-inflammatory neurotransmitters and neuropeptides directed to the activation of Th2 cells and mast cells [108, 109]. Therefore, chronic atopic disorders in the gastrointestinal tract, except for food allergy episodes and anaphylaxis, are rare. Conversely, the gut is a zone of inflammatory autoimmune conditions such as ulcer colitis and Crohn's disease. Damaging mutations have been found in IL-10, IL-10RA, and IL-10RB that lead to profound early-onset any of these inflammatory bowel diseases [100].

IgE-independent gut allergy phenotypes have been reported, such as food protein-induced enterocolitis syndrome, allergic proctocolitis, food-protein induced enteropathy, celiac disease/dermatitis herpetiformis, and cow's milk protein-induced iron deficiency anemia [73]. In particular, cow milk protein-induced non-IgE-mediated allergic colitis has been described in infants and older children with future recovery [110–112]. Soy occupies the second place among culprit food allergens [113]. It was termed food protein-induced enterocolitis syndrome (FPIES), and its pathogenesis is poorly understood but appears to be based on delayed IV type hypersensitivity. The pathology is undoubtedly the most frequent, although the exact prevalence is not well established. In infants with visible rectal bleeding, non-IgE-colitis is causal in up to 60% of cases. Patients with FPIES differ from celiac disease, primary immunodeficiencies, Hirschsprung's disease, and eosinophilic colitis. The following products may be suspected as causative food allergens: avocado, banana, sweet potato, peas, squash, apple, and pear. Peanuts may be a new trigger of acute FPIES, coinciding with an earlier introduction of peanut in infants [114]. However, in most cases, non-IgE-colitis symptoms manifest in infants shortly after introducing cow's milk into the diet, with vomiting, chronic diarrhea, steatorrhea, and features of malabsorption.

The diagnosis of FPIES remains clinical and includes the observation of the resolution of symptoms upon avoidance of offending foods, mainly cow's milk and soy, from the diet. Co-avoidance of banana and avocado is common [115]. In most cases, the main principle is the removal of suspect allergens without broad restrictions on possible triggers. Epinephrine injections should only be prescribed if there is a concomitant severe IgE-mediated food allergy. Naturally, oral AIT has not yet been attempted in non-IgE-colitis.

Key Points

1. The autonomous enteric nervous system (ENS), normal microbiota, pro-tolerogenic neuro molecules, and other factors give particular features to the gastrointestinal tract creating a tolerance zone. The predominant neuro molecules originating from ENS and operating in the gut are serotonin, GABA, CGRP, norepinephrine, and dopamine.
2. Chronic atopic inflammation is not inherent in the gut, whereas persistent food allergies occur in many patients. According to surveys, children and adults' frequent causative food allergens are peanut, hazelnut, seafood, soy, dairy and wheat products, and eggs. Among them, peanut, tree nuts, fish, and shellfish are lifelong and are highly associated with anaphylaxis.
3. Chronic food protein-induced enterocolitis syndrome (FPIES) based on type IV hypersensitivity can develop instead.

Take-Home Messages

1. Write a questionnaire on a family history of a patient who suffers from food allergies.
2. Write a questionnaire on a social patient's history who suffers from food allergies.

3. Write a questionnaire on patients' complaints in food allergies.
4. Write a paragraph about symptoms of food anaphylaxis.
5. Make a flyer about prevalent food allergens.
6. Write a paragraph about non-IgE-colitis.
7. Make a slide presentation on food allergies in children.
8. List causes of urticaria, angioedema, and anaphylaxis.
9. Write a paragraph about food allergies in adults.
10. Write an essay about factors affecting oral tolerance breakdown.
11. Outline enteric nervous system (ENS).
12. Write a paragraph about cross-reactions.

Quiz B

Reading a question, please choose only one right answer.

Question 1

Food allergy is caused by:

1. Inadequate functioning of digestive enzymes.
2. Reactions of the immune system to harmless food.
3. Crohn's disease.
4. Ulcerative colitis.

Question 2

Food intolerance is caused by:

1. Reactions of the immune system to harmless food.
2. Crohn's disease.
3. Ulcerative colitis.
4. Inadequate functioning of digestive enzymes.

Question 3

Innervation of the gastrointestinal tract is provided with:

1. Somatosensory neurons.
2. Somatosensory neurons, enteric nervous system, and vegetative nervous system.
3. Somatosensory neurons and vegetative nervous system.
4. Enteric nervous system.

Question 4

The small intestine contains the following lymphoid aggregates:

1. Peyer's patches.
2. Solitary follicles and appendix.
3. Appendix.
4. Scattered lymphoid elements.

Question 5

A type of gut macrophages suppresses innate and adaptive immunity:

1. Alveolar macrophages.
2. Muscular macrophages.
3. Spleen macrophages.
4. Kupffer's cells.

Question 6

Food protein allergenicity does not depend on:

1. Antigenic structure.
2. Interaction with lipids.
3. Dysbiosis of the gut microbiota.
4. Lymphoid aggregates in the nasopharynx.

Question 7

The intestinal simple columnar epithelium contains:

1. Langerhans cells and $\gamma\delta$T cells.
2. Mucosal macrophages.
3. Neutrophils.
4. B cells.

Question 8

Sensitization and repeated immune response to a food allergen develop in:

1. Intestinal simple columnar epithelium.
2. Submucosa and lymphoid aggregates of the gut.
3. Intestinal lumen.
4. Stomach only.

Question 9

The optimal route of allergen-specific immunotherapy (AIT) in food allergies is:

1. Sublingual.
2. Subcutaneous.
3. Oral.
4. Intralymphatic.

Question 10

Ingestion of food proteins normally leads to:

1. Urticaria.
2. Diarrhea.
3. Anaphylaxis.
4. Immune unresponsiveness (oral tolerance).

Question 11
Factors that are not affecting oral tolerance:

1. Local allergic rhinitis.
2. Inactivation of pTreg cells.
3. Expression of pro-inflammatory cytokines.
4. Predominance of signals from pro-immunogenic neuro molecules.

Question 12
A leading factor predisposing to IgE-dependent food allergies is:

1. Genetically modified food ingredients.
2. Intestinal tract microbiota in atopic individuals.
3. Insufficiency of digestive enzyme secretion.
4. Vegetarian nutrition.

Question 13
Monogenic mutations associated with only food anaphylaxis are revealed:

1. Yes.
2. Maybe.
3. No yet.
4. Unsurely.

Question 14
The most frequent food allergy develops to:

1. Rice.
2. Mutton.
3. Oatmeal.
4. Peanut.

Question 15
Management in patients with food allergies includes:

1. Frequent referrals to an allergist.
2. Strict elimination of the causative food allergen from the diet.
3. Referrals to a gastroenterologist.
4. Physical exam six times per year.

Question 16
The enteric nervous system produces more neuro molecules:

1. Pro-tolerogenic neuro molecules.
2. Pro-immunogenic neuro molecules.
3. Pro-inflammatory cytokines and chemokines.
4. Oxytocin.

References

1. Valenta R, Hochwallner H, Linhart B, Pahr S. Food allergies: the basics. Gastroenterology. 2015;148(6):1120–31. https://doi.org/10.1053/j.gastro.2015.02.006.
2. Carucci L, Coppola S, Luzzetti A, Voto L, Giglio V, Paparo L, Nocerino R, Canani RB. Immunonutrition for pediatric patients with cow's milk allergy: how early interventions could impact long-term outcomes. Front Allergy. 2021;2:676200. https://doi.org/10.3389/falgy.2021.676200.
3. Baker MG, Sampson HA. Phenotypes and endotypes of food allergy: a path to better understanding the pathogenesis and prognosis of food allergy. Ann Allergy Asthma Immunol. 2018;120:245–53. https://doi.org/10.1016/j.anai.2018.01.027.
4. Gupta RS, Warren CM, Smith BM, Jiang J, Blumenstock JA, Davis MM, Schleimer RP, Nadeau KC. Prevalence and severity of food allergies among US adults. JAMA Netw Open. 2019;2(1):e185630. https://doi.org/10.1001/jamanetworkopen.2018.5630.
5. Foong R-X, Dantzer JA, Wood RA, Santos AF. Improving diagnostic accuracy in food allergy. J Allergy Clin Immunol Pract. 2021;9(1):71–80. https://doi.org/10.1016/j.jaip.2020.09.037.
6. Voisin T, Bouvier A, Chiu IV. Neuro-immune interactions in allergic diseases: novel targets for therapeutics. Int Immunol. 2017;29(6):247–61. https://doi.org/10.1093/intimm/dxx040.
7. Ortiz GG, Loera-Rodriguez LH, Cruz-Serrano JA, Torres-Sanchez ED, Mora-Navarro MA, Delgado-Lara DLC, et al. Gut-brain axis: role of microbiota in Parkinson's disease and multiple sclerosis. In: Artis AS, editor. Eat, learn, remember. London: IntechOpen; 2018. p. 11–30. https://doi.org/10.5772/intechopen.79493.
8. Mittal R, Debs LH, Patel AP, Nguyen D, Patel K, O'Connor G, et al. Neurotransmitters: the critical modulators regulating gut-brain axis. J Cell Physiol. 2017;232(9):2359–72. https://doi.org/10.1002/jcp.25518.
9. Klose CSN, Veiga-Fernandes H. Neuroimmune interactions in peripheral tissues. Eur J Immunol. 2021;51:1602–14. https://doi.org/10.1002/eji.202048812.
10. Godinho-Silva C, Cardoso F, Veiga-Fernandes H. Neuro-immune cell units: a new paradigm in physiology. Annu Rev Immunol. 2019;37:19–46. https://doi.org/10.1146/annurev-immunol-042718-041812.
11. Lai NY, Mills K, Chiu IM. Sensory neuron regulation of gastrointestinal inflammation and bacterial host defence. J Intern Med. 2017;282:5–23. https://doi.org/10.1111/joim.12591.
12. Assas BM, Pennock JI, Miyan JA. Calcitonin gene-related peptide is a key neurotransmitter in the neuro-immune axis. Front Neurosci. 2014;8:23. https://doi.org/10.3389/fnins.2014.00023.
13. Auteri M, Zizzo MG, Serio R. GABA and GABA receptors in the gastrointestinal tract: from motility to inflammation. Pharmacol Res. 2015;93:11–21. https://doi.org/10.1016/j.phrs.2014.12.001.
14. Drokhlyansky E, Smillie CS, VanWittenberghe N, Ericsson M, Griffin GK, Eraslan G, et al. The human and mouse enteric nervous system at single-cell resolution. Cell. 2020;182(6):1606–22.e23. https://doi.org/10.1016/j.cell.2020.08.003.
15. Rothenberg ME. An allergic basis for abdominal pain. N Engl J Med. 2021;384:2156–8. https://doi.org/10.1056/NEJMcibr2104146.
16. Carlton SM. Nociceptive primary afferents: they have a mind of their own. J Physiol. 2014;592(16):3403–11. https://doi.org/10.1113/jphysiol.2013.269654.
17. Klimov VV. Skin and mucosal immune system. In: From basic to clinical immunology. Cham: Springer; 2019. https://doi.org/10.1007/978-3-030-0332301_2.
18. Ali A, Tan HY, Kaiko GE. Role of the intestinal epithelium and its interaction with the microbiota in food allergy. Front Immunol. 2020;11:604054. https://doi.org/10.3389/fimmu.2020.604054.
19. Niezgoda M, Kasacka I. Gastrointestinal neuroendocrine cells in various types of hypertension – a review. Prog Health Sci. 2017;7(2):117–25. https://doi.org/10.5604/01.3001.0010.7860.

20. Modasia A, Parker A, Jones E, Stentz R, Brion A, Goldson A, et al. Regulation of enteroendocrine cell networks by the major human gut symbiont Bacteroides thetaiotaomicron. Front Microbiol. 2020;11:575595. https://doi.org/10.3389/fmicb.2020.575595.
21. Walsh KT, Zemper AE. The enteric nervous system for epithelial researchers: basic anatomy, techniques, and interactions with the epithelium. Cell Mol Gastroenterol Hepatol. 2019;8:369–78. https://doi.org/10.1016/j.jcmgh.2019.05.003.
22. Gehart H, van Es JH, Hamer K, Beumer J, Kretzschmar K, Dekkens JF, et al. Identification of enteroendocrine regulators by real-time single-cell differentiation mapping. Cell. 2019;176:1158–73. https://doi.org/10.1016/j.cell.2018.12.029.
23. Chiaranunt P, Tai SL, Ngai L, Mortha A. Beyond immunity: underappreciated functions of intestinal macrophages. Front Immunol. 2021;12:749708. https://doi.org/10.3389/fimmu.2021.749708.
24. Raker VK, Domogalla MP, Steinbrink K. Tolerogenic dendritic cells for regulatory T cell induction in man. Front Immunol. 2015;6:569. https://doi.org/10.3389/fimmu.2015.00569.
25. Tordesillas L, Berin MC. Mechanisms of oral tolerance. Clin Rev Allergy Immunol. 2018;55:107–17. https://doi.org/10.1007/s12016-018-8680-5.
26. Longo G, Berti I, Burks AW, Kraus B, Barbi E. IgE-mediated food allergy in children. Lancet. 2013;382(9905):1656–64. https://doi.org/10.1016/S0140-6736(13)60309-8.
27. Smeekens JM, Immormino RM, Balogh PA, Randell SH, Kulis MD, Moran TP. Indoor dust acts as an adjuvant to promote sensitization to peanut through the airway. Clin Exp Allergy. 2019;49:1500–11. https://doi.org/10.1111/cea.13486.
28. Kulis MD, Smeekens JM, Immormino RM, Moran TP. The airway as a route of sensitization to peanut: an update to the dual allergen exposure hypothesis. J Allergy Clin Immunol. 2021;148(3):689–93. https://doi.org/10.1016/j.jaci.2021.05.035.
29. Han Y, Kim J, Ahn K. Food allergy. Korean J Pediatr. 2012;55(5):153–8. https://doi.org/10.3345/kjp.2012.55.5.153.
30. Jeon YH. Pollen-food allergy syndrome in children. Clin Exp Pediatr. 2020;63(12):463–8. https://doi.org/10.3345/cep.2019.00780.
31. Jeebhay MF, Moscato G, Bang BE, Folleti I, Lipinska-Ojrzanowska LAL, et al. Food processing and occupational respiratory allergy - an EAACI position paper. Allergy. 2019;74:1852–71. https://doi.org/10.1111/all.13807.
32. Pali-Schöll I, Verhoeckz K, Mafra I, Bavaro S, Mills ENC, Monaci L. Allergenic and novel food proteins: state of the art and challenges in the allergenicity assessment. Trends Food Sci Technol. 2019;84:45–8. https://doi.org/10.1016/j.tifs.2018.03.007.
33. Fu L, Cherayil BJ, Shi H, Wang Y, Zhu Y. Allergenicity evaluation of food proteins. In: Food allergy. Singapore: Springer; 2019. p. 93–122. https://doi.org/10.1007/978-981-13-6928-5_5.
34. Hayes M. Allergenicity of food proteins. In: Hayes M, editor. Novel proteins for food, pharmaceuticals and agriculture: sources, applications and advances, Chapter 14. Chichester: Wiley; 2018. https://doi.org/10.1002/9781119385332.ch14
35. De Angelis E, Bavaro SL, Pilolli R, Monaci L. Food and nutritional analysis. Allergenic ingredients. In: Worsfold P, Townshend A, editors. Encyclopedia of analytical science. Amsterdam: Elsevier; 2019. p. 349–73. https://doi.org/10.1016/B978-0-12-409547-2.13957-5.
36. Bannon GA. What makes a food protein an allergen? Curr Allergy Asthma Rep. 2004;4:43–6. https://doi.org/10.1007/s11882-004-0042-0.
37. Verhoeckx KCM, Vissers YM, Baumert JL, Faludi R, Feys M, Flanagan S, et al. Food processing and allergenicity. Food Chem Toxicol. 2015;80:223–40. https://doi.org/10.1016/j.fct.2015.03.005.
38. Francis OL, Wang KY, Kim EH, Moran TP. Common food allergens and cross-reactivity. J Food Allergy. 2020;2(1):17–21. https://doi.org/10.2500/jfa.2020.2.200020.
39. Wang Y-H. Developing food allergy: a potential immunologic pathway linking skin barrier to gut. F1000Res. 2016;5(F1000 Faculty Rev):2660. https://doi.org/10.12688/f1000research.9497.1.

40. Zheng H, Zhang Y, Pan J, Liu N, Qin L, Liu M, Wang T. The role of type 2 innate lymphoid cells in allergic diseases. Front Immunol. 2021;12:586078. https://doi.org/10.3389/fimmu.2021.586078.
41. Wallrapp A, Riesenfeld SJ, Burkett PR, Abdulnour RE, Nyman J, Dionne D, et al. The neuropeptide NMU amplifies ILC2-driven allergic lung inflammation. Nature. 2017;549:351–6. https://doi.org/10.1038/nature24029.
42. Pasha MA, Patel G, Hopp R, Yang Q. Role of innate lymphoid cells in allergic diseases. Allergy Asthma Proc. 2019;40:138–45. https://doi.org/10.2500/aap.2019.40.4217.
43. Abdel-Gadir A, Massoud AH, Chatila TA. Antigen-specific Treg cells in immunological tolerance: implications for allergic diseases. F1000Res. 2018;7:1–13. https://doi.org/10.12688/f1000research.12650.
44. Rivas MN, Burton OT, Rachd R, Chatila TF. Regulatory T cell reprogramming toward a Th2-cell-like lineage impairs oral tolerance and promotes food allergy. Immunity. 2015;42(3):512–23. https://doi.org/10.1016/j.immuni.2015.02.004.
45. Schoos A-MM, Bullens D, Chawes BL, De Vlieger L, DunnGalvin A, Epstein MM, et al. Immunological outcomes of allergen-specific immunotherapy in food allergy. Front Immunol. 2020;11:568598. https://doi.org/10.3389/fimmu.2020.568598.
46. Ramirez DAJ, Bahna SL. Food hypersensitivity by inhalation. Clin Mol Allergy. 2009;7(4):1–6. https://doi.org/10.1186/1476-7961-7-4.
47. Kelleher MM, Tran L, Boyle RJ. Prevention of food allergy - skin barrier interventions. Allergol Int. 2020;69:3–10. https://doi.org/10.1016/j.alit.2019.10.005.
48. van Splunter M, Liu L, van Neerven RJJ, Wichers HJ, Hettinga KA, de Jong NW. Mechanisms underlying the skin-gut cross talk in the development of IgE-mediated food allergy. Nutrients. 2020;12:3830. https://doi.org/10.3390/nu12123830.
49. Shroba J, Barnes C, Nanda M, Chitra CC. Ara h2 levels in dust from homes of individuals with peanut allergy and individuals with peanut tolerance. Allergy Asthma Proc. 2017;38(3):192–6. https://doi.org/10.2500/aap.2017.38.4049.
50. Olivera A, Laky K, Hogan SP, Frischmeyer-Guerreiro P. Editorial: innate cells in the pathogenesis of food allergy. Front Immunol. 2021;2:709991. https://doi.org/10.3389/fimmu.2021.709991.
51. Chinthrajah RS, Hernandes JD, Boyd SD, Galli SJ, Nadeau KC. Molecular and cellular mechanisms of food allergy and food tolerance. J Allergy Clin Immunol. 2016;137(4):984–97. https://doi.org/10.1016/j.jaci.2016.02.004.
52. Sicherer SH, Dampson HA. Food allergy: a review and update on epidemiology, pathogenesis, diagnosis, prevention, and management. J Allergy Clin Immunol. 2018;141(1):41–58. https://doi.org/10.1016/j.jaci.2017.11.003.
53. Canani RB, Paparo L, Nocerino R, Di Scala C, Della Gatta G, Maddalena Y, et al. Gut microbiome as target for innovative strategies against food allergy. Front Immunol. 2019;10:191. https://doi.org/10.3389/fimmu.2019.00191.
54. Iweala OI, Nagler CR. The microbiome and food allergy. Annu Rev Immunol. 2019;37:377–403. https://doi.org/10.1146/annurev-immunol-042718-041621.
55. Mangalam AK, Ochoa-Reparaz JO. Editorial: the role of the gut microbiota in health and inflammatory diseases. Front Immunol. 2020;11:565305. https://doi.org/10.3389/fimmu.2020.565305.
56. Vitetta L, Vitetta G, Hall S. Immunological tolerance and function: associations between intestinal bacteria, probiotics, prebiotics, and phages. Front Immunol. 2018;9:2240. https://doi.org/10.3389/fimmu.2018.02240.
57. Turnbaugh PJ, Ley RE, Hamady M, Fraser-Liggett CM, Knight R, Gordon JI. The human microbiome project. Nature. 2007;449(7164):804–10. https://doi.org/10.1038/nature06244.
58. Shu S-A, Yuen AWT, Woo E, Chu K-H, Kwan H-S, Yang G-X, Yang Y, Leung PSC. Microbiota and food allergy. Clin Rev Allergy Immunol. 2019;57:83–97. https://doi.org/10.1007/s12016-018-8723-y.
59. Palm NW, de Zoete MR, Flavell RA. Immune-microbiota interactions in health and disease. Clin Immunol. 2015;159(2):122–7. https://doi.org/10.1016/j.clim.2015.05.014.

60. Satitsuksanoa P, Jansen K, Głobińska A, van den Veen W, Akdis M. Regulatory immune mechanisms in tolerance to food allergy. Front Immunol. 2018;9:2939. https://doi.org/10.3389/fimmu.2018.02939.
61. Lee KH, Song Y, Wu W, Yu K, Zhang G. The gut microbiota, environmental factors, and links to the development of food allergy. Clin Mol Allergy. 2020;18:2. https://doi.org/10.1186/s12948-020-00120-x.
62. Pascal M, Perez-Gordo M, Caballero T, Escribese MM, Longo MNL, Luengo O, et al. Microbiome and allergic diseases. Front Immunol. 2018;9:1584. https://doi.org/10.3389/fimmu.2018.01584.
63. de Oliveira GLV, Cardoso CRB, Taneja V, Fasano A. Editorial: intestinal dysbiosis in inflammatory diseases. Front Immunol. 2021;12:727485. https://doi.org/10.3389/fimmu.2021.727485.
64. Lo BC, Chen GY, Nuñez G, Caruzo R. Gut microbiota and systemic immunity in health and disease. Int Immunol. 2020;33(4):197–209. https://doi.org/10.1093/intimm/dxaa079.
65. Bryce PJ. Balancing tolerance or allergy to food proteins. Trends Immunol. 2016;37(10):659–67. https://doi.org/10.1016/j.it.2016.08.008.
66. Savidge TC. Epigenetic regulation of enteric neurotransmission by gut bacteria. Front Cell Neurosci. 2016;9:503. https://doi.org/10.3389/fncel.2015.00503.
67. Haahtela T. A biodiversity hypothesis. Allergy. 2019;74(8):1445–56. https://doi.org/10.1111/all.13763.
68. Sikorska-Szaflik H, Sozanska B. Primary prevention of food allergy - environmental protection beyond diet. Nutrients. 2021;13(6):2025. https://doi.org/10.3390/nu13062025.
69. Rosace D, Gomez-Casado C, Fernandez P, Perez-Gordo M, Dominguez MD, Vega A, et al. Profilin-mediated food-induced allergic reactions are associated with oral epithelial remodeling. J Allergy Clin Immunol. 2019;143(2):P681–90.e1. https://doi.org/10.1016/j.jaci.2018.03.013.
70. Keet CA, Wood RA, Matsui EC. Personal and parental nativity as risk factors for food sensitization. J Allergy Clin Immunol. 2012;129(1):169–75. https://doi.org/10.1016/j.jaci.2011.10.002.
71. Jenkinson SE, Whawell SA, Swales BM, Corps EM, Kilshaw PJ, Farthing PM. The aE(CD103) b7 integrin interacts with oral and skin keratinocytes in an E-cadherin-independent manner. Immunology. 2010;132:188–96. https://doi.org/10.1111/j.1365-2567.2010.03352.x.
72. Calvani M, Anania C, Caffarelli C, Martelli A, Miraglia Del Giudice M, Cravidi C, et al. Food allergy: an updated review on pathogenesis, diagnosis, prevention and management. Acta Biomed. 2020;15:91. https://doi.org/10.23750/abm.v91i11-S.10316.
73. Waserman S, Beegin P, Watson W. IgE-mediated food allergy. Allergy Asthma Clin Immunol. 2018;14(2):71–81. https://doi.org/10.1186/s13223-018-0284-3.
74. Eiwegger T, Hung L, San Diego KE, O'Mahony L, Upton J. Recent developments and highlights in food allergy. Allergy. 2019;74(12):2355–67. https://doi.org/10.1111/all.14082.
75. Keet CA, Johnson K, Savage JH, Hamilton RG, Wood RA. Evaluation of *Ara h2* IgE thresholds in the diagnosis of peanut allergy in a clinical population. J Allergy Clin Immunol Pract. 2013;1(1):101–3. https://doi.org/10.1016/j.jaip.2012.08.007.
76. Masthoff LN, Mattsson L, Zuidmeer-Jongjan L, Lidholm J, Andersson K, Akkerdaas JH, et al. Sensitization to *Cor a 9* and *Cor a 14* is highly specific for a hazelnut allergy with objective symptoms in Dutch children and adults. J Allergy Clin Immunol. 2013;132(2):393–9. https://doi.org/10.1016/j.jaci.2013.02.024.
77. Douladiris N, Linhart NB, Swoboda I, Gstottner A, Vassilopolou E, Stolz F, Valenta R, Papadopoulos NG. *In vivo* allergenic activity of a hypoallergenic mutant of the major fish allergen *Cyp c 1* evaluated by means of skin testing. J Allergy Clin Immunol. 2015;136(2):493–5.e8. https://doi.org/10.1016/j.jaci.2015.01.015.
78. Reese G, Schicktanz S, Lauer I, Randow S, Lüttkopf D, Vogel L, Lehrer SB, Vieths S. Structural, immunological and functional properties of natural recombinant *Pen a 1*, the major allergen of Brown Shrimp, *Penaeus aztecus*. Clin Exp Allergy. 2006;36(4):517–24. https://doi.org/10.1111/j.1365-2222.2006.02454.x.

79. Cingolani A, Di Pillo S, Cerasa M, Rapino D, Consilvio NP, Attanasi M, et al. Usefulness of *nBos d 4, 5* and *nBos d 8* specific IgE antibodies in cow's milk allergic children. Allergy Asthma Immunol Res. 2014;6(2):121–5. https://doi.org/10.4168/aair.2014.6.2.121.
80. Chokshi NY, Sicher SH. Molecular diagnosis of egg allergy: an update. Expert Rev Mol Diagn. 2015;15(7):895–906. https://doi.org/10.1586/14737159.2015.1041927.
81. Mumg SHK, Egner W, Shrimpton A, Sargur RB. Using Omega-5 Gliadin (*rTri a 19*) in the diagnosis of anaphylaxis. J Allergy Clin Immunol. 2013;131(I, 2):AB214. https://doi.org/10.1010/j.jaci.2012.12.1434.
82. Koenig JFE, Bruton K, Phelps A, Grydziuszko E, Jimenez-Saiz R, Jordana M. Memory generation and re-activation in food allergy. Immunotargets Ther. 2021;10:171–84. https://doi.org/10.2147/ITT.S284823.
83. Carlson G, Coop C. Pollen food allergy syndrome (PFAS): a review of current available literature. Ann Allergy Asthma Immunol. 2019;123(4):359–65. https://doi.org/10.1016/j.anai.2019.07.022.
84. Leoni C, Volpicella M, Dileo MCD, Gattulli BAR, Ceci LR. Chitinases as food allergens. Molecules. 2019;24(11):2087. https://doi.org/10.3390/molecules24112087.
85. Mansouri M, Rafiee E, Darougar S, Mesdaghi M, Chavoshzadeh Z. Is the atopy patch test reliable in the evaluation of food allergy-related atopic dermatitis? Int Arch Allergy Immunol. 2018;175(1–2):85–90. https://doi.org/10.1159/000485126.
86. Tontini C, Bulfone-Paus S. Novel approaches in the inhibition of IgE-induced mast cell reactivity in food allergy. Front Immunol. 2021;12:613461. https://doi.org/10.3389/fimmu.2021.613461.
87. Chen M, Zhang W, Lee L, Saxena J, Sindher S, Chinthrajah RS, Dant C, Nadeau K. Biologic therapy for food allergy. J Food Allergy. 2020;2(1):86–90. https://doi.org/10.2500/jfa.2020.2.200004.
88. Głobińska A, Boonpiyathad T, Satitsuksanoa P, Kleuskens M, van der Veen W, Sokolowska M, Akdis M. Mechanisms of allergen-specific immunotherapy. Diverse mechanisms of immune tolerance to allergens. Ann Allergy Ashtma Immunol. 2018;121:306–12. https://doi.org/10.1016/j.anai.2018.06.026.
89. Mäntylä J, Thomander T, Hakulinen A, Kukkonen K, Palosuo K, Voutilainen H, Pelkonen A, Kauppi P. The effect of oral immunotherapy treatment in severe IgE mediated milk, peanut, and egg allergy in adults. Immun Inflamm Dis. 2018;6(2):307–11. https://doi.org/10.1002/iid3.218.
90. Nagakura K-I, Sato S, Yanagida N, Nishino M, Asaumi T, Ogura K, Ebisawa M. Oral immunotherapy in Japanese children with anaphylactic peanut allergy. Int Arch Allergy Immunol. 2018;175(3):181–8. https://doi.org/10.1159/000486310.
91. Sampath V, Nadeau KC. Newly identified T cell subsets in mechanistic studies of food immunotherapy. J Clin Invest. 2019;129(4):1431–40. https://doi.org/10.1172/JCI124605.
92. Perkin MR, Logan K, Tseng A, Raji B, Ayis S, Peacock J, et al. Randomized trial of introduction of allergenic foods in breast-fed infants. N Engl J Med. 2016;374(18):1733–43. https://doi.org/10.1056/NEJMoa1514210.
93. Du Toit G, Sampson HA, Plaut M, Burks AW, Akdis CA, Lack G. Food allergy: update on prevention and tolerance. J Allergy Clin Immunol. 2018;141(1):30–40. https://doi.org/10.1016/j.jaci.2017.11.010.
94. Leonard SA. Food allergy prevention, including early food introduction. J Food Allergy. 2020;2(1):69–74. https://doi.org/10.2500/jfa.2020.2.200007.
95. Saidova A, Hershkop AM, Ponce M, Eiwegger T. Allergen-specific T cells in IgE-mediated food allergy. Arch Immunol Ther Exp. 2018;66(3):161–70. https://doi.org/10.1007/s00005-017-0501-7.
96. Valenta R, Karaulov A, Niederberger V, Zhernov Y, Elisyutina O, Campana R, et al. Allergen extracts for *in vivo* diagnosis and treatment of allergy: is there a future? J Allergy Clin Immunol Pract. 2018;6(6):1845–55.e2. https://doi.org/10.1016/j.jaip.2018.08.032.
97. Alcocer MJC, Ares SC, López-Calleja I. Recent advances in food allergy. Braz J Food Technol. 2016;19:e2016047. https://doi.org/10.1590/1981-6723.4716.

98. Poole A, Song Y, O'Sullivan M, Lee KH, Metcalfe J, Guo J, Brown H, Mullins B, Loh R. Children with nut allergies have impaired gene expression of toll-like receptors pathway. Pediatr Allergy Immunol. 2020;31:671–7. https://doi.org/10.1111/pai.13246.
99. Bellanti JA, Settipane RA. Genetics, epigenetics, and allergic disease: a gun loaded by genetics and a trigger pulled by epigenetics. Allergy Asthma Proc. 2019;40(2):73–5. https://doi.org/10.2500/aap.2019.40.4206.
100. Lyons JJ, Milner JD. Primary atopic disorders. J Exp Med. 2018;215(4):1009–22. https://doi.org/10.1084/jem.20172306.
101. Castagnoli R, Lougaris V, Giardino G, Volpi S, Leonardi L, La Torre F, et al. Inborn errors of immunity with atopic phenotypes: a practical guide for allergists. World Allergy Organ J. 2021;14(2):100513. https://doi.org/10.1016/j.waojou.2021.100513.
102. Reber LL, Hernandez JD, Galli SJ. The pathophysiology of anaphylaxis. J Allergy Clin Immunol. 2017;140(2):335–48. https://doi.org/10.1016/j.jaci.2017.06.003.
103. Jiménez-Saiz R, Chu DK, Mandur TV, Walker TD, Gordon ME, Chaudhary R, et al. Lifelong memory responses perpetuate humoral TH2 immunity and anaphylaxis in food allergy. J Allergy Clin Immunol. 2017;140(6):1604–15. https://doi.org/10.1016/j.jaci.2017.01.018.
104. Bruton K, Spill P, Vohra S, Baribeau O, Manzoor S, Gadkar S, et al. Interrupting reactivation of immunological memory reprograms allergy and averts anaphylaxis. J Allergy Clin Immunol. 2021;147(4):1381–92. https://doi.org/10.1016/j.jaci.2020.11.042.
105. Skypala IJ. Food-induced anaphylaxis: role of hidden allergens and cofactors. Front Immunol. 2019;10:673. https://doi.org/10.3389/fimmu.2019.00673.
106. Beck SC, Wilding T, Buka RJ, Baretto RL, Huissoon AP, Krishna MT. Biomarkers in human anaphylaxis: a critical appraisal of current evidence and perspectives. Front Immunol. 2019;10:494. https://doi.org/10.3389/fimmu.2019.00494.
107. Tomar S, Hogan S. Recent advances in mechanisms of food allergy and anaphylaxis. F1000Res. 2020;9:863. https://doi.org/10.12688/f1000research.25638.1.
108. Chen C-S, Barnoud C, Scheiermann C. Peripheral neurotransmitters in the immune system. Curr Opin Physiol. 2021;19:73–9. https://doi.org/10.1016/j.cophys.2020.09.009.
109. Kerage D, Sloan EK, Mattarollo SR, McCombe PA. Interaction of neurotransmitters and neurochemicals with lymphocytes. J Neuroimmunol. 2019;332:99–111. https://doi.org/10.1016/j.jneuroim.2019.04.006.
110. Ozen A, Gulcan EM, Ercan Saricoban H, Ozkan F, Cengizlier R. Food protein-induced non-immunoglobulin E-mediated allergic colitis in infants and older children: what cytokines are involved? Int Arch Allergy Immunol. 2015;168:61–8. https://doi.org/10.1159/000441471.
111. Labrosse R, Graham F, Caubet J-C. Non-IgE-mediated gastrointestinal food allergies in children: an update. Nutrients. 2020;12(7):2086. https://doi.org/10.3390/nu12072086.
112. Díaz JJ, Espín B, Segarra O, Domínguez-Ortega G, Blasco-Alonso J, Cano B, Rayo A, Moreno A. Food protein-induced enterocolitis syndrome. J Pediatr Gastroenterol Nutr. 2019;68:232–6. https://doi.org/10.1097/MPG.0000000000002169.
113. Agyemang A, Novak-Wegrzyn A. Food protein-induced enterocolitis syndrome: a comprehensive review. Clin Rev Allergy Immunol. 2019;57(2):261–71. https://doi.org/10.1007/s12016-018-8722-z.
114. Freeman CM, Murillo JC, Hines BT, Wright BL, Schroeder SR, Bauer CS. Learning early about peanut-triggered food protein-induced enterocolitis syndrome. J Food Allergy. 2021;3(1):32–6. https://doi.org/10.2500/jfa.2021.3.210003.
115. Maciag MC, Bartnikas LM, Sicherer SH, Herbert LJ, Young MC, Matney F, et al. A slice of FPIES (food protein-induced enterocolitis syndrome): insights from 441 children with FPIES as provided by caregivers in the International FPIES Association. J Allergy Clin Immunol Pract. 2020;8(5):1702–9. https://doi.org/10.1016/j.jaip.2020.01.030.

Allergen-Specific Immunotherapy (AIT) 8

Contents

Didactics
Knowledge. Upon successful completion of this chapter, students should be able to:

1. Explain the mechanisms of action of allergen-specific immunotherapy (AIT).
2. Be familiar with the allergen nomenclature.
3. Describe the allergic skin tests and other methods for allergy diagnosis.
4. Outline the main AIT's protocols.
5. Describe indications, contraindications, and side effects of AIT.

Acquired Skills. Upon successful completion of this chapter, students should demonstrate the following skills:

1. Interpret the knowledge related to atopic diseases and their treatment.
2. Critically evaluate the clinical literature about allergens and AIT.
3. Discuss the scientific articles from the current research literature to criticize experimental and clinical data and formulate new hypotheses in allergy.

Supplementary Information The online version contains supplementary material available at [https://doi.org/10.1007/978-3-031-04309-3_8].

V. V. Klimov, *Textbook of Allergen Tolerance*,
https://doi.org/10.1007/978-3-031-04309-3_8

4. Obtain a patient's history, including the history of present illness, past medical history, social, family, and occupational history, and review of systems.
5. Perform a patient's physical examination thoroughly.
6. Explain the rationale for the choice of AIT in a patient.
7. Execute the allergen administration using the simulator.
8. Have a clear perception of the presented immunology definitions expressed orally and in written form.
9. Formulate the presented immunology terms.
10. Correctly answer the quiz questions.

Attitude and Professional Behaviors. Students should be able to:

1. Have the readiness to be hard-working.
2. Behave professionally at all times.
3. Recognize the importance of studying and demonstrate a commitment.
4. Demonstrate the consideration of the patient's feelings, ethnic, religious, cultural, and social background, and display empathy.

8.1 Introduction

▶ **Definition** Allergen-specific immunotherapy (AIT) is a highly effective method of interventional immunology intended to treat atopic diseases.

Allergen-specific immunotherapy (AIT), invented by outstanding British researcher Leonard Noon has been used in healthcare for over 100 years [1]. AIT is not homeopathy. In contrast, this method consists of achieving allergen tolerance in IgE-dependent disorders. AIT helped millions of atopic patients, children, females, and males, and created novel unexpectable trends in medicine. However, some problems remain. First of all, medications for AIT require improvements to significantly shorten such long protocols, with no loss of efficacy. Second, AIT, irrespective of the route of administration, must become completely safe. In the future, AIT medicines will be based on component resolved diagnosis and innovated using modified allergens, a combination of allergens with immunostimulatory adjuvants and biologics, synthetic hypoallergenic peptides, allergens encapsulated in liposomes and VLP (virus-like particles), cell therapy, nucleic acid-based vaccines, recombinant allergen-specific antibodies (for passive immunization), etc. [2–4]. Unfortunately, AIT's impact on the immune system, particularly the neuroimmune network and neurogenic inflammation, remains incompletely understood.

8.2 History of the Invention

Leonard Noon was the only boy in a family of four: his father was a mathematics master at Charterhouse School, and his mother was the sister of a famous housemaster of the same school, and had a sister, Dorothy. To study medicine, Noon (see Fig. 8.1) went up to Cambridge. He had a brilliant career at Cambridge, where he

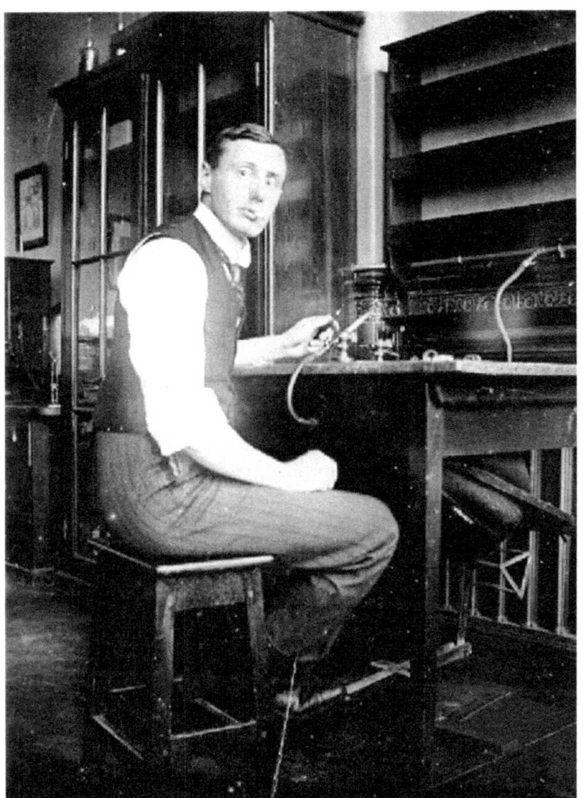

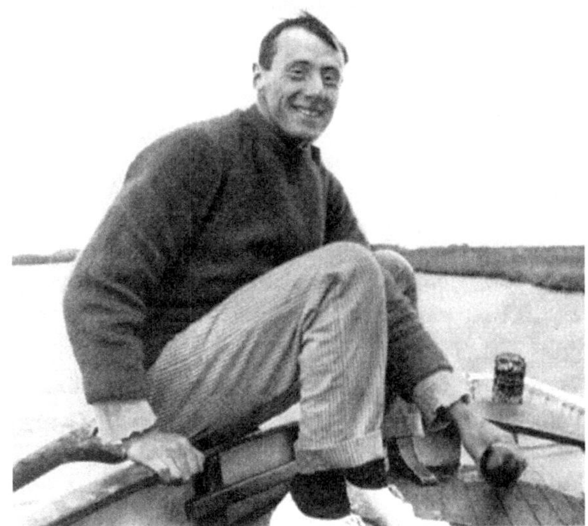

Fig. 8.1 Leonard Noon (1877–1913)

obtained a first-class in both parts of the Natural Science Tripos in 1898 and 1900 and a major scholarship for advanced physiology at Trinity College in 1899. From there, he went for his hospital work at St. Bartholomew's Hospital in London [5]. Then, for the winter of 1905–1906, he worked in the laboratory of Professor Borrel in the winter course on pathogenic bacteria and molds in the Pasteur Institute in Paris.

Together with his friend and coworker, J. Freeman Noon started working hours to immunize guinea pigs against glanders. Professor Borrel surprisingly tolerated this rather unsuitable and dangerous research after he had closely watched this technique. French students were surprised at this method.

When Noon was back in London again, he left his work at St. Bartholomew's and moved to Almroth Wright's laboratory at St. Mary's Hospital. He fell ill with tuberculosis but, having got a taste for research work, did not get away from the laboratory till past midnight and often worked on till three or four in the morning and sometimes till dawn. Noon's interests were very distinct: he was fond of small boat sailing, rowing, rock climbing, and rifle shooting, and was interested in photography and aviation [5]. Noon proved himself a most capable pathologist during the short span of life allotted to him. His work was almost wholly connected with immunity and was of a general theoretical character opening up broad inquiry fields rather than a direct practical application.

However, ideas for possible research on immunization, including treating midsummer hay fever, were very alluring in Almroth Wright's laboratory at that time. His sister, Dorothy Noon, collected grass pollen for him. After some tentative but vital experiments on the specificity of grass pollen for true hay fever, he amply confirmed the initial idea of the immunization. Noon felt worse, began to lose weight, and developed a cough with night temperature; then, he spat up tubercle bacilli and had an acute hemorrhage. After 2 years of bedrest, when he published his remarkable revolutionary article "Prophylactic inoculation against hay fever" in "Lancet" [6], he died in 1913. Long before anti-allergy medications appeared, Noon demonstrated that preventive subcutaneous immunization with grass pollen relieved immediate conjunctival sensitivity to grass pollen. This idea was developed over the following 100 years, and millions of people worldwide were effectively treated for atopic allergic diseases.

In 1930, J. Freeman published the first rush immunotherapy protocol [7], and, in 1954, W. Frankland performed the first controlled clinical trial of pollen immunotherapy [8].

8.3 Rationale of Allergen-Specific Therapy and Future Perspectives

Twenty years ago, the WHO position paper on immunotherapy classified AIT as a treatment form with the highest level of evidence-based medicine and made recommendations regarding the composition and dosing of products for subcutaneous AIT. AIT is a well-documented, safe, effective treatment option for all types of atopic diseases. In contrast to pharmacotherapy, AIT addresses the basic immunopathological mechanisms responsible for disease-modifying and preventing allergic disorders. Therefore, it is the main rationale for allergen-specific immunotherapy in atopic patients.

There are at least seven described routes of allergen administration into the body: subcutaneous [9–11], sublingual [12–14], oral [15–17], epicutaneous [18–20], intradermal [21], intralymphatic [18, 22], and intravaginal (see Chap. 9). Nowadays, two main, well-studied routes of AIT are in use, subcutaneous immunotherapy [9] and sublingual immunotherapy [12]. The third route, oral AIT, has been developing. In World Allergy Organization (WAO) position papers in 2009 and 2014, sublingual AIT was stated to be as effective as subcutaneous AIT but with a better safety profile [23, 24].

So far, we already see the potential future prospects in AIT, such as alternative application routes, immune-modulating adjuvants, allergoids, recombinant vaccines, recombinant allergen-specific antibodies [2, 3, 4, 25, 26], containers for allergens, and cell therapy [27, 28].

Adjuvants, including nanoparticles [29], modify the properties of allergen vaccines modulating allergen delivery and acting as a cumulation depot. Besides, they upregulate Th1-dependent IgG immune responses and limit undesired side effects [26, 30, 31]. The lack of allergenicity of allergoids employed for AIT for a long time allows their recruitment in accelerated up-dosing schemes, shortening the immunotherapeutic protocol [32, 33].

Recombinant hypoallergenic vaccines are engineered to reduce the presence of allergen-specific T cell epitopes and maintain the derivatives' capacity to induce competing IgG antibodies [34, 35]. In the experiment, a hypoallergenic *Ara h 2* mutant with abolished IgE binding and anaphylactogenic ability but retained T cell activation was generated. The approach included the removal of linear and conformational IgE epitopes and the generated mutant did not induce anaphylaxis in peanut-sensitized mice [36].

Passive immunization with recombinant allergen-specific IgG antibodies supported by experimental animal studies allows competition with pathogenic IgE antibodies to reduce allergic inflammation [37]. The principle of virus-like particles (VLPs) uses the intrinsic ability of some viral capsid and envelope proteins to self-organize in VLP without other viral components, including the viral genome [38, 39]. Liposomes are spherical bilipid-layer vesicles engaged for medications, vaccines, and nutrients delivery in the body [40].

Application of novel approaches in creating medications for AIT sometimes excludes allergens themselves. Does it raise an ironic question is the allergen needed in allergy immunotherapy? [41]. Allergens produced by recombinant DNA technology can be used in AIT as unmodified recombinant allergens or hypoallergenic variants with lower IgE reactivity [35]. The classification of major and minor allergens will be outdated since the new molecular era of allergology is commencing [42]. The choice of allergens for AIT will little by little become molecular by the component resolved diagnosis (CRD) contrasted to skin prick testing (SPT) [4, 43].

The oral route of AIT in food allergies is currently at the cutting-edge. The regular oral administration of small but gradually increasing amounts of food allergens is conducted under medical supervision. During the initial dose-escalation, up-dosing every 1–2 weeks, an allergen is taken with food, and physical activity is avoided for 2 h [44]. When the up-dosing period is completed, a daily maintenance dose may be taken at home. However, the oral route induces desensitization, irrespective of whether achievement of persistent tolerance is not yet evident. In the course of oral AIT, mild and moderate adverse reactions are frequent, for example, mouth or throat itching, abdominal pain, but the risk of anaphylaxis and eosinophilic esophagitis exists. At present, oral AIT has not been standardized beyond studies ongoing with peanuts [15, 16, 17, 44, 45]. However, the first publications about the use of allergenic molecules in oral AIT have occurred [46]. In 2020, Food and Drug Administration (FDA) approved the first licensed OIT product for peanut allergy—Palforzia® (Peanut (*Arachis hypogaea*) Allergen Powder-dnfp) [47]. The European Academy of Allergy and Clinical Immunology (EAACI) prepared the guidelines on AIT for IgE-dependent food allergy. Trials have found substantial benefits for cow's milk, hen's eggs, and peanut allergies. AIT with food allergens should only be performed in research or clinical centers with extensive experience in such immunotherapy that patients should frequently visit during up-dosing. Patients must also make an informed decision about the therapy [48].

Epicutaneous immunotherapy is based on the high density of specialized antigen-presenting Langerhans cells in the epidermis that load with an allergen to impact immunity significantly. Simultaneously, it is possible to deliver both allergens and tolerogenic adjuvants [18]. The method may consist of daily exposure to allergens in a new skin patch for maintenance dosing [19]. Since the epidermis is not vascularized, the risk of systemic adverse events is lower than in routine AIT. Epicutaneous AIT demonstrated a more prolonged treatment effect in food allergies. A study of peanut allergic subjects aged 4–25 years showed that treatment with peanut patches was safe and resulted in a modest response after 52 weeks. An increase in peanut-specific IgG_4 levels was observed in peanut-sensitized patients, along with trends toward reduced basophil activation and peanut-specific Th2 cytokines [49].

Intradermal AIT has the potential to the sensitization to inhalant allergens and therefore is not recommended [21].

Intralymphatic immunotherapy includes merely three ultrasound-guided injections of indoor, pollen, and animal allergens at 4-week intervals to the inguinal lymph nodes, making it possible to receive the entire treatment within 2 months. In total, AIT typically requires treatment periods of approximately 3 years [22]. Continuously increasing numbers of published intralymphatic trials are promising, but there is currently insufficient evidence to support its routine use [50].

Subcutaneous immunotherapy [9–11] is the classical therapeutic method in atopic diseases used for over 100 years. There is enormous potential for development in combinations of allergens or allergoids with biologics like omalizumab and a lot of various adjuvants such as recombinant allergens, hypoallergenic variants, conformational variants, deletion mutants, allergen fragmentations, allergen oligomers, and hybrid allergens/mosaic antigens [33, 51]. Although clinical developments were mainly focused on sublingual AIT, increasingly innovative medication developments with the subcutaneous route of administration retake place over the past decade.

Sublingual AIT is mainly indicated for the treatment of respiratory allergies and atopic dermatitis. It exists in the form of tablets and liquid formulations (drops). Both allergen forms are administered under the tongue and held there until swallowed or spat out. The potential for development of sublingual AIT is associated with safety and a low risk of systemic adverse reactions, the provision of long-term posttreatment benefits, expanded list of indications, and absence of necessity to visit the hospital and consult allergists frequently [12, 13]. Therefore, it may quickly expand any modifications with the allergen composition. After 30 years of clinical trials, practical use, and rapid evolution, sublingual AIT remains a good precision medicine paradigm [24].

8.4 Clinical Aspects of AIT's Protocols

▶ **Definition** An adverse reaction is a side effect, which may occur in AIT and require/not require proper treatment and even AIT's discontinuation. Tolerability is the degree to which a person can accept overt adverse effects.

Allergen-specific immunotherapy with regulated standardized allergen extracts is a highly effective and disease-modifying therapeutic method, which can induce long-term remission of atopic conditions. So far, evidence of AIT efficacy and safety have been demonstrated for HDM, grass, birch, ragweed, Japanese cedar, and peanuts. AIT can be administered for 3–5 years with continuing relief of symptoms for years after discontinuation, whereas pharmacotherapy must be continued since it has no disease-modifying activity [52]. It even showed that persons suffering from allergic rhinitis with polysensitization obtained the same benefits and improved quality of life after AIT's 3–5 yearly protocol [53].

These are the following indications of AIT in atopic diseases [9, 24, 53]:

- Pharmacotherapy unable to control the symptoms effectively.
- Serious side effects caused by drug treatment.
- Patients are reluctant to accept continuous or long-term pharmacotherapy.

These are the following contraindications to AIT in atopic diseases:

- Recurrence of atopic allergic conditions
- Uncontrolled, severe asthma
- Severe cardiovascular disorder
- Severe systemic autoimmune diseases
- Psychoses
- Malignant tumors
- Pregnancy at the start of immunotherapy
- Acute infections

Table 8.1 Adverse reactions in the course of AIT by WAO classification [54–58]

Subcutaneous route		Sublingual route	
Grade 0	No side symptoms	Grade I (mild)	Minimal side effects with no troublesome
Grade I	Symptoms present in a single organ like skin itch, non-generalized urticaria, etc.	Grade II (moderate)	Local side effects require symptomatic treatment
Grade II	Symptoms present in more than a single organ like severe cough, chest tightness, etc.	Grade III (severe)	Side effects require the discontinuation of AIT
Grade III	Severe systemic reactions like asthmatic attack, laryngeal edema, etc.		
Grade IV	Anaphylaxis		
Grade V	Death		

In most patients, adverse reactions occur commonly within 30 min after the injection and, depending on severity, can require treatment (see Table 8.1). If they appear or acute infection happens, the allergen's dose must be decreased, or the therapy even temporarily discontinued.

From 2008 to 2013, online surveying elicited information on two fatal reactions in 28.9 million subcutaneous AIT injection visits, and now the rate of systemic reactions has remained steady (0.02%) [52]. Safety continues to be monitored [59].

There were described three cases of severe adverse reactions during AIT [60]. Patients had the cosensitization to *D. pteronissinus* and *L. destructor* (storage mite) defined by the component resolved diagnosis (CRD) study of blood samples; extracts with major HDM allergens (*Der p 1*, *Der p 2*, *Der p 10*, and *Der p 23*) additionally contained the major *L. destructor* allergen, *Lep d 2*. So, the cosensitization to some mites species may play a possible negative role as a risk factor in the course of AIT.

There was an evaluation of 12,546 subcutaneous AIT injections for the 2010–2015-period in 773 atopic patients, Mexico. According to the WAO classification system, 30% of persons had grade I adverse reactions, 67.5% exhibited grade II, and one patient (2.5%) developed grade III adverse effects. No fatal reactions occurred [61].

Starting AIT is commonly recommended for children in different countries from 3 to 5 years [9, 53]. The efficacy of AIT and relevant patient benefit is proven and evident [62]. Unfortunately, low treatment compliance in some children and their parents leads to the destruction of conventional AIT protocols and the achievement of desirable treatment efficacy [63, 64]. Hopefully, the improvement of the intended AIT medicine's quality will significantly shorten the treatment, with no loss of effectiveness. Any medication must not exceed the tolerability of patients, i.e., the degree to which the person can accept overt adverse effects.

Quiz A

Reading a question, please choose only one right answer.

Question 1

Allergen-specific immunotherapy (AIT) is:

1. Homeopathic method.
2. Immunosurgical method for treatment of atopic diseases.
3. Method of interventional immunology intended to treat atopic diseases.
4. Method of pharmacotherapy.

Question 2

AIT currently has a high level of:

1. Expectations.
2. Evidence-based medicine.
3. Tolerability.
4. Noneffectiveness.

Question 3

The purpose of the AIT's future development in atopic diseases is not:

1. To move pharmacotherapy instead.
2. To create a better adverse effect profile.
3. To spread AIT in developing countries.
4. To shorten existing long protocols with no loss of efficacy significantly.

Question 4

The optimal route of AIT in food allergies is:

1. Subcutaneous.
2. Intralymphatic.
3. Sublingual.
4. Oral.

Question 5

Limitations of the oral route of AIT are:

1. Noneffectiveness.
2. A high frequency of adverse effects.
3. A low level of tolerability.
4. Not standardized medicines except for peanuts.

Question 6
Allergen-specific immunotherapy (AIT) was invented by:

1. J. Freeman.
2. L. Noon.
3. C.R. Richet.
4. D. Bovet.

Question 7
An indication to AIT is:

1. Psychoses.
2. Uncontrolled, severe allergic asthma.
3. COVID-19.
4. Atopic disease in remission.

Question 8
A contraindication to AIT is:

1. A low level of compliance.
2. Drug treatment.
3. Malignant tumors.
4. Effective control of the symptoms.

Question 9
Grade II adverse reactions in subcutaneous AIT:

1. Skin itch and non-generalized urticaria.
2. Anaphylaxis.
3. Severe systemic reactions like an asthmatic attack.
4. Severe cough and chest tightness.

Question 10
The most popular route of AIT is currently:

1. Subcutaneous.
2. Intralymphatic.
3. Sublingual.
4. Oral.

Question 11
The potential for the development of sublingual AIT is associated with:

1. A high level of tolerability.
2. A high level of expectations.

3. Encouraging management.
4. Safety and a low risk of systemic adverse reactions.

Question 12
Potential future perspectives in AIT development exist:

1. Yes.
2. No.
3. Possibly.
4. No way.

Question 13
The method AIT has the purpose of achieving:

1. A short-term clinical remission.
2. Relief in an asthmatic attack.
3. Transfer of perennial allergic rhinitis to seasonal form.
4. Allergen tolerance.

Question 14
Are international position papers related to AIT:

1. No.
2. Not yet.
3. Yes.
4. Expected.

Question 15
AIT is commonly recommended for children in different countries:

1. Over 7 years.
2. 3–5 years.
3. From 2 years.
4. In adults only.

Question 16
The desirable duration of AIT is:

1. 2 years.
2. 10 years.
3. 1 year.
4. 3–5 years.

8.5 Protocols of Executing Allergen-Specific Immunotherapy

▶ **Definition** AIT's protocol executes according to AIT established by the international or national position papers.

Previously, a healthcare professional (allergist) prescribes medicine, a route of administration, and a schedule. Before the beginning, patients must make an informed decision about the therapy through discussion with patients, physicians, and caregivers, which is critical for balancing potential therapeutical benefits, compliance, and the risk of AIT-related adverse reactions [47]. At the transition time, before integrating allergenic molecules in practice, only standardized allergen extracts should be used for AIT. A trained nurse executes subcutaneous injections in the allergist's office [52]. After that, a patient must remain under qualified medical observation for at least 30 min before discharge. Monthly patient visits to the hospital for these procedures are mandatory.

Unlike the conventional scheme, there is an alternative regimen of AIT. A high-dose, accelerated escalation schedule is described for the subcutaneous route as well-tolerated in adults and children [65]. If an allergoid is in use, the accelerated schedule consists of repeated high-dose injections with increasing amounts of allergen extracts at intervals of 1 week over a period of 2 weeks at the beginning of an up-dosing period [65]. Cluster, rush, and ultra-rush schedules are modifications of the accelerated escalation scheme, and rush/ultra-rush regimens are more rapid than cluster schedules [56, 66, 67]. These schedules provide significant time benefits over conventional immunotherapy for the patients, are recommended for venom AIT in high-risk people, but have potentially more systemic adverse reactions [67].

Sublingual formulations (drops or tablets) are carried out by a patient at home daily. In the case of adverse effects, the patient should inform the allergist about them.

See some medicines and procedures of executing AIT in Figs. 8.2, 8.3, and 8.4 and Tables 8.2, 8.3, 8.4, and 8.5. There are pictures of demonstration items.

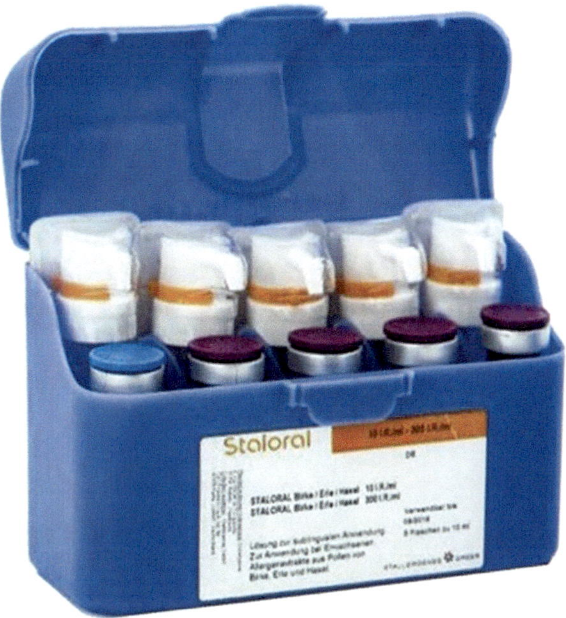

Fig. 8.2 Staloral® sublingual immunotherapy. Birch/Alder/Hazel Allergen extract

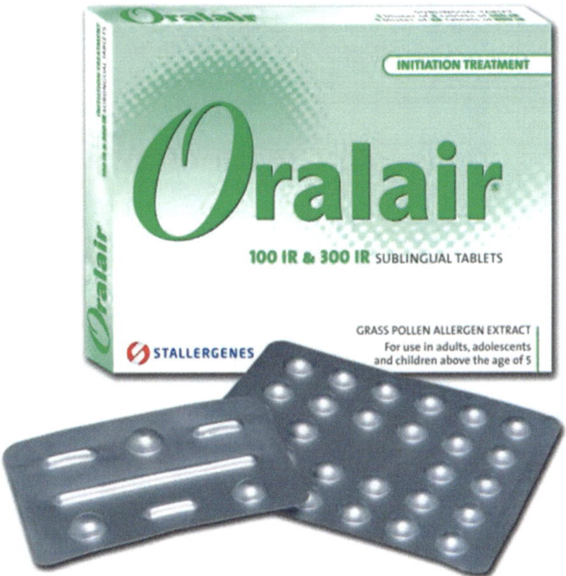

Fig. 8.3 Oralair® Grass Pollen Sublingual extract

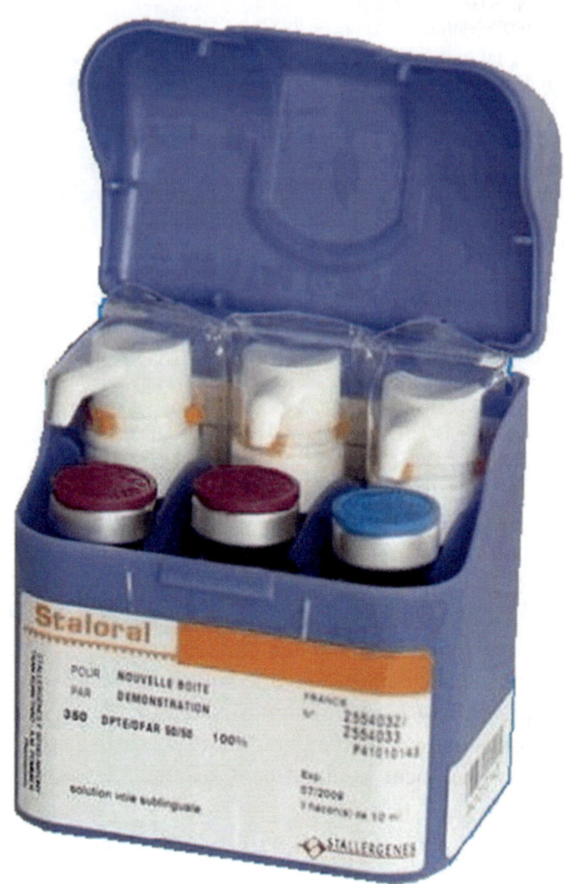

Fig. 8.4 Staloral® sublingual/oral immunotherapy. House Dust Mite allergen extract

Table 8.2 Initial subcutaneously set of ALUSTAL®—House Dust Mite allergen extract [56, 68][a]

ALUSTAL	№ injection	Content	Vial
Initial set	1 2 3 4	Commonly, initial allergen-specific therapy will be weekly injections lasting for about 14 weeks. This will be of the allergen to which a patient is sensitized to in increasing concentrations up to the highest dose he/she can tolerate. Alustal® is given as an injection under the skin (subcutaneously). It is not injected intramuscularly or into a blood vessel. Alustal® in each concentration is injected in the following order: 0.1 mL, 0.2 mL, 0.4 mL, 0.8 mL, depending on the tolerance	0.1 IR/mL (IC/mL) (Yellow cap)
	5 6 7 8		1 IR/mL (IC/mL) (Green cap)
	9 10 11 12 13 14		10 IR/mL (IC/mL) (Blue cap)

IR/mL means the *index of reactivity* per mL (IC/mL is the *index of concentration* per mL)
This AIT protocol is approximate only and may be adapted to the reactivity of each individual
For very sensitive patients, AIT could be initiated with a lower concentration
[a]The protocol description is based on accessible reference sources and presented for educational purposes only

Table 8.3 Maintenance subcutaneously set of ALUSTAL®—House Dust Mite allergen extract [56, 68][a]

ALUSTAL	№ injection	Content	Vial
Maintenance set	15	Maintenance allergen-specific therapy will be one time per 2 weeks, then monthly injections of the highest concentration that the patient can tolerate comfortably. The interval between injections must not exceed 6 weeks. Alustal® is given as an injection under the skin (subcutaneously). It is not injected intramuscularly or into a blood vessel. For example, it is injected by 0.4 mL, 0.5 mL, or 0.6 mL, individually, depending on the tolerance	10 IR/mL (IC/mL) (Blue cap)
	16		
	17		
	18		
	19		
	20		
	21		
	22		
	23		
	24		
	25		
	26		
	27		
	28		
	29		
	30		
	31		
	32		

This AIT protocol is approximate only and may be adapted to the reactivity of each individual
For very sensitive patients, AIT could be initiated with a lower concentration
[a]The protocol description is based on accessible reference sources and presented for educational purposes only

Table 8.4 Maintenance subcutaneously set of ALUSTAL® (ending) [56, 68][a]

ALUSTAL	№ injection	Content	Vial
Maintenance set	33	Maintenance allergen-specific therapy will be of monthly injections of the highest concentration that the patient can tolerate comfortably. The interval between injections must not exceed 6 weeks. Alustal® is given as an injection under the skin (subcutaneously). It is not injected intramuscularly or into a blood vessel. Maintenance AIT should continue for 3–5 years, depending on the severity of the allergy and response to AIT	10 IR/mL (IC/mL) (Blue cap)
	34		
	35		
	36		
	37		
	38		
	39		
	40		
	41		
	42		
	43		
	44		
	45		
	46		
	47		
	48		
	49		
	50		
	51		
	52		
	53		

This AIT protocol is approximate only and may be adapted to the reactivity of each individual
For very sensitive patients, AIT could be initiated with a lower concentration
[a]The protocol description is based on accessible reference sources and presented for educational purposes only

Table 8.5 Initiated and maintenance phases of sublingual AIT with STALORAL® [56, 69][a]

STALORAL	Day	Pressures	Content	Vial
Initial (titration) set	1 2 3 4 5	1 2 3 4 5	Allergen-specific immunotherapy is initiated with a 9-day titration phase with increasing number of pressures, depending on the tolerance, daily. Patients are instructed to deposit the prescribed dose directly under the tongue and keep it there for 2 min before swallowing. 1 pressure (0.2 mL) = 2 IR	10 IR/mL (IC/mL) (Blue cap)
	6 7 8 9	1 2 3 4	Then patients took from 1 to 8 pressures of the 300 IR/mL concentration once daily. Later, AIT is continuing on a perennial schedule. 1 pressure (0.2 mL) = 60 IR	300 IR/mL (IC/mL) (Violet cap)
Maintenance set	Recommended dose of 2–4 pressures daily with the 300/mL IR concentration, i.e., 120–240 IR per day			300 IR/mL (IC/mL) (Violet cap)

This AIT protocol is approximate only and may be adapted to the reactivity of each individual

For very sensitive patients, AIT could be initiated with a lower concentration

[a]The protocol description is based on accessible reference sources and presented for educational purposes only

8.6 Constituting the Allergen Tolerance During AIT

▶ **Definition** The tolerogenic response is an immunologic process leading to the establishment of allergen tolerance.

In developing atopic disease, an adaptive Th2-regulated IgE-mediated response with the participation of innate immunity takes place, resulting in allergen tolerance breakdown. After that, we can see Th2 polarization, constant IgE production, and persistent allergic inflammation. In the recurrence of this disease, the allergen tolerance remains broken down.

In short words, AIT triggers in the immune system tolerogenic response to the causative allergen leading to the Th2 allergen tolerance, IgE antibodies production stopping-off, re-switching to IgG_4 and IgA_2 blocking or competing antibodies [70–73], and forming allergen-specific memory pTregs, T cells, and B cells (see Fig. 8.5)

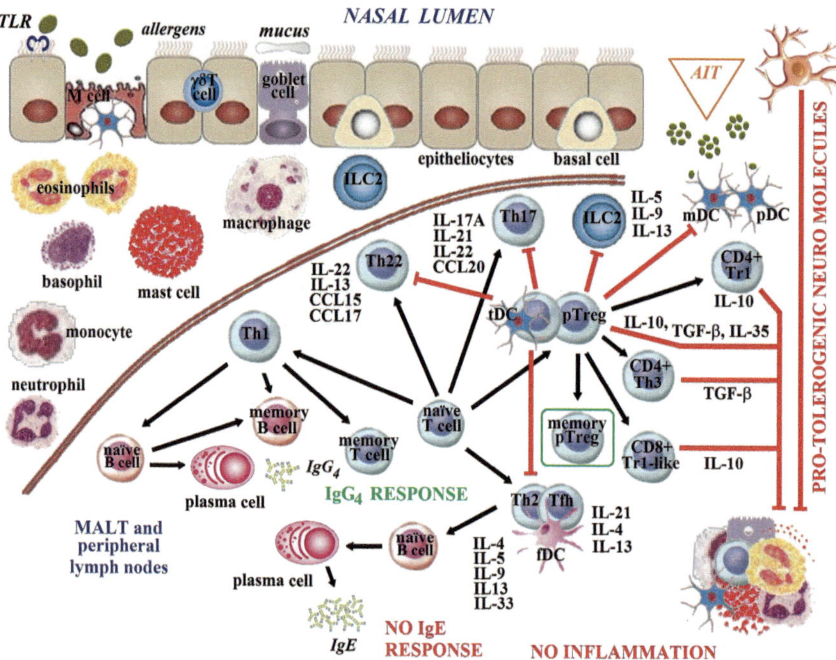

Fig. 8.5 Constituting the allergen tolerance during AIT. At the beginning of AIT, when the allergen doses are low, only tDCs and pTreg occur. Next, all spectrum of pro-tolerogenic cells and molecules, including pTregs subsets, get involved in the process, signs of clinical efficacy appear, and allergen tolerance plus the memory pTreg, B cells, and T cells establish. Finally, all types of helper T cells, ILC2, and inflammatory cells are suppressed, a shift of Th2 to Th1 in part of the control for IgG_4 and IgA_2 synthesis proceeds instead. ILC2 group 2 innate lymphoid cell, mDC myeloid dendritic cell, pDC plasmacytoid DC, tDC tolerogenic DC, Tfh follicular helper T cell, fDC follicular DC, pTreg peripheral Treg cell, Tr1 type 1 regulatory T cell, Th3 type 3 helper T cell

[74, 75]. Notably, AIT's allergen/allergens type does not significantly influence AIT immunologic monitoring [76, 77].

Th2a cells with the unique pathway, or pathogenic (pro-allergic) Th2 cells have recently been identified [78]; they are targeted explicitly by AIT and proposed as a biomarker of successful AIT outcome. It has been found in AIT that pro-allergic Th2a cells are deleted, allowing concurrent downregulating T cell responses to emerge [79]. Another new subset, ILCreg, suppressing T cell activation is demonstrated as a possible promoting factor of AIT-induced tolerance [80].

For the first time, a balance of follicular helper (Tfh) T cells and T follicular regulatory (Tfr) cells in AIT has been studied [81]. Tfh cells are known as pro-immunogenic regulatory cells responsible for the germinal center formation and IgE synthesis maintenance. In contrast, Tfr originated from nTreg cells suppress the germinal centers, Tfh cells, and, accordingly, IgE production. It was found that AIT inhibited Tfh cells and induced Tfr cell population. Furthermore, circulating Tfr cells in patients with allergic rhinitis showed a specific defect in suppressing IgE secretion [82], but this defect and Tfr function improved after AIT.

The sequence of changing immunologic parameters in AIT is the following. In the beginning, partial allergen tolerance is already forming due to the transitory increase in two principal pro-tolerogenic cells, tDCs and pTregs, that may be characterized as a low-dose T-dependent tolerance with the absence of any clinical efficacy [83]. The whole spectrum of pro-tolerogenic cells and molecules is little by little commencing to turn on to mid-year [84–90], causing the stimulation of Th1 cells in a part of upregulating re-switching antibody isotype from IgE to IgG_1, IgG_4, and IgA_2. In responsive persons, the IgE level is initially elevated but returns to the baseline after the first year of the immunotherapy. The IgG_4 is enhanced, but an increase in IgG_4 stabilizes after the second year [87]. However, early insignificantly increased blocking antibody titers do not correlate with clinical AIT efficacy yet [71].

By the first year-end and later, immunosuppressive cytokines, IL-10, TGF-β, IL-27, IL-35, and IL-10-secreting Bregs have been increasing, inhibiting Th2, Tfh, Th17, and ILC2 cells. Notably, Bregs enhance earlier than pTregs [91], reaching the maximum after the second year [87]. On the other hand, a medium level of pTregs is observed after 30-week immunotherapy, continuing to increase, slightly declining by the end of the third year of AIT [87].

Thus, during shaping allergen tolerance in AIT, blocking IgG_4 antibodies increase to 12 months and stabilize after the second year, whereas IgE antibodies initially enhance and diminish after the first year. Regulatory B (Bregs) cells reach a high level at the end of the second year, but regulatory T (pTregs) cells significantly increase from the 30-week therapy and for the second and third years, slightly declining by the third year-end [87].

Monitoring immunologic parameters in AIT showed a slight difference between the response to *Der p 1* and *Der p 2*. From baseline to the first year-end, a statistically significant increase in serum IL-10 was observed, but IL-4, IL-13, and IFN-γ remained unchanged [77]. In another group of researchers, the serum IFN-γ level was increased after 1-, 6-, and 12-month subcutaneous but not sublingual AIT, and, conversely, the IL-10 value did not change [92]. In the third group, it has been found that *Der p 1*-specific IL-10 and IL-22 responses increased after 30 weeks [93].

In addition, three types of allergen-specific memory cells are shaped when AIT is completed [74, 75]:

1. memory pTregs,
2. memory T cells upregulating IgG/IgA synthesis, and
3. memory B cells responsible for the proliferation of daughter plasma cells secreting IgG/IgA.

During the AIT course, an analysis of the systemic innate immune cell composition has been performed. In the first year, the repertoire of immature dendritic cells changed, namely an increase in CD141+mDC-1 and pDC was observed, whereas CD1c+mDC-2 level was reduced. Group 2 ILC decreased and group 1 ILC enhanced replacing ILC2 after 12 months of AIT. This ILC subsets change remained stable even in the third year. In addition, AIT did not affect the content of circulating NK cells, diminished HLA-DR++ nonclassical monocytes, and increased the level of HLA-DR^{lo} intermediate monocytes [94]. It is known that monocytes are currently divided into classical (80–90%), intermediate (5–10%), and nonclassical (5–10%) subsets [95], and all of them can take part in allergic inflammation.

The research on neuro molecules in AIT has not been carried out yet, but protolerogenic neurotransmitters and neuropeptides may also participate in the tolerogenic process [96], exerting the following known effects. Norepinephrine suppresses Th2, ILC2, and eosinophils; CGRP downregulates ILC2 inactivating alarmins, IL-25, IL-31, TSLP; oxytocin and VIP inhibit macrophages; serotonin downregulates Th17, ILC2, and macrophages; GABA inhibits Th17.

From a theoretical viewpoint, after completing AIT, the established allergen tolerance, a form of immune tolerance, may be characterized as the long-term T cell dependent state [83, 86, 97], the unresponsiveness to the causative allergen.

In the AIT experiment, a first group of mice was sensitized with *rMet e 1* (shrimp allergen) orally with a high dose, a second group received a medium dose, and a third group got a low dose. All groups were desensitized, regardless of the dose, but mice in the first group experienced severe systemic reactions during AIT. In the second and third groups, the *FoxP3 gene* was expressed, and pTregs and associated cytokines upregulated [98].

The problem of biomarkers of successful AIT remains unsolved but known and new parameters were proposed for this purpose [99–102]. However, most researchers postulate no reliable and invariable biomarkers predicting AIT efficacy [103, 104].

Shamji et al. [87, 105] substantiated the following group of biomarkers of successful AIT:

1. specific IgE/total IgE ratio,
2. IgG-subclasses such as $sIgG_1$ and $sIgG_4$, including $sIgE/IgG_4$ ratio,
3. serum inhibitory activity for IgE: IgE-blocking factor (IgE-BF) and IgE-facilitated antigen binding to B cells (IgE-FAB),
4. basophil activation test,
5. cytokines and chemokines,
6. cellular markers (Tregs, Bregs, and DCs), and
7. *in vivo* biomarkers such as provocation tests.

In a study however the levels of IgE-blocking factor (IgE-BF) and IgE-facilitated antigen binding to B cells (IgE-FAB) did not correlate with clinical improvements after subcutaneous AIT [106]. So the reliability of this biomarker appeared to be inconsistent.

An interesting study has been carried out. CD25+CD71+CD73$^-$ Breg cells secreting IL-10 are increased following AIT inhibiting allergen-specific CD4+ T cells within the next weeks of the up-dosing period (the first year of AIT), whereas FoxP3+ pTreg cells are expected to enhance in a significant amount only after 3 years of AIT. At the same time, the known tolerance biomarker, ratio of Th17/pTreg, was changing to convert Th17 into the transitory phenotype FoxP3+IL-17$^-$, and later fully pTreg cells [91]. The ratio of Th17/Breg taken after the up-dosing period might be a new prognostic biomarker correlating with AIT success. This new biomarker is awaiting to be validated in larger cohorts. Therefore, there is still no answer to the question of whether this marker is helpful. Hopefully, this parameter will serve as predicting biomarkers of AIT's efficacy [91].

The enhanced serum LTA_4H level was identified as a new diagnostic candidate biomarker for predicting AIT outcomes in patients with *Artemisia* sensitization. Proteomics analysis and ELISA were used in persons evaluated on a uniform standard. The LTA_4H level increased in a more effective AIT and diminished at risk for AIT failure [101]. Another study considered fundamental relevant aspects, including the molecular IgE-repertoire, the potency of effector cells, the kinetics of allergen degradation and absorption, allergen-specific T cell reactivity capacity, genes/methylations, and the state of the gut microbiome [102]. In the third study, the authors developed a new application of computational approaches to select relevant biomarkers in AIT in peanut and cow's milk allergies [107].

A typically lifelong allergic disease requires some form of immunologic memory. For the first time, using single B cell technology, the cellular and clonal origin of IgE memory responses following mucosal allergen administration in sublingual AIT was studied. It found that on mucosal allergen exposure, allergen-specific IgE memory resides in allergen-specific IgG+ memory B cells. By necessity, B cells rapidly switch isotype and expand into short-lived IgE+ plasmablasts. Of course, it may explain an initial increase in IgE at the beginning of AIT. However, this event is unexpected and can serve as a potential target and new biomarker for sublingual AIT [108].

In the last decade, innovative approaches to AIT have overcome existing problems in standardization, safety, long protocol duration, efficacy, and costs, but some challenges remain. AIT modifies allergen-specific memory T cells and B cells, regulates allergen-specific IgE and IgG production, involves regulatory T (Treg) cells, and changes mast cell and basophil activation thresholds as well as dendritic cell phenotypes [80]. Immunoglobulin and T cell receptor transcript repertoires and epigenetic changes may be a source of new predictive biomarkers for AIT monitoring, and omic technologies drive the identification of these new biomarkers [109].

Key Points

1. Over 100 years ago, Dr. L. Noon invented allergen-specific immunotherapy (AIT), which became the most promising therapeutic method for atopic diseases. AIT is classified as a treatment modality with the highest level of evidence-based medicine.
2. Nowadays, AIT efficacy and safety are demonstrated in double-blind, multicenter, placebo-controlled studies, and protocols of executing this immunotherapy and clinical comments were established and approved in the international position papers. Subcutaneous and sublingual AIT methods are used worldwide, whereas oral, epicutaneous, and intralymphatic routes of allergen administration have been developing and accumulating evidence for their routine use. The advantages of AIT exceed those in pharmacotherapy.
3. AIT constitutes the long-term T cell-dependent allergen tolerance and allergen-specific memory regulatory T cells in patients with almost all kinds of atopic conditions. During AIT, an increase in IgG_4 blocking antibodies, pTregs, and Bregs and a decrease in IgE occur.

Take-Home Messages

1. Write an essay about Leonard Noon.
2. Write a flyer about allergens' routes of administration.
3. Write an essay about innovations in AIT.
4. Make a slide presentation about subcutaneous AIT protocol.
5. Make a slide presentation about sublingual AIT protocol.
6. Write a paragraph about indications of AIT in atopic diseases.
7. Write a paragraph about contraindications to AIT in atopic diseases.
8. List possible adverse reactions in the course of AIT.
9. Write a flyer about the frequency of allergen uptake depending on a route of administration.
10. Write a paragraph about allergen extracts and allergenic molecules for AIT.
11. List biomarkers before and after AIT completion.

Quiz B

Reading a question, please choose only one right answer.

Question 1

Allergen-specific immunotherapy (AIT) was invented by:

1. C.R. Richet.
2. J. Freeman.
3. L. Noon.
4. D. Bovet.

Question 2

The purpose of the AIT's development in atopic diseases is not:

1. To spread AIT in developing countries.
2. To create a better adverse effect profile.
3. To move pharmacotherapy instead.
4. To shorten existing long protocols with no significant loss of efficacy.

Question 3

AIT currently has a high level of evidence-based medicine:

1. Not yet.
2. Yes.
3. It has been expected.
4. No way.

Question 4

This route of AIT is not recommended for use:

1. Subcutaneous.
2. Intradermal.
3. Sublingual.
4. Oral.

Question 5

The oldest, to a more significant extent, studied route of AIT is:

1. Oral.
2. Intralymphatic.
3. Sublingual.
4. Subcutaneous.

Question 6

An indication to AIT is:

1. Atopic disease in remission.
2. Uncontrolled, severe allergic asthma.
3. Malignant tumors.
4. Severe systemic autoimmune diseases.

Question 7

A contraindication to AIT is:

1. Patients are reluctant to accept continuous or long-term pharmacotherapy.
2. Serious side effects caused by drug treatment.
3. Acute infections.
4. Pharmacotherapy unable to control the symptoms effectively.

Question 8

Grade III adverse reactions in subcutaneous AIT:

1. Anaphylaxis.
2. Skin itch and non-generalized urticaria.
3. Severe systemic reactions like an asthmatic attack.
4. Severe cough and chest tightness.

Question 9

During the maintenance phase of subcutaneous AIT, subcutaneous injections are executed:

1. Daily.
2. Monthly.
3. Weekly.
4. Bimonthly (one time per 2 months).

Question 10

During the maintenance phase of sublingual AIT, administration of allergen is executed:

1. Two times per day.
2. Monthly.
3. Weekly.
4. Daily.

Question 11

Immunologic efficacy of AIT is associated with:

1. Establishing allergen-specific memory Treg cells.
2. Th2-dependent response.
3. Immunoregulation by Tfh cells.
4. Inhibiting Th3 cells.

Question 12
Immunosuppressive cytokines are:

1. IL-10, IL-27, IL-35, and TGF-β.
2. IFN-γ, TNF-β, and IL-2.
3. TNF-β, IL-1, and GM-CSF.
4. IL-4, IL-5, and IL-13.

Question 13
The most potent immunosuppressive cytokine is:

1. IL-35.
2. TGF-β.
3. IL-27.
4. IL-10.

Question 14
The tolerogenic response is:

1. Immunologic process is characterized by sensitization.
2. Immunologic process leading to forming allergen tolerance.
3. Inhibition of pTreg cells.
4. Inhibition of tDCs.

Question 15
Allergen-specific immunotherapy (AIT) is:

1. Method of pharmacotherapy.
2. Immunosurgical method for treatment of atopic diseases.
3. Method of interventional immunology intended to treat atopic diseases.
4. Homeopathic method.

Question 16
In AIT, Th1 cells operate with re-switching antibody isotype from IgE to:

1. IgD.
2. IgM.
3. IgD and IgM.
4. IgG4 and IgA2.

References

1. Durham S, Nelson H. Allergen immunotherapy: a centenary celebration. World Allergy Organ J. 2011;4(6):104–6. https://doi.org/10.1097/WOX.0b013e3182218920.
2. Pfaar O, Lou H, Zhang Y, Klimek L, Zhang L. Recent developments and highlights in allergen immunotherapy. Allergy. 2018;73:2274–89. https://doi.org/10.1111/all/13652.
3. Gunawardana NC, Durham SR. New approaches to allergen immunotherapy. Ann Allergy Asthma Immunol. 2018;121:293–305. https://doi.org/10.1016/j.anai.2018.07.014.
4. Akinfenwa O, Rodriguez-Dominguez A, Vrtala S, Valenta R, Campana R. Novel vaccines for allergen-specific immunotherapy. Curr Opin Allergy Clin Immunol. 2021;21(1):86–99. https://doi.org/10.1097/ACI.0000000000000706.
5. Freeman J. Leonard Noon. Int Arch Allergy Appl Immunol. 1953;4:282–4.
6. Noon L, Cantab BC. Prophylactic inoculation against hay fever. Lancet. 1911;177(4580):1572–3. https://doi.org/10.1016/s0140-6736(00)78276-6.
7. Freeman J. Rush inoculation with special reference to hay fever treatment. Lancet. 1930;1:744.
8. Frankland AW, Augustin R. Prophylaxis of summer hayfever and asthma: controlled trial comparing crude grass pollen extracts with isolated main protein component. Lancet. 1954;1:1055.
9. Klimek L, Brehler R, Hamelmann E, Kopp M, Ring J, Treudler R, et al. Development of subcutaneous allergen immunotherapy (part 2): preventive aspects and innovations. Allergo J Int. 2019;28:107–19. https://doi.org/10.1007/s40629-019-0097-z.
10. Vogelberg C, Brueggenjuergen B, Richter H, Jutel M. Impact of subcutaneous allergoid AIT on patients with allergic rhinitis and/or asthma: a retrospective real-life, long-term cohort analysis. Eur Respir J. 2020;56:243. https://doi.org/10.1183/13993003.congress-2020.243.
11. Castro-Almarales RL, Ronquillo-Díaz M, Álvarez-Castelló M, Rodríguez-Canosa J, González-León M, Enríquez-Domínguez I, et al. Subcutaneous allergen immunotherapy for asthma: a randomized, double-blind, placebo-controlled study with a standardized *Blomia tropicalis* vaccine. World Allergy Organ J. 2020;13:100098. https://doi.org/10.1016/j.waojou.2020.100098.
12. Ohashi-Doi K, Lund K, Mitobe Y, Okamiya K. State of the art: development of a sublingual allergy immunotherapy tablet for allergic rhinitis in Japan. Biol Pharm Bull. 2020;43(1):41–8.
13. Caffarelli C, Mastrorilli C, Procaccianti M, Santoro A. Use of sublingual immunotherapy for aeroallergens in children with asthma. J Clin Med. 2020;9:3381. https://doi.org/10.3390/jcm9103381.
14. Lin SY, Erekosima N, Kim JM, Ramanathan M, Suarez-Cuervo Y, Yohalakshmi C, Ward D, Segal JB, et al. Sublingual immunotherapy for the treatment of allergic rhinoconjunctivitis and asthma: a systematic review. JAMA. 2013;309(12):1278–88. https://doi.org/10.1001/jama.2013.2049.
15. Głobińska A, Boonpiyathad T, Satitsuksanoa P, Kleuskens M, van der Veen W, Sokolowska M, Akdis M. Mechanisms of allergen-specific immunotherapy. Diverse mechanisms of immune tolerance to allergens. Ann Allergy Asthma Immunol. 2018;121:306–12. https://doi.org/10.1016/j.anai.2018.06.026.
16. Mäntylä J, Thomander T, Hakulinen A, Kukkonen K, Palosuo K, Voutilainen H, Pelkonen A, Kauppi P. The effect of oral immunotherapy treatment in severe IgE mediated milk, peanut, and egg allergy in adults. Immun Inflamm Dis. 2018;6(2):307–11. https://doi.org/10.1002/iid3.218.
17. Nagakura K-I, Sato S, Yanagida N, Nishino M, Asaumi T, Ogura K, Ebisawa M. Oral immunotherapy in Japanese children with anaphylactic peanut allergy. Int Arch Allergy Immunol. 2018;175(3):181–8. https://doi.org/10.1159/000486310.
18. Wang Y, Kong Y, Wu MX. Innovative systems to deliver allergen powder for epicutaneous immunotherapy. Front Immunol. 2021;12:647954. https://doi.org/10.3389/fimmu.2021.647954.

19. Liu G, Liu M, Wang J, Mou Y, Che H. The role of regulatory T cells in epicutaneous immunotherapy for food allergy. Front Immunol. 2021;12:660974. https://doi.org/10.3389/fimmu.2021.660974.
20. Chow TG, Parrish C, Bird JA. Food allergy: epicutaneous immunotherapy. J Food Allergy. 2020;2(1):81–5. https://doi.org/10.2500/jfa.2020.2.200016.
21. Slovick A, Douiri A, Muir R, Guerra A, Tsioulos K, Hay E, et al. Intradermal grass pollen immunotherapy increases TH2 and IgE responses and worsens respiratory allergic symptoms. J Allergy Clin Immunol. 2017;139:1830–9.e13. https://doi.org/10.1016/j.jaci.2016.09.024.
22. Senti G, Freiburghaus A, Larenas-Linnemann D, Hoffmann HJ, Patterson AM, Klimek L, et al. Intralymphatic immunotherapy: update and unmet needs. Int Arch Allergy Immunol. 2019;178:141–9. https://doi.org/10.1159/000493647.
23. Canonica GW, Bousquet J, Casale T, Lockey RF, Baena-Cagnani CE, Pawankar R, et al. Sublingual immunotherapy: World Allergy Organization Position Paper. Allergy. 2009;64(Suppl 91):1–59. https://doi.org/10.1111/j.1398-9995.2009.02309.x.
24. Passalacqua G, Bagnasco D, Canonica GW. 30 years of sublingual immunotherapy. Allergy. 2020;75:1107–20. https://doi.org/10.1111/all.14113.
25. Machado OLT, Campos-Mesquita DM, Pacheco-Soares T. Antihistaminic treatment, allergen-specific immunotherapy, and blockade of IgE as alternative allergy treatments. In: Athari SS, editor. Allergen, Chapter 4. London: IntechOpen; 2017. p. 67–75. https://doi.org/10.5772/intechopen.69912.
26. Jensen-Jarolim E, Roth-Walter F, Jordakieva G, Pali-Schöll I. Allergens and adjuvants in allergen immunotherapy for immune activation, tolerance, and resilience. J Allergy Clin Immunol. 2021;9(5):1780–9. https://doi.org/10.1016/j.jaip.2020.12.008.
27. Baranyi U, Farkas AM, Hock K, Mahr B, Linhart B, Gattringer M, et al. Cell therapy for prophylactic tolerance in immunoglobulin E-mediated allergy. EBioMedicine. 2016;7:230–9. https://doi.org/10.1016/j.ebiom.2016.03.028.
28. Esmaeilzadeh E, Tahmasebi S, Athari SS. Chimeric antigen receptor - T cell therapy: applications and challenges in treatment of allergy and asthma. Biomed Pharmacother. 2020;123:109685. https://doi.org/10.1016/j.biopha.2019.109685.
29. Johnson L, Duschl A, Himly M. Nanotechnology-based vaccines for allergen-specific immunotherapy: potentials and challenges of conventional and novel adjuvants under research. Vaccine. 2020;8:237. https://doi.org/10.3390/vaccines8020237.
30. Klimek L, Schmidt-Weber CB, Kramer MF, Skinner MA, Heath MD. Clinical use of adjuvants in allergen-immunotherapy. Expert Rev Clin Immunol. 2017;13(6):599–610. https://doi.org/10.1080/1744666X.2017.1292133.
31. Kirtland ME, Tsitoura DC, Durham SR, Shamji MH. Toll-like receptor agonists as adjuvants for allergen immunotherapy. Front Immunol. 2020;11:599083. https://doi.org/10.3389/fimmu.2020.599083.
32. Oliver CE. The use of allergoids and adjuvants in allergen immunotherapy. Arch Asthma Allergy Immunol. 2017;1:040–60. https://doi.org/10.29328/journal.haard.1001006.
33. Klimek L, Fox GC, Thum-Oltmer S. SCIT with a high-dose house dust mite allergoid is well tolerated: safety data from pooled clinical trials and more than 10 years of daily practice analyzed in different subgroups. Allergo J Int. 2018;27(5):131–9. https://doi.org/10.1007/s40629-018-0059-x.
34. Valenta R, Campana R, Focke-Tejkl M, Niederberger V. Vaccine development for allergen-specific immunotherapy based on recombinant allergens and synthetic allergen peptides: lessons from the past and novel mechanisms of action for the future. J Allergy Clin Immunol. 2016;137(2):351–7. https://doi.org/10.1016/j.jaci.2015.12.1299.
35. Nandy A, Creticos PS, Häfner D. Recombinant allergens in specific immunotherapy. In: Kleine-Tebbe J, Jakob T, editors. Molecular allergy diagnostics. Cham: Springer; 2017. https://doi.org/10.1007/978-3-319-42499-6_26.
36. Tsheppe A, Palmberger D, van Rijt L, Kalic T, Mayr V, Palladino C, et al. Development of a novel Ara h 2 hypoallergen with no IgE binding or anaphylactogenic activity. J Allergy Clin Immunol. 2019;145(1):229–38. https://doi.org/10.1016/j.jaci.2019.08.036.

37. Orengo JM, Radin AR, Kamat V, Badithe A, Ben LH, Bennett BL, et al. Treating cat allergy with monoclonal IgG antibodies that bind allergen and prevent IgE engagement. Nat Commun. 2018;9:1421. https://doi.org/10.1038/s41467-018-03636-8.
38. Klimov VV. Vaccination. In: From basic to clinical immunology. Cham: Springer; 2019. https://doi.org/10.1007/978-3-030-0332301_8.
39. Klimek L, Kündig T, Kramer M, Guethoff S, Jensen-Jarolim E, Schmidt-Weber C, et al. Virus-like particles (VLP) in prophylaxis and immunotherapy of allergic diseases. Allergo J Int. 2018;27(8):245–55. https://doi.org/10.1007/s40629-018-0074-y.
40. López RR, Ocampo I, Sánchez L-M, Alazzam A, Bergeron K-F, Camacho-León S, et al. Surface response based modeling of liposome characteristics in a periodic disturbance mixer. Micromachines (Basel). 2020;11(3):235. https://doi.org/10.3390/mi11030235.
41. Kündig TM, Klimek L, Schendzielorz P, Renner WA, Senti G, Bachmann MF. Is the allergen really needed in allergy immunotherapy? Curr Treat Options Allergy. 2015;2:72–82. https://doi.org/10.1007/s40521-014-0038-5.
42. Caraballo L, Valenta R, Acevedo N, Zakzuk J. Are the terms major and minor allergens useful for precision allergology? Front Immunol. 2021;12:651500. https://doi.org/10.3389/fimmu.2021.651500.
43. Matricardi PM, Dramburg S, Potapova E, Skevaki C, Renz H. Molecular diagnosis for allergen immunotherapy. J Allergy Clin Immunol. 2018;143(3):P831–43. https://doi.org/10.1016/j.jaci.2018.12.1021.
44. Feuille E, Nowak-Wegrzyn A. Allergen-specific immunotherapies for food allergy. Allergy Asthma Immunol Res. 2018;10(3):189–206. https://doi.org/10.4168/aair.2018.10.3.189.
45. Schoos A-MM, Bullens D, Chawes BL, De Vlieger L, DunnGalvin A, Epstein MM, et al. Immunological outcomes of allergen-specific immunotherapy in food allergy. Front Immunol. 2020;11:568598. https://doi.org/10.3389/fimmu.2020.568598.
46. Fuhrmann V, Huang H-J, Akarsu A, Shilovskiy I, Elisyutina O, Khaitov M, et al. From allergen molecules to molecular immunotherapy of nut allergy: a hard nut to crack. Front Immunol. 2021;12:742732. https://doi.org/10.3389/fimmu.2021.742732.
47. Sood AK, Scurlock AM. Food allergy oral immunotherapy. J Food Allergy. 2020;2(1):75–80. https://doi.org/10.2500/jfa.2020.2.200005.
48. Pajno GB, Fernandez-Rivas M, Arasi S, Roberts G, Akdis CA, Alvaro-Lozano M, et al. EAACI guidelines on allergen immunotherapy: IgE-mediated food allergy. Allergy. 2018;73(4):799–814. https://doi.org/10.1111/all.13319.
49. Jones SM, Sicherer SH, Burks AW, et al. Epicutaneous immunotherapy for the treatment of peanut allergy in children and young adults. J Allergy Clin Immunol. 2017;139(4):1242–52.e9. https://doi.org/10.1016/j.jaci.2016.08.017.
50. Lee SP, Choi SJ, Joe E, Lee SM, Lee MW, Shim JW, et al. A pilot study of intralymphatic immunotherapy for house dust mite, cat, and dog allergies. Allergy Asthma Immunol Res. 2017;9:272–7. https://doi.org/10.4168/aair.2017.9.3.272.
51. Tonti E, Larché M. Concepts and perspectives on peptide-based immunotherapy in allergy. Allergo J Int. 2016;25:144–53. https://doi.org/10.1007/s40629-016-0121-5.
52. Wise SK, Lin SY, Toskala E, Orlandi RR, Akdis AA, Alt JA, et al. International consensus statement on allergy and rhinology: allergic rhinitis. Int Forum Allergy Rhinol. 2018;8(2):108–352. https://doi.org/10.1002/alr.22073.
53. Bao Y, Chen J, Cheng L, Guo Y, Hong S, Kong W, et al. Chinese guideline on allergen immunotherapy for allergic rhinitis. J Thorac Dis. 2017;9(11):4607–50. https://doi.org/10.21037/jtd.2017.10.112.
54. Robertson K, Montazeri N, Shelke U, Jeimy S, Kim H. A single centre retrospective study of systemic reactions to subcutaneous immunotherapy. Allergy Asthma Clin Immunol. 2020;16:93. https://doi.org/10.1186/s13223-020-00491-5.
55. Cox L, Larenas-Linnemann D, Lockey RF, Passalacqua G. Speaking the same language: The World Allergy Organization subcutaneous immunotherapy systemic reaction grading system. J Allergy Clin Immunol. 2010;125(3):569–74.e1–7. https://doi.org/10.1016/j.jaci.2009.10.060.

56. Cox L, Nelson H, Lockey R, Contributors W. Allergen immunotherapy: a practice parameter third update. J Allergy Clin Immunol. 2011;127(suppl 1):S1–55. https://doi.org/10.1016/j.jaci.2010.09.034.
57. Epstein TG, Calabria C, Cox LS, Dreborg S. Current evidence on safety and practical considerations for administration of sublingual allergen immunotherapy (SLIT) in the United States. J Allergy Clin Immunol Pract. 2017;5(1):34–40.e2. https://doi.org/10.1016/j.jaip.2016.09.017.
58. Lim CE, Sison CP, Ponda P. Comparison of pediatric and adult systemic reactions to subcutaneous immunotherapy. J Allergy Clin Immunol Pract. 2017;5(5):1241–7.e2. https://doi.org/10.1016/j.jaip.2017.01.014.
59. Huang Y, Wang C, Wang X, Zhang L, Lou H. Efficacy and safety of subcutaneous immunotherapy with house dust mite for allergic rhinitis: a meta-analysis of randomized controlled trials. Allergy. 2019;74(1):189–92. https://doi.org/10.1111/all.13583.
60. Arroabarren E, Echechipía S, Galbete A, Lizaso MT, Olaguibel JM, Tabar AI. Association between component-resolved diagnosis of house dust mite allergy and efficacy and safety of specific immunotherapy. J Investig Allergol Clin Immunol. 2019;29(2):164–7. https://doi.org/10.18176/jiaci.0359.
61. Molina-Sáenz MM, Villa-Arango AM, Cardona-Villa R. Safety of subcutaneous immunotherapy with tyrosine-adsorbed house dust mite extracts in patients with allergic disease. Rev Alerg Mex. 2017;64:52–65.
62. Blome C, Hadler M, Karagiannis E, Kirsch J, Neht C, Kressel N, Augustin M. Relevant patient benefit of sublingual immunotherapy with birch pollen allergen extract in allergic rhinitis: an open, prospective, non-interventional study. Adv Ther. 2020;37:2932–45. https://doi.org/10.6084/m9.figshare.12091017.
63. Novak NM, Buhl T, Pfaa O. Adherence during early allergen immunotherapy and strategies to motivate and support patients. Eur Med J. 2018;3(3):21–9.
64. Aytekin ES, Soyer Ö, Şekerel BE, Şahiner ÜM. Subcutaneous allergen immunotherapy in children: real life compliance and effect of COVID-19 pandemic on compliance. Int Arch Allergy Immunol. 2021;182:631–6. https://doi.org/10.1159/000514587.
65. Bovermann X, Ricklefs I, Vogelberg C, Klimek L, Kopp MV. Accelerated dose escalation with 3 injections of an aluminum hydroxide-adsorbed allergoid preparation of 6 grasses is safe for children and adolescents with moderate to severe allergic rhinitis. Int Arch Allergy Immunol. 2021;182:524–34. https://doi.org/10.1159/000512561.
66. Martínez FJS, Piñana VL, González-Mancebo E, Villajos IS-G, García-González F, Sánchez-Hernández C, et al. Observational study on the tolerability of cluster subcutaneous immunotherapy in patients with rhinoconjunctivitis with or without asthma sensitized to pollen: The SIMO study. Saf Health. 2018;4:6. https://doi.org/10.1186/s40886-018-0074-0.
67. Fokkens W, van Maaren M, Wolvers M, van Wijk RG. Rush immunotherapy with multiple aeroallergens is safe in an adult population. Rhinol Online. 2018;1:35–7. https://doi.org/10.4193/RHINOL/18.019.
68. Alustal House Dust Mites Extract initial treatment set. 2019. https://www.healthdirect.gov.au/medicines/brand/amt,63041000168103/alustal-house-dust-mites-extract-initial-treatment-set.
69. Staloral. Evidence is difference. Sublingual solution of allergen extracts for immunotherapy. Monograph. Stallergenes; 2011. p. 1–68.
70. Acosta GS, Kinaciyan T, Kitzmüller C, Möbs C, Pfützner W, Bohle B. IgE-blocking antibodies following SLIT with recombinant *Mal d 1* accord with improved apple allergy. J Allergy Clin Immunol. 2020;146(4):894–900.e2. https://doi.org/10.1016/j.jaci.2020.03.015.
71. Huber S, Lang R, Steiner M, Aglas L, Ferreira F, Wallner M, et al. Does clinical outcome of birch pollen immunotherapy relate to induction of blocking antibodies preventing IgE from allergen binding? A pilot study monitoring responses during first year of AIT. Clin Transl Allergy. 2018;8:39. https://doi.org/10.1186/s13601-018-0226-7.

72. Hoh RA, Joshi SA, Liu Y, Wang C, Roskin KM, Lee J-Y, et al. Single B-cell deconvolution of peanut-specific antibody responses in allergic patients. J Allergy Clin Immunol. 2016;137(1):157–67. https://doi.org/10.1016/j.jaci.2015.05.029.
73. Gotoh M, Kaminuma O. Sublingual immunotherapy: how sublingual allergen administration heals allergic diseases; current perspective about the mode of action. Pathogens. 2021;10:147. https://doi.org/10.3390/pathogens10020147.
74. Gratz IK, Campbell DJ. Organ-specific and memory Treg cells: specificity, development, function, and maintenance. Front Immunol. 2014;5:333. https://doi.org/10.3389/fimmu.2014.00333.
75. Yao Y, Wang N, Chen C-L, Pan L, Wang Z-C, Yunis J, et al. CD23 expression on switched memory B cells bridges T-B cell interaction in allergic rhinitis. Allergy. 2020;75(10):2599–612. https://doi.org/10.1111/all.14288.
76. Rhyou H-I, Nam Y-H. Efficacy of allergen immunotherapy for allergic asthma in real world practice. Allergy Asthma Immunol Res. 2020;12(1):99–109. https://doi.org/10.4168/aair.2020.12.1.99.
77. Justicia JL, Padrò C, Roger A, Moreno F, Rial MJ, Parra A, et al. Immunological parameters as biomarkers of response to microcrystalline tyrosine-adjuvanted mite immunotherapy. World Allergy Organ J. 2021;14(6):1000545. https://doi.org/10.1016/j.waojou.2021.100545.
78. Wambre E, Bajzik V, DeLong JH, O'Brien K, Nguyen Q-A, Speake C, et al. A phenotypically and functionally distinct human TH2 cell subpopulation is associated with allergic disorders. Sci Transl Med. 2017;9(401):eaam9171. https://doi.org/10.1126/scitranslmed.aam9171.
79. Wambre E. Effect of allergen-specific immunotherapy on CD4+ T cells. Curr Opin Allergy Clin Immunol. 2015;15(6):581–7. https://doi.org/10.1097/ACI.0000000000000216.
80. Komlósi ZI, Kovács N, Sokolowska M, van de Veen W, Akdis M, Akdis CA. Mechanisms of subcutaneous and sublingual aeroallergen immunotherapy. What is new? Immunol Allergy Clinics. 2020;40(1):P1–14. https://doi.org/10.1016/j.iac.2019.09.009.
81. Schulten V, Tripple V, Seumois G, et al. Allergen-specific immunotherapy modulates the balance of circulating Tfh and Tfr cells. J Allergy Clin Immunol. 2018;141(2):775–7.e6. https://doi.org/10.1016/j.jaci.2017.04.032.
82. Yao Y, Wang Z-C, Wang N, Zhou P-C, Chen C-L, Song J, et al. Allergen immunotherapy improves defective follicular regulatory T cells in patients with allergic rhinitis. J Allergy Clin Immunol. 2019;144(1):118–28. https://doi.org/10.1016/j.jaci.2019.02.008.
83. Matsuoka T, Shaji MH, Durham SR. Allergen immunotherapy and tolerance. Allergol Int. 2013;62:403–13. https://doi.org/10.2332allergolint.13-RAI-0650.
84. Steveling-Klein EH. Allergen-specific immunotherapy. Eur Med J. 2016;1(4):78–87.
85. Akdis M, Akdis CA. Mechanisms of allergen-specific immunotherapy: multiple suppressor factors at work in immune tolerance to allergens. J Allergy Clin Immunol. 2014;133:621–31. https://doi.org/10.1016/j.jaci.2013.12.1088.
86. Kucuksezer UC, Ozdemir C, Cevhertas L, Ogulur I, Akdis M, Akdis CA. Mechanisms of allergen-specific immunotherapy and allergen tolerance. Allergol Int. 2020;69(4):549–60. https://doi.org/10.1016/j.alit.2020.08.002.
87. Drazdauskaitè G, Layhadi JA, Shamji MH. Mechanisms of allergen immunotherapy in allergic rhinitis. Curr Allergy Asthma Rep. 2021;21:2. https://doi.org/10.1007/s11882-020-00977-7.
88. Wisniewski J, Agrawal R, Woodfolk JA. Mechanisms of tolerance induction in allergic disease: integrating current and emerging concepts. Clin Exp Allergy. 2013;43(2):164–76. https://doi.org/10.1111/cea.12016.
89. Calzada D, Baos S, Cremades-Jimeno L, Cardaba B. Immunological mechanisms in allergic diseases and allergen tolerance: the role of Treg cells. J Immunol Res. 2018;2018:6012053. https://doi.org/10.1155/2018/6012053.
90. van de Veen W, Akdis M. Tolerance mechanisms of allergen immunotherapy. Allergy. 2019;75(5):1017–8. https://doi.org/10.1111/all.14126.
91. Zissler UM, Schmidt-Weber CB. Predicting success of allergen-specific immunotherapy. Front Immunol. 2020;11:1826. https://doi.org/10.3389/fimmu.2020.01826.

92. Xian M, Feng M, Dong Y, Su Q, Li J. Changes in CD4+CD25+FoxP3+ regulatory T cells and serum cytokines in sublingual and subcutaneous immunotherapy in allergic rhinitis with or without asthma. Int Arch Allergy Immunol. 2020;181(1):71–80. https://doi.org/10.1159/000503143.
93. Boonpiyathad T, Sokolowska M, Morita H, Ruckert B, Kast JI, Wawrzyniak M, et al. Der p 1-specific regulatory T-cell response during house dust mite allergen immunotherapy. Allergy. 2019;74(5):976–85. https://doi.org/10.1111/all.13684.
94. Eljaszewicz A, Ruchti F, Radzikowska U, Globinska A, Boonpiyathad T, Gschwend A, et al. Trained immunity and tolerance in innate lymphoid cells, monocytes, and dendritic cells during allergen-specific immunotherapy. J Allergy Clin Immunol. 2021;147:1865–77.
95. Guilliams M, Mildner A, Yona S. Developmental and functional heterogeneity of monocytes. Immunity. 2018;49:595–613. https://doi.org/10.1016/j.immuni.2018.10.005.
96. Kerage D, Sloan EK, Mattarollo SR, McCombe PA. Interaction of neurotransmitters and neurochemicals with lymphocytes. J Neuroimmunol. 2019;332:99–111. https://doi.org/10.1016/j.jneuroim.2019.04.006.
97. Zouali M. Immunological tolerance: mechanisms. In: eLS. Paris: Wiley; 2007. p. 1–9. https://doi.org/10.1002/9780470015902.a0000950.pub2.
98. Leung NYH, Wai CYY, Shu SA, Chang CC, Chu KH, Leung PSC. Low-dose allergen-specific immunotherapy induces tolerance in a murine model of shrimp allergy. Int Arch Allergy Immunol. 2017;174:86–96. https://doi.org/10.1159/000479694.
99. Ciprandi G, Silvestri M. Serum specific IgE: a biomarker of response to allergen immunotherapy. J Investig Allergol Clin Immunol. 2014;24(1):35–9.
100. Kouser L, Kappen J, Walton RP, Shamji MH. Update on biomarkers to monitor clinical efficacy response during and post treatment in allergen immunotherapy. Curr Treat Options Allergy. 2017;4:43–53. https://doi.org/10.1007/s40521-017-0117-5.
101. Ma T-T, Cao M-D, Yu R-L, Shi H-Y, Yan W-J, Liu J-G, et al. Leukotriene A4 hydrolase is a candidate predictive biomarker for successful allergen immunotherapy. Front Immunol. 2020;11:559748. https://doi.org/10.3389/fimmu.2020.559746.
102. Czolk R, Klueber J, Sørensen M, Wilmes P, Codreanu-Morel F, Skov PS, et al. IgE-mediated peanut allergy: current and novel predictive biomarkers for clinical phenotypes using multi-omics approaches. Front Immunol. 2021;11:594350. https://doi.org/10.3389/fimmu.2020.594350.
103. Sindher SB, Long A, Acharya S, Sampath V, Nadeau KC. The use of biomarkers to predict aero-allergen and food immunotherapy responses. Clin Rev Allergy Immunol. 2018;55:190–204. https://doi.org/10.1007/s12016-018-8678-z.
104. Hardy LC, Smeekens JM, Kullis MD. Biomarkers in food allergy immunotherapy. Curr Allergy Asthma Rep. 2019;19(12):61. https://doi.org/10.1007/s11882-019-0894-y.
105. Shamji MH, Kappen JH, Akdis M, Jensen-Jarolim E, Knol E, Kleine-Tebbe J, et al. Biomarkers for monitoring clinical efficacy of allergen immunotherapy for allergic rhinoconjunctivitis and allergic asthma: an EAACI position paper. Allergy. 2017;72(8):1156–73. https://doi.org/10.1111/all.13138.
106. Wang W, Yin J, Wang X, Ma T, Lan T, Song Q, Guo Y. Relationship between serum inhibitory activity for IgE and efficacy of Artemisia pollen subcutaneous immunotherapy for allergic rhinitis: a preliminary self-controlled study. Allergy Asthma Clin Immunol. 2020;16:18. https://doi.org/10.1186/s13223-020-0416-4.
107. van Bilsen JHM, Verschuren L, Wagenaar L, Vonk MM. A network-based approach for identifying suitable biomarkers for oral immunotherapy of food allergy. BMC Bioinformatics. 2019;20(1):206. https://doi.org/10.1186/s12859-019-2802-9.
108. Hoof I, Schulten V, Layhadi JA, Stranzl T, Christensen LH, de la Mata SH, et al. Allergen-specific IgG+ memory B cells are temporally linked to IgE memory responses. J Allergy Clin Immunol. 2020;146(1):180–91. https://doi.org/10.1016/j.jaci.2019.11.046.
109. van Zelm MC, McKenzie CI, Varese N, Rolland JM, O'Hehir RE. Recent developments and highlights in immune monitoring of allergen immunotherapy. Allergy. 2019;74:2342–54. https://doi.org/10.1111/all.14078.

Allergen Tolerance in the Genitourinary Tract

9

Contents

Didactics

Knowledge. Upon successful completion of this chapter, students should be able to:

1. List the clinical types of sperm allergic reactions.
2. Be familiar with the definitions of allergic inflammation in the vagina.
3. Differentiate these definitions.
4. Describe innervation of the genitourinary tract in both females and males.
5. Draw clinical symptoms of sperm allergies.
6. List the prevalent forms of allergic disorders in the female genitourinary tract.
7. Describe allergic inflammation in sperm allergies.
8. List clinical symptoms of vulvodynia.

Acquired Skills. Upon successful completion of this chapter, students should demonstrate the following skills:

Supplementary Information The online version contains supplementary material available at [https://doi.org/10.1007/978-3-031-04309-3_9].

V. V. Klimov, *Textbook of Allergen Tolerance*,
https://doi.org/10.1007/978-3-031-04309-3_9

1. Interpret the knowledge related to the neuroimmune system of the vagina and penis.
2. Critically evaluate the clinical literature about sperm allergy.
3. Discuss the scientific articles from the current research literature to criticize clinical data concerning sperm allergy.
4. Obtain a patient's history, including the history of present illness, past medical history, social, family, and occupational history, and review of systems of patients with food allergy.
5. Perform a patient's physical examination thoroughly.
6. Explain the rationale for the choice of diagnosis of chronic vulvovaginitis in a patient.
7. Have a clear perception of the presented allergology definitions expressed orally and in written form.
8. Formulate the presented immunology and allergy terms.
9. Correctly answer the quiz questions.

Attitude and Professional Behaviors. Students should be able to:

1. Have the readiness to be hard-working.
2. Behave professionally at all times.
3. Recognize the importance of studying and demonstrate a commitment.
4. Demonstrate the consideration of the patient's feelings, ethnic, religious, cultural, and social background, and display empathy.

9.1 Introduction

The vagina and penis are target organs for allergic inflammation and adaptive immune responses to both allergens and infectious agents. In atopic individuals, an allergic reaction in these peripheral genital organs is often accompanied by other allergic manifestations throughout the body, like asthma, allergic rhinitis, etc. Innervation peculiarities in the vagina and penis predispose to allergic inflammation plus "neurogenic inflammation" and painful intercourse. Microbiota of genitals of both genders plays an essential role either in the immune homeostasis or in microbial imbalance that involves pathogen-associated molecular patterns (PAMPs) via toll-like receptors (TLRs) in processes in this area, facilitates allergen tolerance breakdown, and evokes such uncommon regional disorders as sperm allergy, vulvodynia, chronic vulvovaginitis, etc.

9.2 Neuroimmune System of the Genitourinary Tract

The mucosal immune system of the genitourinary tract has some peculiarities, as follows [1, 2]:

- The absence of organized lymphoid follicles in the distal part of the genitourinary tract
- The predominance of IgG over sIgA in lumen's secretions *(IgG > sIgA)*
- Regulatory influence of sex hormones

The proximal part is supported by the gut-associated lymphoid tissue (GALT).

Normal vaginal microbiota includes Döderlein's flora, which consists of *Lactobacteria spp*, including *Lactobacillus acidophilus* [3, 4]. *Lactobacteria* are the most important mutualistic microbes producing lactic acid and hydrogen peroxide that decrease vaginal pH and protect the female genitourinary tract against the colonization of pathogenic species, performing the tolerogenic function. In healthy females, *Lactobacteria* must make up 10^8–10^{12} CFU/mL or not less than 80–95% of the vaginal microbial mass. If this parameter is lower, bacterial vaginosis occurs. In female urethra, *Lactobacillus spp*, *Prevotella spp*, and *Streptococcus spp* are predominant [5].

In uncircumcised men, normal urethral microbiota contains *Prevotella spp*, *Porphyromonas spp*, *Anaerococcus spp*, *Streptococcus spp*, and *Finegoldia spp*; in circumcised men, normal urethral microbiota includes *Corynebacterium spp*, *Staphylococcus spp*, and *Gardnerella spp* (less anaerobic bacteria) [6]. Regardless of circumcision, *Prevotella spp*, *Streptococcus spp*, and *Corynebacterium spp* are prevalent in male urethra [5]. The composition of penile microbiota can influence the incidence of bacterial vaginosis in female sex partners [7].

The lumens of the vagina, cervix, and urethra represent the secretory effector sites of the mucosal immune system (see Fig. 9.1). A non-keratinized stratified squamous epithelium covers distal parts of the genitourinary tract in women and uncircumcised men. CD8aa+ γδT cells are in-built in the epithelium, which expresses TLR. This type of epithelium enables the production of mucus as a factor of innate immunity [1–3]. Autonomic efferent innervation to the upper two-thirds of the vagina proceeds through the uterovaginal plexus (sympathetic and parasympathetic fibers). Autonomic efferent innervation to the lower vagina is carried via the pudendal nerve [8].

A keratinized stratified squamous epithelium covers the glans penis in circumcised men, exhibiting another factor of innate immunity, keratinization. Uncircumcised males lack this protective factor. If keratinization is taken into consideration, the foreskin is the "Achilles' heel" of male innate immunity. Under the epithelial cover, there are many immune system cells, including macrophages, NK

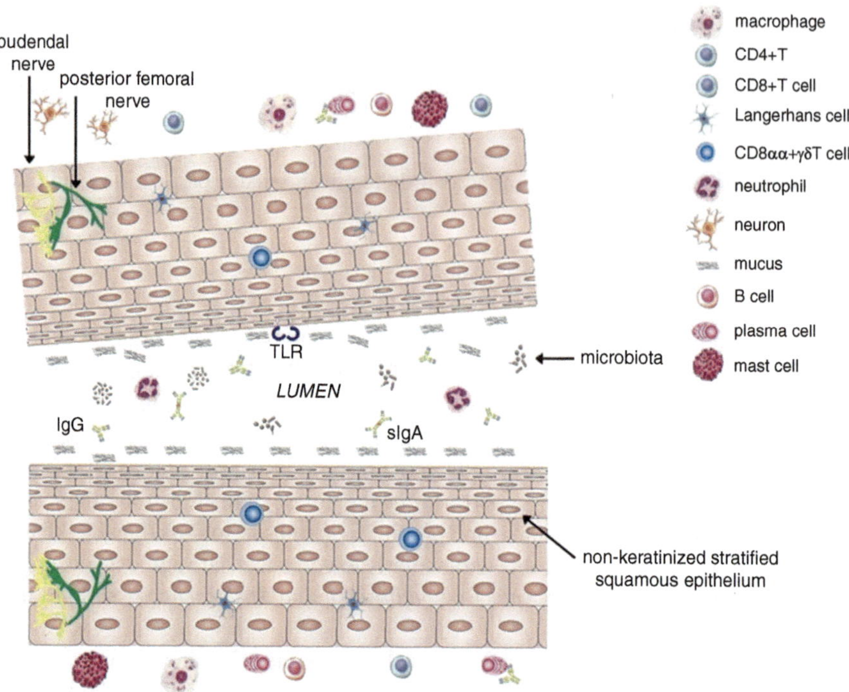

Fig. 9.1 Neuroimmune system of the vagina. The vaginal walls are covered by non-keratinized stratified squamous epithelium, contain immune cells, and are innervated by the uterovaginal plexus and pudendal nerve. The vaginal lumen is rich in microbiota, mainly Döderlein's flora, mucus, antimicrobial peptides, IgG, and sIgA, expressed by epithelium pattern recognition receptors (PRRs), including toll-like receptors (TLRs)

cells, dendritic cells, CD4+ T cells, CD8+ T cells, etc., which take part in immune processes. It is the inductive site of the genitourinary tract. The cells function here and may migrate to the draining inguinal lymph nodes [1, 2]. The penis is innervated by the dorsal nerve, pudendal nerve, and cavernous nerve.

In women and men, the genitourinary neuroimmune system is coordinated by the same neuro molecules: neurotransmitters (dopamine, serotonin, norepinephrine, and GABA), neuropeptides (opioids), neurohormones (vasopressin and oxytocin), and neurotrophins, including the nerve growth factor (NGF) [8–11].

From a clinical viewpoint, any imbalances in the mucosal immune system, in both females and males, promote various genitourinary tract diseases. Bacterial vaginosis in women increases the transmission risk of sexually transmitted infections, including *HIV*, and the risk of preterm birth in pregnant women. More severe problems are chronic recurrent colpitis, cervicitis, and pelvic inflammatory disease, including abscesses. There may be an elevated transmission risk of sexually transmitted infections to sexual partners in males, chronic recurrent urethritis, prostatitis, epididymitis, and oligozoospermia.

9.3 Allergic Reactions to Sperm Allergens

▶ **Definition** Sperm allergy means the different allergic disorders caused by sperm allergens accumulated in the vagina or affected glans penis.

The first publication about sperm allergy was written in 1958 in the Dutch language [12]. Atopic individuals, females, heterosexual males, and males who have sex with men may respond to allergens of the seminal plasma [13–17]. It is known that they develop the following rare disorders:

1. Acute local reactions (burning semen syndrome, skin rash, localized urticaria, etc.) [18, 19]
2. Postorgasmic illness syndrome [20–23]
3. Generalized urticaria and angioedema [13, 15, 24]
4. Anaphylaxis [15, 24]

They are mainly IgE-dependent, but in local allergic reactions to sperm, both IgE-mediated and type IV hypersensitivity mechanisms may happen [25]. A possible link was reported between localized semen allergy and type IV hypersensitivity [26]. Defining type I hypersensitivity to seminal fluid-free spermatozoa is performed by skin prick testing (SPT) [27]. However, most cases of allergic diseases in the genital area remain undetected [28].

The prevalence, incidence, pathophysiology, and prognosis of sperm allergy are unrecognized and are not studied [14, 29]. The local allergic response to sperm commonly occurs within 30 min post-coitus and presents frequently the *early-phase* atopy manifested by the following symptoms: vaginal burning, itching, local urticaria, and redness in females, and glans penis burning in males. Notably, allergy to one's own sperm exists in males. Attempts of AIT with autologous sperm in sexual partner pairs with *semen burning syndrome* (Gulf War veterans' families) were published [18].

Patients can also show systemic reactions such as wheezing, shortness of breath, severe cough, dizziness, and anaphylaxis [15, 24]. A case history of a patient who developed anaphylaxis after anal intercourse has been published, although this patient never manifested sperm allergies after vaginal coitus. SPT with sperm showed a highly positive result. This case exhibits that the route of exposure to sperm may play a role in developing allergen tolerance or sperm allergies, including anaphylaxis [30].

Postorgasmic illness syndrome presents combining of both the *early-phase* atopy and *late-phase* atopy inflammation-based conditions in males. Symptoms can begin right away after ejaculation, include flu-like syndrome, headache, myalgia, local allergic reactions in the eyes, nose, and throat, and last for 2–7 days [20–23, 31]. Successful AIT attempts with diluted autologous sperm in males are described [32, 33].

The seminal fluid and spermatozoa contain an extensive array of glycoproteins, which take part in multiple functions. One group of the seminal proteins is engaged in metabolism, regulating osmotic pressure and pH of seminal plasma, transport of ions, lipid, and hormones. The second group is involved in immune responses mainly directed against female's immunity that is essential for spermatozoa survival and fertilization. However, the allergenicity properties of seminal proteins are not studied [34, 35]. Schjenken and Robertson [36] suppose that semen in the female oviduct has one more function, signaling to choose the best father. The pool of pTregs is expanded that assists implantation by suppressing inflammation, mediating tolerance to male transplantation antigens, and promoting uterine vascular adaptation and placental development.

On the other hand, semen, particularly in HIV-positive males, is a mixture containing anti-inflammatory (TGF-β and IL-10) and pro-inflammatory cytokines (IL-8, CCL-2 (MCP-1), and CCL-5 (RANTES)), prostaglandin E_2 and enzymes with the potential to alter the immune environment of the lower female reproductive tract. Cervicovaginal epithelial cells respond with significantly elevated levels of IL-6, IL-8, TNF-β, and CCL2 (MCP-1), create genital inflammation and predisposition to any pathology [37].

In atopic individuals, some sperm proteins may trigger allergic sensitization and subsequent clinical manifestation. The main criteria for the diagnosis of sperm allergy is the absence of allergic symptoms when condoms, particularly made of lambskin, are used during intercourse, determination of negative skin prick testing with suspect allergens, and a low concentration of allergen-specific serum IgE [15]. Sperm allergy in women may also be evoked by a male's consumption of food allergic products or drug allergens if a female is atopic and sensitized to these allergens.

To define the possible allergen as causative in a case of sperm allergy, Weidinger et al. [38] carried out the study of samples of female's blood and male's seminal plasma and spermatozoa, and SPTs, and assessed the results.

Initially, total serum IgE to seminal plasma was 1412 kU/L. SPTs showed positive reactions to 1:2, 1:4, 1:16, and 1:160 dilutions of her husband's seminal plasma, but not to the spermatozoa. After a subcutaneous AIT attempt, specific serum IgE against seminal plasma was 4.27 kU/L, positive SPT reactions against seminal plasma could be observed up to a dilution of 1:10. However, at this time, clinical manifestations took place. By Western blotting, prostate-specific antigen (PSA) has been separated from seminal plasma. After additional lab procedures, the results strongly demonstrated that PSA was selectively recognized by IgE antibodies contained in the patient's serum. Together, PSA could be identified as the causative allergen as strongly indicated by positive SPT, immunoblotting, cellular antigen stimulation, and basophil activation test. Therefore, human PSA may be a key culprit in IgE-mediated vaginal reactions to semen [38]. Interestingly, PSA carries a high homology to the canine prostatic kallikrein (*Can f 5*) [16]. Later in Japan, clinically relevant cross-reactivity has been described between *Can f 5* (serum specific IgE was 28.1 kU/L) and human PSA in atopic women [39].

An immunologic study was carried out on 19 women with semen allergy, localized and systemic forms. Skin prick testing (SPT) with medium-molecular weight seminal plasma proteins (SSP) was positive. In female blood, increased IgE to male SPP, higher in systemic reactions, was revealed. The whole seminal plasma-derived PSA, the known sperm allergen, significantly inhibited binding IgE to whole seminal plasma only in systemic reactions, demonstrating the presence of functional SPP-specific IgE in women with systemic reactions [40].

The link between sexual behaviors and IgE-dependent hypersensitivity may account for unusual or unexplained allergic reactions like sperm allergies. Human organic fluids (saliva, sweat, and sperm) frequently act as carriers of potential culprit allergens and may cause skin and respiratory allergic manifestations. Unfortunately, this problem is underestimated [25].

Despite this, the proper treatment of local reactions must be prescribed during the avoidance of contact with seminal fluid through either abstinence, coitus interruptus, or prophylactic antihistamines. For systemic reactions, after emergency measures, AIT via subcutaneous, sublingual, intralymphatic, or intravaginal administration [14, 15, 32, 41] with the partner's seminal plasma or PSA may be considered [13]. As some patients refuse AIT, the most common and most effective preventive method for sperm allergy is to use condoms during intercourse [14].

In addition, 52 cases of suspected hypersensitivity to cervicovaginal fluid in both localized and systemic forms were identified in men. In contrast to semen hypersensitivity, the pathogenesis of this new allergic manifestation remains unstudied [42].

The history of allergies related to the genitourinary tract in females and males is long and underestimated [12, 43].

9.4 Allergen Tolerance Breakdown in the Genitourinary Tract and Painful Coitus

9.4.1 Vulvodynia

▶ **Definition** Vulvodynia is a chronic pain syndrome in the vagina caused by immunopathologic mechanisms.

Vulvodynia occurs in young women who are unable to have vaginal sex with men. Some women cannot even insert in the vagina their first tampon and do not overcome a light touch (allodynia). Other women feel pain from any penis penetration, and this pain may be either more strong, like knife-sharp, or weak in the limited vagina's areas [44].

The etiology, prevalence, and incidence of vulvodynia are unknown. So far, no causative factor has yet been identified exactly. In vulvar biopsies taken from patients there were found the following:

- Infiltration of T cells and fibroblasts
- Overexpression of all types TLRs on fibroblasts in the subepithelial area [45]
- Degranulation of mast cells
- Hyperinnervation [46]

The pudendal nerve innervating the distal part of the genitourinary tract carries sympathetic fibers, including motor and sensory fibers [47]. By molecular biological methods, the production of pro-inflammatory cytokines, IL-1, IL-6 [45, 48], and TNF-α [44], and neuropeptides, substance P, and calcitonin-gene-related peptide (CGRP) [49] is revealed.

The survey of 662 women showed the presence of urticaria, insect allergy, and seasonal allergic rhinitis in the past medical history and reported vulvodynia in 78% (pain on contact), including in 33% knife-like pain, and in 22% vulvar burning [48]. As vaginal mucosa is a target organ capable of exhibiting an allergic response similar to the nose, eyes, lungs, and skin, vulvodynia appears to be the allergic and "neurogenic inflammation" around the pudendal nerve. Interestingly, similar symptoms (male dyspareunia, pudendal neuralgia) sometimes occur in males.

The therapy for vulvodynia includes the direct administration of local corticosteroids with the anti-inflammatory aim, applying capsaicin (Qutenza®) patch to relieve pain and diminish allergic inflammation. In the experiment, capsaicin exerted antioxidant and anti-inflammatory effects in food allergies and painkiller and anticarcinogenic action [50]. In vulvodynia, sublingual AIT is used if the atopic sensitization is proven.

9.4.2 Chronic Vulvovaginitis

▶ **Definition** Chronic vulvovaginitis is the recurrent allergic inflammation in the vagina combined with systemic symptoms based on many pathogenic factors.

Chronic vulvovaginitis is a combination of (1) allergic atopic or contact inflammation in the vagina, often accompanied by extra organic atopies, (2) "neurogenic inflammation" similar to vulvodynia, and (3) systemic reaction caused by pro-inflammatory cytokines, IL-1, IL-6, and TNF-α [51]. The disease manifests in atopic females caused partly by a mainly unusual group of allergens: inhalant type, including HDM and pet's allergens, bits of food products, latex, sperm, and *Candida albicans* [52] (see Fig. 9.2). The vaginal mucosa is a target organ, able to exert an allergic response similar to the other organs. The vagina may be an essential route for the entrance of any allergens with induction of local or even severe systemic reactions [19]. A strong association has been shown between atopy and some recurrent vulvovaginal disorders; therefore, atopy can be an essential causative factor in the pathogenesis of recurrent vulvovaginitis [53].

Alternatively, there is allergic contact dermatitis of the vulva based on type IV hypersensitivity in which women complain of typical vulvovaginitis symptoms.

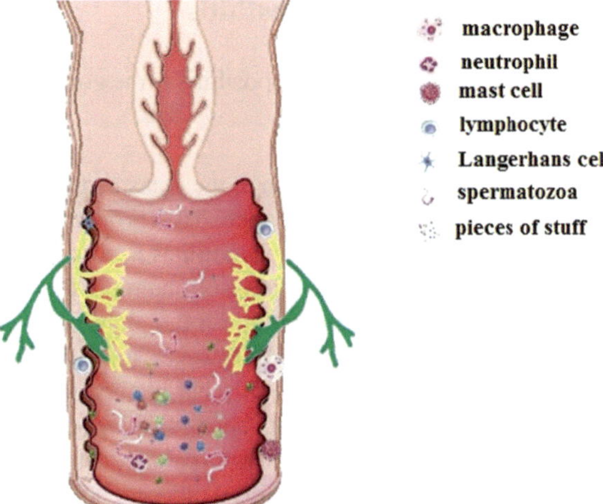

Fig. 9.2 Accumulation of spermatozoa and tiny pieces of stuff in the vagina. The vagina accumulates not only the proteins of seminal plasma and spermatozoa required for the fertilization. Various small pieces can get into the vaginal lumen, among which there are sources of allergens: HDMs, pet's scales and dander, bits of food products, latex, mold, etc., which create the prerequisites for allergic inflammation

This pathology corresponds to chronic vulvovaginitis [54] and is its pathogenic counterpart, including "neurogenic inflammation" and possible systemic reactions. Methylisothiazolinone is the organic compound used in many cosmetic and personal care products, which frequently causes IV type hypersensitivity-based contact allergy in the vulvovaginal area [55].

Simultaneously, we can find an imbalance of microbiota with expanded growth of *Gardnerella vaginalis* leading to symptoms of bacterial vaginosis [4] and the following manifestations: vaginal discharge, itching and pain, extra organic allergies, fever, insomnia, gastrointestinal disorders, and common discomfort. A study of 248 *HIV*-uninfected women's menstrual cup supernatants was undertaken to detect the bacterial vaginosis biomarkers. There was observed recent semen exposure to PSA, correlated with bacterial vaginosis prevalence and a significant increase in an inflammatory chemokine CCL3 (MIP-1α) [56].

In chronic vulvovaginitis, there is a decrease in central GABA activity and an increase in serotonin potency. The imbalance of these neurotransmitters causes the development of "neurogenic inflammation" and the overproduction of mentioned powerful pro-inflammatory cytokines, IL-1, IL-6, and TNF-α, which result in fever, insomnia, and the "acute phase" of inflammation [51], up to "cytokine storm."

The pathogenic peculiarity of chronic vulvovaginitis requires treatment with psychotropic medications and immunology intervention:

- GABA-ergic amplification
- Antidepressants
- Antihistamines
- Probiotics
- AIT by various routes, including subcutaneous [52].

9.4.3 Allergic Balanoposthitis

▶ **Definition** Allergic balanoposthitis is the group of different allergic disorders of the glans penis and prepuce.

Balanitis is the inflammation of the glans penis, and balanoposthitis is the inflammation of both glans and prepuce. This process may have a different origin, but namely, allergic inflammation sometimes occurs in children and adult men.

If a male takes a drug like any sulfonamide, the drug can get into semen and be a source of local allergic reaction on the glans penis (allergic balanoposthitis) and vagina (allergic vulvovaginitis). However, this disorder may be both IgE-dependent and IgE-independent. The use of local medications (cream, ointment, lotion, etc.) applied on the glance penis, latex condoms, or oral intercourse [57] may lead to the same allergic reaction. So, allergic balanoposthitis is frequently associated with drug/chemical allergies. Sometimes, allergic balanitis and urethritis may be caused by both IgE allergy and IV type hypersensitivity [58].

If a male suffers from atopic dermatitis, the inflammatory process may exclusively localize on the glans penis (circumpenile atopic dermatitis) and penile shaft. In this case, a physician observes typical symptoms of atopic dermatitis: lichenification, local itch, erythema, papulation, excoriations, crusts, and dryness, and must differentiate the disorder from scabies [59]. Such disease is more common in uncircumcised males.

Naturally, in such conditions, coitus would be painful and undesirable.

9.5 Preventive Benefit of Male Circumcision

▶ **Definition** Circumcision is the surgical removal of the prepuce on the penis.

Because uncircumcised males cannot perfectly maintain the cleanliness of the penis even in the highest level of hygiene, some problems, e.g., anaerobic microbiota, remain. Notably, the penis' prepuce may accumulate allergenic pieces of stuff and induce allergic reactions in atopic females or males who have sex with men. These tiny pieces of stuff are the following:

- Slight remains of semen
- Smegma
- *Candida albicans*
- Latex particles
- Feces of house dust mites (HDM)
- Topical medications, soaps, and detergents
- Textile dyes

In this case, male circumcision has an anti-allergic purpose and is a new challenge for healthcare professionals, which is not published yet and requires discussion.

Additionally, it is known that in adults, the non-keratinized glans epithelium accepts and transmits such infections as *HIV* and *HPV* creating an infectious and oncologic risk for a sexual partner [6, 60, 61]. Circumcision significantly reduces the prevalence of anaerobic bacteria that diminishes the threat of the inflammatory process in the penis and the risk of bacterial vaginosis in a female sexual partner [6]. Besides, the glans penis inflammation predisposes to allergic reactions in both partners. Centers for Disease Control and Prevention (USA) published a position paper regarding male circumcision [62]. In boys, circumcision prevents the penis from microtraumas, balanitis, balanoposthitis, phimosis, paraphimosis, and various urinary infections [63].

Key Points

1. The peripheral genital organs are target organs for allergic inflammation and adaptive immune responses to both allergens and infectious agents. They may play an essential role in the entrance of any allergens with induction of local or even severe systemic manifestations.
2. Allergen tolerance breakdown in the genitourinary tract results in sperm allergic reactions, vulvodynia, chronic vulvovaginitis, and male problems.
3. The preventive benefit of male circumcision has a new context from an allergy viewpoint.

Take-Home Messages

1. Describe the structure of the female genitourinary tract.
2. Describe the structure of the male genitourinary tract.
3. Write an essay about the epithelial cover of genitals and the benefits of different types of epithelium.
4. Write a paragraph about Döderlein's flora.
5. Write a flyer about the pudendal nerve.
6. Write a paragraph about pieces of stuff accumulated under the foreskin.
7. Write a flyer about the CDC position regarding male circumcision.
8. List pathogenic parts of chronic vulvovaginitis.
9. List pathogenic variants of sperm allergy.
10. List possible AIT routes of administration in females.
11. Write a paragraph about the pathogenesis of postorgasmic illness syndrome.
12. Write a paragraph about the allergic drug balanoposthitis.

Quiz

Reading a question, please choose only one right answer.

Question 1

Autonomic efferent innervation to the lower vagina is provided with:

1. Enteric nervous system.
2. Pudendal nerve.
3. Vagus nerve.
4. Uterovaginal plexus.

Question 2

Walls of distal parts of the genitourinary tract in women covers:

1. Keratinized stratified squamous epithelium.
2. Non-keratinized stratified squamous epithelium.
3. Simple columnar epithelium with microvilli.
4. Pseudostratified columnar epithelium.

Question 3

Glans penis in uncircumcised men covers:

1. Transitional epithelium.
2. Non-keratinized stratified squamous epithelium.
3. Simple columnar epithelium with microvilli.
4. Keratinized stratified squamous epithelium.

Question 4

Glans penis in circumcised men covers:

1. Stratisfied columnar epithelium.
2. Non-keratinized stratified squamous epithelium.
3. Simple columnar epithelium with microvilli.
4. Keratinized stratified squamous epithelium.

Question 5

This immunoglobulin is prevalent in the vagina's lumen:

1. SIgA.
2. IgG.
3. IgM.
4. IgE.

Question 6

Non-severe allergic reaction to sperm is:

1. Anaphylaxis.
2. Generalized urticaria.
3. Burning semen syndrome.
4. Generalized angioedema.

Question 7

Postorgasmic illness syndrome occurs in:

1. Males.
2. Females.
3. Males and females.
4. Only males who have sex with men.

Question 8

For a male, an allergy to own sperm exists:

1. It is impossible.
2. Yes.
3. No way.
4. Never.

Question 9

A protein in semen is the potential allergen:

1. Prostaglandin E_2.
2. Fertilization antigen-1.
3. Cleavage signal protein-1.
4. Prostate-specific antigen (PSA).

Question 10

Human organic fluids are carriers of potential allergens and may cause allergic manifestation:

1. Cerumen and tear.
2. Secretion of the stomach.
3. Saliva, sweat, and sperm.
4. Blood and lymph.

Question 11

In chronic vulvovaginitis, a combination of pathologic factors does not include:

1. "Neurogenic inflammation."
2. Allergic inflammation in the vagina.
3. Chronic pharyngitis.
4. Systemic reaction caused by pro-inflammatory cytokines.

Question 12
It has been found these neurotransmitters play a role in chronic vulvovaginitis:

1. GABA, serotonin.
2. Acetylcholine.
3. Norepinephrine.
4. Glycine, L-glutamate.

Question 13
Allergic balanoposthitis may not be associated with:

1. Drug/chemical allergies.
2. Mild atopic dermatitis.
3. Severe atopic dermatitis.
4. Crohn's disease.

Question 14
May allergen-specific immunotherapy (AIT) be used in sperm allergy:

1. It is possible.
2. No.
3. No way.
4. Never.

Question 15
Benefit of male circumcision is linked with:

1. Prevention of allergic reactions as the prepuce discontinues accumulating allergens.
2. Improvement of intercourse.
3. Improvement of penis appearance.
4. Ancient tradition.

Question 16
Sperm allergy may manifest in other organs not related to the genitourinary tract:

1. No.
2. Yes.
3. It is impossible.
4. Never.

References

1. Martell JAO. Immunology of urinary tract infections. GMS Infect Dis. 2020;8:Doc21. https://doi.org/10.3205/id000065.
2. Klimov VV. Skin and mucosal immune system. In: From basic to clinical immunology. Cham: Springer; 2019. https://doi.org/10.1007/978-3-030-0332301_2.
3. Al-Nasiry S, Ambrosino E, Schlaepfer M, Morré SA, Wieten L, Willem J, et al. The interplay between reproductive tract microbiota and immunological system in human reproduction. Front Immunol. 2020;11:378. https://doi.org/10.3389/fimmu.2020.00378.
4. Aldunate M, Srbinovski D, Hearps A, Latham CF, Ramsland PA, Gugasyan R, Cone RA, Tachedjian G. Antimicrobial and immune modulatory effects of lactic acid and short chain fatty acids produced by vaginal microbiota associated with eubiosis and bacterial vaginosis. Front Physiol. 2015;6:164. https://doi.org/10.3389/fphys.2015.00164.
5. Pohl HG, Groah SL, Petez-Losada M, Ljungberg I, Sprague BM, Crandal N, Caldovic L, Hsieh M. The urine microbiome of healthy men and women differs by urine collection method. Int Neurourol J. 2020;24(1):41–51. https://doi.org/10.5213/inj.1938244.122.
6. Onywera H, Williamson A-L, Ponomarenko J, Meiring TL. The penile microbiota in uncircumcised and circumcised men: relationships with HIV and Human Papillomavirus infections and cervicovaginal microbiota. Front Med. 2020;7:383. https://doi.org/10.3389/fmed.2020.00383.
7. Mehta SD, Zhao D, Green SJ, Agingu W, Otieno F, Bhaumik R, Bhaumik D, Bailey RC. The microbiome composition of a man's penis predicts incident bacterial vaginosis in his female sex partner with high accuracy. Front Cell Infect Microbiol. 2020;10:433. https://doi.org/10.3389/fcimb.2020.00433.
8. Graziottin A, Giraldi A. Anatomy and physiology of women's sexual function. In: H Porst, J Buvat, editors. Standard practice in sexual medicine, Chapter 19. Oxford: Blackwell; 2006. p. 289–304.
9. Barth C, Villringer A, Sacher J. Sex hormones affect neurotransmitters and shape the adult female brain during hormonal transition periods. Front Neurosci. 2015;9:37. https://doi.org/10.3389/fnins.2015.00037.
10. Calabrò RS, Cacciola A, Bruschetta D, Milardi D, Quattrini F, Sciarrone F, et al. Neuroanatomy and function of human sexual behavior: a neglected or unknown issue? Brain Behav. 2019;9:e01389. https://doi.org/10.1002/brb3.1389.
11. Hull EM, Dominguez JM, Muschamp JW. Neurochemistry of male sexual behavior. In: Lajtha A, Blaustein JD, editors. Handbook of neurochemistry and molecular neurobiology. Boston: Springer; 2007. p. 37–94. https://doi.org/10.1007/978-0-387-30405-2_2.
12. Specken JLH. Een merkwaardig geval van allergie in de gynecologie. Ned Tijdschr Verloskunde. 1958;380:314–9.
13. Lema VM. Allergy to human seminal plasma: case report and literature review. Women's Health Gynecol. 2017;3(3):1–4.
14. Nishihara Y, Shimizu T, Ichihara S, Suekata Y, Maeda K. Seminal plasma allergy: a literature review. J Gen Fam Med. 2015;16(4):265–70.
15. Allam J-P, Haidl G, Novak N. Semen allergy. Hautarzt. 2015;66(12):919–23. [In German]. https://doi.org/10.1007/s00105-015-3710-1.
16. Liccardi G, Caminati M, Senna G, Calzetta L, Rogliani P. Anaphylaxis and intimate behaviour. Curr Opin Allergy Clin Immunol. 2017;17(5):350–5. https://doi.org/10.1097/ACI.0000000000000386.
17. Lavery WJ, Stevenson M, Bernstein JA. An overview of seminal plasma hypersensitivity and approach to treatment. J Allergy Clin Immunol Pract. 2020;8(9):2937–42. https://doi.org/10.1016/j.jaip.2020.04.067.
18. Bernstein JA, Perez A, Floyd R, Bernstein L. Is burning semen syndrome a variant form of seminal plasma hypersensitivity? Obstet Gynecol. 2003;101(1):93–102. https://doi.org/10.1016/s0029-7844(02)02318-9.

19. Moraes PSA, Taketomi EA. Allergic vulvovaginitis. Ann Allergy Asthma Immunol. 2000;85:253–67.
20. Le TV, Nguyen HMT, Hellstrom WJG. Postorgasmic illness syndrome: what do we know so far? J Rare Dis Res Treat. 2018;3(2):29–33.
21. Nguyen HMT, Bala A, Gabrielson AT, Hellstrom WJG. Post-orgasmic illness syndrome: a review. Sex Med Rev. 2018;6(1):11–5. https://doi.org/10.1016/j.sxmr.2017.08.006.
22. Abdessater M, Elias S, Mikhael E, Alhammadi A, Beley S. Post orgasmic illness syndrome: what do we know till now? Basic Clin Androl. 2019;29:13. https://doi.org/10.1186/s12610-019-0093-7.
23. Strashny A. First assessment of the validity of the only diagnostic criteria for postorgasmic illness syndrome (POIS). Int J Impot Res. 2019;31(5):369–73. https://doi.org/10.1038/s41443-019-0154-7.
24. Wolthers OD. A five-year followup of human seminal plasma allergy in an 18-year-old woman. Case Rep Med. 2012;2012:257246. https://doi.org/10.1155/2012/257246.
25. Caminaty M, Giorgis V, Palterer B, Racca F, Salvottini C, Rossi O. Allergy and sexual behaviours: an update. Clin Rev Allergy Immunol. 2019;56:269–77. https://doi.org/10.1007/s12016-017-8618-3.
26. Calogiuri G, Nettis E, DiLeo E, Foli C, Vacca A. Is the localized seminal plasma hypersensitivity the mucosal aspect of protein contact dermatitis? J Allergy Clin Immunol. 2015;135(4):P1090–1. https://doi.org/10.1016/j.jaci.2014.11.041.
27. Carrol M, Horne G, Anrobus R, Fitzgerald C, Brison D, Helbert M. Testing for hypersensitivity to seminal fluid-free spermatozoa. Hum Fertil (Camb). 2013;16(2):128–31. https://doi.org/10.3109/14647273.2013.800238.
28. Marfatia YS, Patel D, Menon DS, Naswa S. Genital contact allergy: a diagnosis missed. Indian J Sex Transm Dis AIDS. 2016;37(1):1–6. https://doi.org/10.4103/0253-7184.180286.
29. Sublett JW, Bernstein JA. Seminal plasma hypersensitivity reactions: an updated review. Mt Sinai J Med. 2011;78(5):803–9. https://doi.org/10.1002/msj.20283.
30. Martí-Garrido J, López-Salgueiro R, Bartolomé-Zavala B, Perales-Chordá C, Hernández-Fernández de Rojas D. Anaphylaxis after anal intercourse with tolerance by vaginal route. Ann Allergy Asthma Immunol. 2019;122(3):346–7. https://doi.org/10.1016/j.anai.2018.10.006.
31. Suarez PJ, Maya WDC. Postorgasmic illness syndrome: semen allergy in men. Actas Urol Esp. 2013;37:593. https://doi.org/10.1016/j.acuro.2013.03.002.
32. Kim TB, Shim YS, Lee SM, Son ES, Shim JW, Lee SP. Intralymphatic immunotherapy with autologous semen in a Korean man with post-orgasmic illness syndrome. J Sex Med. 2018;6:174–9. https://doi.org/10.1016/j.esxm.2017.12.004.
33. Waldinger MD, Meinardi MM, Zwinderman AH, Schweitzer DH. Postorgasmic illness syndrome (POIS) in 45 Dutch Caucasian males: clinical characteristics and evidence for an immunogenic pathogenesis (part 1). Sex Med. 2011;8:1164–70. https://doi.org/10.1111/j.1743-6109.2010.02166.x.
34. Pilch B, Mann M. Large-scale and high-confidence proteomic analysis of human seminal plasma. Genome Biol. 2006;7(5):R40. https://doi.org/10.1186/gb-2006-7-5-r40.
35. Perumal P. Seminal plasma proteins. Nat Proc. 2012. Presentation from 19 March; https://doi.org/10.1038/npre.2012.7001.1.
36. Schjenken JE, Robertson SA. The female response to seminal fluid. Physiol Rev. 2020;100(3):1077–117. https://doi.org/10.1152/physrev.00013.2018.
37. Rametse CL, Adefuye A, Oliver AJ, Curry L, Gamieldien H, Burgers WA, et al. Inflammatory cytokine profiles of semen influence cytokine responses of cervicovaginal epithelial cells. Front Immunol. 2018;9:2721. https://doi.org/10.3389/fimmu.2018.02721.
38. Weidinger S, Mayerhofer A, Raemsch R, Ring J, Köhn F-M. Prostate-specific antigen as allergen in human seminal plasma allergy. J Allergy Clin Immunol. 2005;117(1):213–5. https://doi.org/10.1016/j.jaci.2005.09.040.
39. Tanaka M, Nakagawa Y, Kotobuki Y, Katayama I. A case of human seminal plasma allergy sensitized with dog prostatic kallikrein, *Can f 5*. Allergol Int. 2019;68:259–60. https://doi.org/10.1016/j.alit.2018.08.003.

40. Ghosh D, Bernstein JA. Systemic and localized seminal plasma hypersensitivity patients exhibit divergent immunologic characteristics. J Allergy Clin Immunol. 2014;134(4):P969–72. https://doi.org/10.1016/j.jaci.2014.05.016.
41. Resnick DJ, Chen L, Low J, Lee-Wong MF. Seminal plasma hypersensitivity and successful intravaginal graded challenge. Int J Asthma Allergy Immunol. 2014;10(1):1–6.
42. Jankowski M, Kodyra E, Kaszubowska J, Czajkowski R. Characterization of patients with suspected hypersensitivity to cervicovaginal fluid. J Eur Acad Dermatol Venereol. 2018;32(1):86–90. https://doi.org/10.1111/jdv.14550.
43. Köhn F-M. Suspected hypersensitivity to cervicovaginal fluid - what can we learn from the seminal plasma allergy story? J Eur Acad Dermatol Venereol. 2018;32(1):10. https://doi.org/10.1111/jdv.14762.
44. Bohm-Starke N. Medical and physical predictors of localized provoked vulvodynia. Acta Obstet Gynecol Scand. 2010;89(12):1504–10. https://doi.org/10.3109/00016349.2010.528368.
45. Falsetta ML, Foster DC, Woeller CF, Pollock SJ, Bonham AD, Piekns-Przybylska D, et al. Toll-like receptor signaling contributes to proinflammatory mediator production in localized provoked vulvodynia. J Low Genit Tract Dis. 2018;22(1):52–7. https://doi.org/10.1097/LGT.0000000000000036.
46. Bernstein J, Goldschmid N, Sabo E. Hyperinnervation and mast cell activation may be used as histopathologic diagnostic criteria for vulvar vestibulitis. Gynecol Obstet Investig. 2004;58(3):171–8. https://doi.org/10.1159/000079663.
47. Wadhwa V, Hamid AS, Kumar Y. Pudendal nerve and branch neuropathy: magnetic resonance neurography evaluation. Acta Radiol. 2017;58(6):726–33. https://doi.org/10.1177/0284185116668213.
48. Harlow BL, He W, Nguyen R. Allergic reactions and risk of vulvodynia. Ann Epidemiol. 2009;19(11):771–7. https://doi.org/10.1016/j.annepidem.2009.06.006.
49. Kiettisanpipop P, Panyakhamlerd K, Taweepolcharoen C, Bongsebandhu-Phubhakdi S, Triratanachat S, Chaikittisilpa S, et al. The differences of pain receptor and pain-related neurotransmitters in the vagina of pre- and post-menopausal women. J Med Assoc Thai. 2021;104(3):375–82. https://doi.org/10.35755/jmedassocthai.2021.03.11430.
50. Antunes MM, Coelho BSL, Cichi TM, de Castro IC, Leite JIA, Teixeira LG. Oral supplementation with capsaicin reduces oxidative stress and IL-33 on a food allergy murine model. World Allergy Organ J. 2019;12(7):100045. https://doi.org/10.1016/j.waojou.2019.100045.
51. Theodoropoulos DS, Michalopoulou AP, Cullen NA, Stockdale CK. Neuromodulation in the management of allergic chronic vaginitis. Reprod Syst Sex Disord. 2016;5(4):1000197. https://doi.org/10.4172/2161-038X.1000197.
52. Bernstein JA, Seidu L. Chronic vulvovaginal *Candida* hypersensitivity: an underrecognized and undertreated disorder by allergists. Allergy Rhinol (Providence). 2015;6(1):44–9. https://doi.org/10.2500/ar.2015.6.0113.
53. Ozturk S, Caliskaner Z, Karaayvaz M, Dede M, Gulec M. Hypersensitivity to aeroallergens in patients with recurrent vulvovaginitis of undetermined etiology. J Obstet Gynaecol Res. 2007;33(4):496–500. https://doi.org/10.1111/j.1447-0756.2007.00578.x.
54. Woodruff CM, Trivedi MK, Botto N, Kornik R. Allergic contact dermatitis of the vulva. Dermatitis. 2018;29(5):233–43. https://doi.org/10.1097DER.0000000000000339.
55. Eubel J, Diepgen TL, Weisshaar E. Allergic diseases in the genital area. Hautarzt. 2015;66(1):45–52. [In German]. https://doi.org/10.1007/s00105-014-3561-1.
56. Mngomezulu K, Mzobe GF, Mtshali A, Osman F, Liebenberg LJP, Garrett N, et al. Recent semen exposure impacts the cytokine response and bacterial vaginosis in women. Front Immunol. 2021;12:695201. https://doi.org/10.3389/fimmu.2021.695201.
57. Marasca C, Cappello M, Patruno C, Marasca D, Squillace L, Megna M. Petechia of the penis: sexual habits or adverse drug reaction? Curr Urol. 2018;12(3):167–8. https://doi.org/10.1159/000489438.
58. El-Reshaid KA, Sallam HT. Male genital allergy. J Drug Deliv Ther. 2021;11(3):4–6. https://doi.org/10.22270/jddt.v11i3.4699.

59. Grillo E, Jimenez N, Miguel-Morrondo A, Vano-Galvan S. Resistant itchy lesions in a young man. Aus Fam Physician. 2012;41(12):951–3.
60. Pintye J, Baeten JM. Benefits of male circumcision for MSM: evidence for action. Lancet. 2019;7:e388–9. https://doi.org/10.1016/S2214-109X(19)30038-5.
61. Morris BJ, Hankins CA, Lumbers ER, Mindel A, Klausner JD, Krieger JN, Cox G. Sex and male circumcision: women's preferences across different cultures and countries: a systematic review. Sex Med. 2019;7:145–61. https://doi.org/10.1016/j.esxm.2019.03.003.
62. Centers for Disease Control and Prevention. Male circumcision. https://www.cdc.gov/hiv/risk/male-circumcision.html. Accessed 4 Oct 2018
63. Morris B, Krieger JN. Male circumcision protects against urinary tract infections. In: Bjerklund Johansen TE, Wagenlehner FME, Matsumoto T, Cho YH, Krieger JN, Shoskes D, Naber KG, editors. Urogenital infections and inflammations. Duesseldorf: German Medical Science GMS Publishing House; 2017. https://doi.org/10.5680/lhuii000015.

Allergies in COVID-19 and Post-COVID Syndrome

10

Contents

Didactics

Knowledge. Upon successful completion of this chapter, students should be able to:

1. List the risk groups in COVID.
2. Be familiar with the definitions related to *SARS-CoV-2* and COVID-19.
3. List proteins of *SARS-CoV-2*.
4. Describe reactions and responses of the immune system in COVID-19.
5. List risk factors in COVID-19.
6. List the severe forms of pulmonary diseases in COVID-19, which may be fatal.
7. Describe "cytokine storm."
8. List clinical symptoms in COVID-19.

Acquired Skills. Upon successful completion of this chapter, students should demonstrate the following skills:

1. Interpret the knowledge related to the COVID-19 pandemic.
2. Critically evaluate the clinical literature about COVID-19.

Supplementary Information The online version contains supplementary material available at [https://doi.org/10.1007/978-3-031-04309-3_10].

V. V. Klimov, *Textbook of Allergen Tolerance*,
https://doi.org/10.1007/978-3-031-04309-3_10

3. Discuss the scientific articles from the current research literature to criticize clinical data concerning *SARS-CoV-2* and COVID-19.
4. Obtain a patient's history, including the history of present illness, past medical history, social, family, and occupational history, and review of systems of patients with COVID-19.
5. Perform a study case history of a patient with COVID-19.
6. Describe the management of COVID-19 with accompanying allergies.
7. Have a clear perception of the presented allergology definitions expressed orally and in written form.
8. Formulate the presented immunology and allergy terms.
9. Correctly answer the quiz questions.

Attitude and Professional Behaviors. Students should be able to:

1. Have the readiness to be hard-working.
2. Behave professionally at all times.
3. Recognize the importance of studying and demonstrate a commitment.
4. Demonstrate the consideration of the patient's feelings, ethnic, religious, cultural, and social background, and display empathy.

10.1 Introduction

▶ **Definition** COVID-19 is the pandemic infection caused by the coronavirus *SARS-CoV-2* and has spread worldwide since 2019.

SARS-CoV-2 means "severe acute respiratory syndrome-related coronavirus 2." It is very contagious in humans displaying a high rate of mortality. A higher likelihood of death has been found among COVID-19 patients who suffered from preexisting comorbid cardiovascular diseases, immune and metabolic disorders, respiratory, cerebrovascular, renal and hepatic diseases, and any types of cancers [1]. The World Health Organization declared on 11 March 2020 a pandemic, COVID-19, caused by *SARS-CoV-2*.

SARS-CoV-2 has four proteins: the S Protein (spike), including S1 and S2 subunits, E Protein (envelope), M Protein (membrane), and N protein (nucleocapsid) (see Fig. 10.1). The nucleocapsid holds the single-stranded (ssRNA) RNA genome.

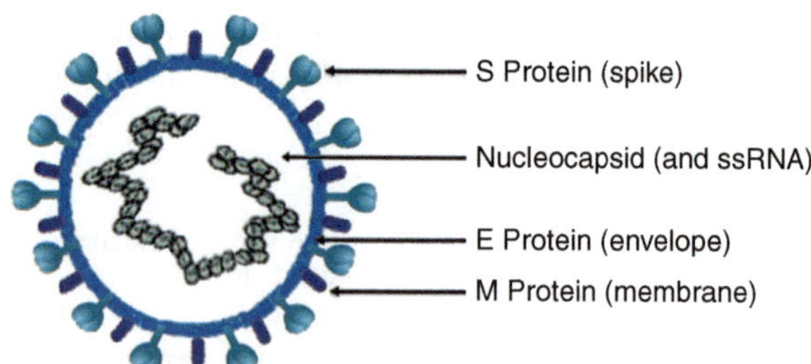

Fig. 10.1 Structure of *SARS-CoV-2*. *SARS-CoV-2* contains ssRNA and four structural proteins: S (spike), N (nucleocapsid), E (envelope), and M (membrane). S Protein is required for entry into a host cell

The spikes are responsible for allowing the virus to attach to a host cell membrane, binding to the angiotensin-converting enzyme 2 (ACE2) receptor [2]. The host transmembrane serine protease-2 (TMPRSS2) cleaves S Protein and modifies it, facilitating binding to ACE2 and entering a host cell. Furin and ADAM-17 are additional molecules required to promote uptake of the virus.

The virus then fuses with the host membrane, releases its RNA into the cell, and makes the cell produce copies of virions. Virions infect other cells disseminating throughout the body. Transmission of the infection occurs via the unified airway, skin, and indirect contact if contaminated subjects are used. The incubation period is uncertain yet. There is also a lack of knowledge about reinfection and long-term immune memory [3].

10.2 Immune Responses to *SARS-CoV-2*

The upper airway is the main port of entry for *SARS-CoV-2*. The infection can eventually progress into hyperinflammation in the lungs, and in severe cases into acute respiratory distress syndrome and respiratory insufficiency. It is accompanied by the release of damage-associated molecular patterns (DAMPs) coming from dying and already dead ACE2+ epithelial cells [4]. Upon entry to the human body, including the unified airway, *SARS-CoV-2* triggers:

1. Reactions of innate immunity leading to the activation via PRR of inflammasome NLRP3, production of pro-inflammatory cytokines such as TNF-α, IL-6, IL1-β, and a process of pyroptosis and, in immunocompromised persons, a "cytokine storm" [5, 6].
2. An adaptive CD8+ T cell-mediated immune response, which will allow destroying viruses through apoptosis by cytotoxic T cells and forming of possible long-term memory in the future [7] plus a CD4+ T cell-mediated response, which eventually acts via immune inflammation.
3. An advanced adaptive B cell-mediated immune response, which will be mainly valuable as a source of two types of antibodies, anti-S and anti-N [8].

Paradoxically, it has been found that an increased myeloid-derived suppressor (MDSCs) cells count correlates with disease severity. It is known that MDSCs suppress T cell responses, drive the hyperinflammatory process due to activating innate immunity, and diminish the lymphocyte count [9]. It has also been reported that an elevated level of IL-10 in severe cases of COVID-19 corresponds to the nonclassical pro-inflammatory effect of this immunosuppressive cytokine in the face of systemic inflammation [10].

Mucosal-associated invariant T (MAIT) cells were explored by single-cell transcriptomic technology in severe and moderate cases of COVID-19. The MAIT cells were consistent with disease severity and demonstrated more clonal expansions in severe cases, displaying increased pyroptotic MAIT cells. Therefore, it has been supposed that pyroptosis is a leading cause of MAIT cell deaths during *SARS-CoV-2* infection [11].

In patients with comorbid atopic diseases, allergen tolerance or allergen tolerance breakdown exist in parallel to immune responses against the virus. This intriguing subject remains unstudied.

The immunogenicity of viral proteins is different. S Protein is a potent inducer of T cell antiviral Th1 response, whereas nucleocapsid protein (N protein) is smaller than S Protein immunogenic [12]. But only anti-S protein antibodies (especially those targeting the ACE2 receptor-binding domain region) are neutralizing and protective. Anti-N protein antibodies are detected as weakly binding antibodies [8]. Seroconversion commonly appears between 7 and 14 days after the first clinical symptoms, and antibody titers persist in the weeks following virus clearance. IgG antibodies reach a maximal value by the 21st day [13, 14]. A multiplex-based assay, analyzing IgG, IgM, and IgA antibodies against the receptor-binding domain (RBD) of S1 Protein depending on the week of the COVID-19 course, and the specificity and sensitivity of anti-N Protein antibodies study were set up. A significant increase in IgM, IgG, and IgA antibodies against RBD was observed between the first and the third weeks of disease, and isotype switching appeared earlier for IgA than for IgG [15].

In previously healthy persons, immune responses to *SARS-CoV-2* proceed by adequate pathways, but in immunocompromised patients, the immune system cannot respond appropriately [7]. In a normal antiviral response due to controlling innate immunity (pro-inflammatory cytokines, IFNs, NK cells, M1 macrophages, and pyroptosis), T cell response (cytotoxic CD8+ T cells, and apoptosis), and B cell response (neutralizing specific IgG antibodies), the immune system eliminates the virus with no further tissue damage.

In immunocompromised patients, elderly persons, and persons suffering comorbid pathologies, immune responses are abnormal, weakened, and inadequately hyperinflammatory. Because of the "cytokine storm," coagulopathy and secondary damage at the systemic endothelial level as well as at the alveolar level are developing [7, 13]. Lymphopenia is the most frequently described prognostic marker in COVID-19, and it occurs to predict morbidity and mortality even at early stages [13]. Besides, the viral evolution in immunocompromised patients may be caused by known mutations: B.1.1.7α, B.1.351β, P.1γ, and B.1.617.2δ [16].

The analysis of HLA polymorphism showed that—regardless of race and ethnic groups—HLA class II molecules polymorphism influenced the development of protective immunity after *SARS-CoV-2* infection and after vaccination at the individual level [17].

In total, previous, current observations show that *SARS-CoV-2* has particularly adapted to escape from immune responses at the early stage of infection. Most immune system mechanisms are associated with inadequate type 1 IFN responses, weak functioning NK cells, increased pro-inflammatory cytokine production up to a "cytokine storm," and massive damage to tissues [18].

The lungs are the main target organ during *SARS-CoV-2* infection because the unified airway is the main entrance for the virus and has a high concentration of ACE2 in type II pneumocytes. People at the most significant risk of mortality from COVID-19 tend to be those with underlying conditions, such as those with a weakened immune system, comorbid heart or lung pathology, obesity, or the elderly [19]. The lung pathology related to risk factors includes preexisting chronic obstructive pulmonary disease (COPD) and severe bronchial asthma. However, the other atopic diseases do not impact the severity of COVID-19 in hospitalized patients [20].

10.3 Preexisting Comorbid Atopic Diseases in COVID-19

▶ **Definition** A comorbid disease is a pathologic condition, which accompanies the course of the main disease.

It is known that allergies in the unified airway are linked to an increased frequency of viral respiratory tract infections, allergic rhinitis, and non-severe allergic asthma seem not to be a risk factor for COVID-19 or disease severity [21]. As a possible explanation for this observation, researchers reported a negative correlation between ACE2 mRNA expression and IgE and Th2 cytokine activity, i.e., atopy does not predispose to the entry of *SARS-CoV-2* to the body [22, 23]. Another report found that ACE2 expression was significantly negatively associated with IL-13, whereas transmembrane serine protease-2 (TMPRSS2) expression was significantly positively linked to this cytokine (see Fig. 10.2) [24]. TMPRSS2 is needed for S Protein cleavage on the viral S2 subunit and the host receptor ACE2.

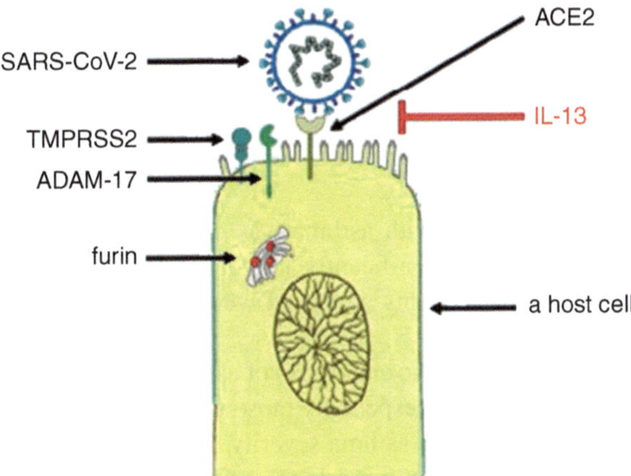

Fig. 10.2 IL-13 inhibits ACE2. Host cells express the angiotensin-converting enzyme 2 (ACE2) receptor required for attachment to viral S Protein when *SARS-CoV-2* must get into the cell. The host transmembrane serine protease-2 (TMPRSS2) cleaves S Protein and modifies it, facilitating binding to ACE2 and entering the host cell. Furin, a serine protease located in the Golgi apparatus, induces proteolytic cleavage of S Protein chains, changes their conformation to improve cell membrane fusion. ADAM-17, a disintegrin and metalloprotease 17 or "sheddase," facilitates the host cell's uptake of the viral particle. Host IL-13 inhibits ACE2 expression that decreases *SARS-CoV-2* entry into the cells

In the lower airway epithelium, increased ACE2 expression occurs in older adults and males, whereas decreased ACE2 expression arises in patients with atopic asthma and reduced furin and, paradoxically, enhanced ADAM-17 expressions. Furin and ADAM-17 are needed to promote the uptake of the virus [25]. Sputum furin expression levels were closely associated with neutrophilic inflammation and inflammasome activation. It might indicate the cause of a greater morbidity and mortality outcome from COVID-19 in the Th2-low/IL-17/neutrophilic severe asthma endotype [26].

An online survey was undertaken to reach out to the worldwide allergy community in 78 countries of all continents [27]. The questionnaire contained 24 questions covering clinical practice and subjects related to COVID-19 accompanying allergies. The main audience consisted of 635 allergists with long-term professional experience. Most of them who were managing allergic patients during the pandemic agreed that patients had no increased risk of contacting *SARS COV-2* or developing COVID-19.

A systematic review and meta-analysis assessed the prevalence and mortality risk of preexisting comorbidities among patients with identified asthma as a preexisting comorbid disease in patients with COVID-19 [1, 28]. Although the mortality risk in COVID-19 patients with respiratory pathology was almost two times higher than those with no respiratory diseases, Th2-high/eosinophilic endotypes of asthma were not found to be a significant contributor to this category [29]. Another systemic review and meta-analysis reported a lack of increase in the risk of mortality, hospitalization, intensive care unit admission, or length of hospitalization between 389 patients with asthma and with COVID-19 infection compared with patients without asthma [30].

It suggests that atopic individuals with allergic asthma who have Th2-high/eosinophilic endotypes may have some degree of defense against COVID-19, perhaps due to some asthma-related features such as the inhibition of the ACE-2 receptor by IL-13 and conventional asthma pharmacotherapy.

A case history of a patient with asthma was described as being infected with *SARS-CoV-2* and exhibited a significantly longer intubation time before the first symptoms [31]. The atopic patients who died were elderly and had comorbidities such as obesity [32].

The Th2-low/Th17/neutrophilic endotypes of asthma may serve as a likely target to treat patients with COVID-19, especially those with an IL-17 prevalent response. Since IL-17 levels correlate with asthma severity, it means that severe asthma was identified as constituting a potential risk factor for COVID-19 severity [29]. A “cytokine storm” frequently occurs in the Th2-low/Th17/neutrophilic endotypes of asthma accompanying COVID-19. FDA approved JAK2 inhibitor fedratinib for reducing mortality of patients with these immune profiles [33].

In a large population-based cohort study, patients with nonallergic asthma were at a higher risk of severe COVID-19 when compared with allergic asthma [34]. One possible explanation for this could be the reduced ACE2 expression in allergic asthma, potentially making the unified airway less significant to viral invasion. Conversely, targeting IL-17 in severe COVID-19 patients with acute respiratory distress syndrome is an enlightened option considering its role in the induction of IL-1β, IL-6, TNF-α, GM-CSF, and neutrophil recruitment, which are known to drive the pathogenesis of acute respiratory distress syndrome [28].

It was found that preexisting eosinophilia protected against COVID-19-associated admission, and development of eosinophilia during hospitalization was linked with decreased mortality if allergic asthma was comorbid pathology. Furthermore, a Th2-high/eosinophilic asthma endotype might predict diminished COVID-19 morbidity and mortality [35]. Conversely, low eosinophil levels correlate with poor outcomes in critically ill patients [36]. In re-positive *SARS-CoV-2* patients, eosinophil counts decreased significantly as well as during the initial diagnosis, whereas they increased normally in persons who had not COVID-19 recurrence [37]. It is known that the ability of eosinophilia to exert both pro-inflammatory and antiviral effects may alter the course of COVID-19 [28].

An epidemiologic study of COVID-19 with asthma was carried out in New York and Dublin, Ireland [38]. In contrast with Wuhan, China, a slightly higher prevalence of current adult asthma was found in New York; the reported rate of comorbid asthma was higher in adults in Ireland. Among patients with allergic asthma, males, African Americans, and persons with diabetes mellitus have increased ACE2 and TMPRSS2 expression in their sputum cells that can be associated with a poor prognosis when infected with the *SARS-CoV-2*. So, asthma may worsen the disease course of COVID-19 [39]. There remains a need for more extensive and more detailed epidemiologic studies for specifying to what extent COVID-19 poses a risk to patients of defined asthma severity [38].

The clinical history of a 55-year-old woman with severe asthma treated for 3 years with mepolizumab (anti-IL-5 monoclonal antibodies) has been described [40]. When she visited the allergic clinic, she came into contact with a patient with COVID. At this time, she had adverse effects from mepolizumab such as elevated liver enzyme levels. The fact that COVID-19 did not progress and underlying asthma did not worsen the comorbid disease suggested that the biological agents used in treating respiratory diseases might have protective effects on the course of COVID-19. Another clinical report about efficacy treatment of patients with severe asthma accompanying COVID-19 using benralizumab (an anti-IL-5Rα monoclonal antibody) has also been published [41].

There are controversial data concerning the predisposition of allergic and nonallergic rhinitis to *SARS-CoV-2* infection. An increased likelihood has been described of *SARS-CoV-2* contagion and poor clinical outcomes; contrary to the above, another research group observed that rhinosinusitis was associated with a lower risk of hospitalization and mild course of COVID-19 [42]. In a case-controlled randomized study of 125 patients, it was found that allergic rhinitis did not affect the severity of COVID-19 [43]. In total, there is limited knowledge about the relationship between susceptibility to *SARS-CoV-2* infection, the risk of severe COVID-19 development, and allergic rhinitis as the precise role of ACE2 in nasal diseases has not yet been elucidated. The nasal cavity serves as the first barrier, protecting the lower part of the unified airway and undergoing the initial impact. However, most reports demonstrated that nasal conditions such as allergic rhinitis and chronic rhinosinusitis do not appear to be at high risk for COVID-19 [44].

It has been shown that patients with atopic dermatitis did not have a significantly increased risk for *SARS-CoV-2* infection, including those on corticosteroid medications (prednisone), methotrexate, and other immunosuppressive drugs [45]. Though patients with atopic dermatitis have an increased infection risk, biologic dupilumab blocking the shared α chain receptor for IL-4 and IL-13, does not enhance the risk of *SARS-CoV-2* contagion [46]. Atopic dermatitis is linked with other atopic diseases such as allergic rhinitis and asthma, in which the risk of respiratory infections is increased. Limited studies evaluated the efficacy of systemic medications and biologics in atopic dermatitis if COVID-19 occurred, but it is expected that systemic immunomodulatory and biologic treatments might protect patients from worsening *SARS-CoV-2* outcomes [47].

10.4 Immunity and Allergies in COVID-19 Convalescents

▶ **Definition** Post-COVID syndrome (long COVID) is a pathologic condition, which develops in half of COVID convalescents, manifests by clinical symptoms, such as cough, fatigue, memory loss, and pain, and lasts for several months.

There are different viewpoints on whether *SARS-CoV-2* reinfections are possible, and there is an urgent need to develop a *SARS-CoV-2* vaccine for convalescents. For example, it has been described that in the long-term *SARS-CoV-2* can impact the homeostasis of CD4+ T cells in convalescents who suffered from a severe course of COVID-19 [48]. The World Health Organization (WHO) on October 6, 2021, published a definition of long COVID for the first time, seeking to clarify one of the poor understood aspects of the coronavirus pandemic. Here is how the U.N. health agency has defined long COVID as "post COVID-19 condition," the name proposed by WHO's International Classification of Diseases. The WHO estimated that 10–20% of COVID-19 patients experienced prolonged symptoms for months following infection. These symptoms commonly include cough, persistent fatigue, headache, cognitive dysfunction, and depressive disorder [49].

A study of protective antibodies in COVID-19 convalescents was carried out to substantiate the urgent need to develop a *SARS-CoV-2* vaccine. It has been found that a natural *SARS-CoV-2* infection does not induce a protective antibody response inhibiting the virus-ACE2 receptor interaction in all convalescents, and therefore *SARS-CoV-2* vaccines are required. The molecular interaction assays could help identify subjects with developed protective antibodies and screen candidate vaccines to induce antibodies that inhibit the virus-ACE2 receptor interaction [50].

However, antibodies are not the essential protective factor of the immune system in viral infections compared with cytotoxic CD8+ T cells [51].

The available studies on the immunology of *SARS-CoV-2* infection converge in indicating that it generates a robust and persistent immunity. This statement does not differ from respiratory viruses known so far: in naturally appearing viral respiratory infections, reinfections are exceptional [52]. The modern analytical strategy developed beyond earlier findings by identifying many epitopes recognized by CD8+ T cells that spanned different viral proteins in COVID-19 convalescent subjects who recovered from the severe ill condition. The unmanipulated phenotypic profiles of these cells were simultaneously revealed. These new findings can be employed to further guide epitope selection for rationally designed vaccine candidates and vaccine test strategies [53, 54].

The course of comorbid atopic diseases after experiencing COVID-19 at follow-up is almost unexplored [55]. Patients with severe asthma were studied during the spring 2020 COVID-19 outbreak in Paris, France. All patients ($n = 37$, 70% females) were identified by an expert team of asthma specialists in a large university hospital hosting a severe asthma clinic, allowing systematic analysis of required information and thorough follow-up. Interestingly, mild pneumonia during the COVID-19 course tended to be more frequent in asthmatic patients with higher doses of inhaled corticosteroids than in control. Asthma therapy was unchanged in all patients, including biologics. There were two deaths as outcomes of COVID-19. At a 1-month follow-up, experience of COVID-19 pneumonia was not associated with asthma exacerbation in patients who did not modify their asthma treatment [56]. This means that proper therapy is important.

The trend of allergic rhinitis post-COVID-19 pandemic incidence was studied in 128 patients aged 5–65 years. There was a reported statistically significant decrease in allergic rhinitis post-pandemic incidence that could probably be related to the diminished pollution due to lockdown and an increase in indoor activities [57].

Many patients who experienced COVID-19 have disease-related symptoms for several weeks or months after the acute phase. The so-called *post-COVID syndrome* includes persistent symptoms caused by organ damage, residual inflammation, an effect from prolonged mechanical ventilation, and an impact on preexisting health disorders [58]. The full range of the duration and severity of post-COVID syndrome is not currently studied.

The following has been found exploring a cohort of 277 patients in a Mediterranean region 3 months after hospitalization [59]. A post-COVID syndrome was detected in half of the COVID-19 survivors. Radiological and spirometric changes were mild and observed in less than 25% of patients. Chronic respiratory diseases, including asthma, were revealed in 18.1% [59]. The reason for a lower prevalence of the post-COVID syndrome in patients with asthma could refer to a lower *SARS-CoV-2* infection in asthmatic patients. There was an impact of Th2-cytokines on ACE2 [24] and corticosteroid therapy, which almost all patients received. In fact, *in vitro* studies have shown that inhaled corticosteroids reduce the replication of *SARS-CoV-2* in the unified airway epithelium [60].

A cough, a common symptom of the post-COVID syndrome and a neuronal reflex, persists for weeks or months after acute *SARS-CoV-2* infection, with cognitive disorder, fatigue, memory loss, insomnia, and pain. In a pooled analysis, the prevalence of persistent cough was found in 18% of convalescents 6 weeks through 4 months who were earlier hospitalized [61]. The post-COVID syndrome might result from "neurogenic inflammation" and reactions of the neuroimmune system [61, 62]. According to the concept of "neurogenic inflammation," neurons can damage the tissue they innervate, and a cough resembles this case. In the peripheral nervous system, inflammatory cells, including macrophages and dendritic cells, infiltrate nerves and neuronal tissues to participate in inflammatory processes, which may become chronic. This "neurogenic inflammation" would be expected to dramatically alter sensory neuron activity and potentially cause a persistent cough [61].

If the cough is associated with allergic atopic background, modified management must be considered. There are no contraindications for the basic medication treatment in atopic diseases. Wearing a face mask reduces the transmission risk of the *SARS-CoV-2* virus, but it also reduces allergic rhinitis manifestation [63]. Regardless of acute *SARS-CoV-2* infection, executing AIT may be done under strict safety protocols in *Hymenoptera* venom allergy. In all other cases, AIT is performed via the subcutaneous or sublingual route of allergen administration in convalescents only. Ongoing mite and pollen AIT allows reducing allergic symptoms such as coughing and sneezing during post-COVID syndrome [64].

As for vaccination, mass vaccination planned globally can limit the current COVID-19 pandemic by protecting individuals. People vaccinated against the *SARS-CoV-2* decrease the risk of viral transmission to individuals who have not been vaccinated [65, 66].

Key Points

1. *SARS-CoV-2* triggers the innate immunity and adaptive immune responses in a different manner depending on health status, comorbid pathology, including distinct endotypes of atopic diseases. COVID-19 outcomes are determined by the same factors plus the quality of treatment and care.
2. The Th2-high/eosinophilic endotypes of asthma due to Th2-profile cytokines reduce ACE2 expression and do not predispose to *SARS-CoV-2* entry in the unified airway epithelium. Conversely, the Th2-low/Th17/neutrophilic endotypes are prone to viral contagion and severity of both asthma and COVID-19.
3. In post-COVID syndrome, exacerbations in atopic patients occur rarely compared to the appearance of a cough. Such a cough as a neuronal reflex may result from "neurogenic inflammation" and reactions of the neuroimmune system affected by the virus.

Take-Home Messages

1. List the proteins of *SARS-CoV-2*.
2. Write a flyer about a ligand and receptor when the virus enters a host cell.

3. Write an essay about comorbid atopic diseases in COVID-19.
4. Make a slide presentation about adaptive immune responses in COVID-19.
5. Make a slide presentation about reactions of innate immunity in COVID-19.
6. Write a paragraph about antibodies in COVID-19.
7. Write a paragraph about IL13 inhibition of *SARS-CoV-2* uptake by a host cell.
8. List symptoms of the post-COVID syndrome.
9. Write a paragraph about endotypes of asthma.
10. Write a paragraph about eosinophils in COVID-19.
11. Write a paragraph about cough in post-COVID syndrome.

Quiz

Reading a question, please choose only one right answer.

Question 1

A *SARS-CoV-2* protein required for entry in a host cell is:

1. M Protein.
2. S Protein.
3. N Protein.
4. E Protein.

Question 2

The main receptor-binding *SARS-CoV-2* Protein S is:

1. TMPRSS2.
2. Furin.
3. ADAM-17.
4. ACE2.

Question 3

Cytokine inhibiting ACE2 expression is:

1. TNF-α.
2. IL-13.
3. IFN-α.
4. IL-6.

Question 4

A comorbid disease does not predispose to COVID-19 severe cases:

1. Atopy.
2. Heart pathology.
3. Obesity.
4. Elderly age.

Question 5
The incubation period of *SARS-CoV-2* infection is:

1. 1 day.
2. 1 week.
3. Uncertain yet.
4. 2 weeks.

Question 6
Asthma's endotype or phenotype predisposing to COVID-19 severe cases is:

1. Th1/Th17/neutrophilic asthma.
2. Th2/eosinophilic asthma.
3. Asthma in young people.
4. Asthma in children.

Question 7
An adaptive immune response is essential for defense against *SARS-CoV-2*:

1. Simple B cell mediated response.
2. Advanced B cell-mediated response.
3. CD8+ T cell-mediated response.
4. CD4+ T cell-mediated response.

Question 8
A reaction of innate immunity is essential for defense against *SARS-CoV-2*:

1. Phagocytosis.
2. Interferons and NK cells.
3. Proteins of the acute phase.
4. Complement activation.

Question 9
SARS-CoV-2 escapes from immune responses at the early stage of infection:

1. No.
2. Unknown.
3. No way.
4. Yes.

Question 10
Cytokines taking part in "cytokine storm":

1. IL-10, IL-35, and TGF-β.
2. IFN-γ, IL-2, and IL3.

3. IL-1β, IL-6, and TNF-α.
4. IL-4, IL-5, and IL-13.

Question 11
A severe syndrome is a frequent cause of COVID-19 mortality:

1. Acute respiratory distress syndrome.
2. Post-COVID syndrome.
3. Myalgic encephalomyelitis/chronic fatigue syndrome.
4. Acute coronary syndrome.

Question 12
In COVID-19, blood eosinophils correlate with:

1. Poor outcome if a low level.
2. Poor outcome if a high level.
3. No correlation.
4. Positive outcome if a low level.

Question 13
Eosinophils exert:

1. Pro-inflammatory effect.
2. Antiviral effect.
3. Pro-inflammatory and antiviral effects.
4. Anti-inflammatory effect.

Question 14
Post-COVID syndrome occurs in:

1. Little of the COVID-19 survivors.
2. Half of the COVID-19 survivors.
3. Does not occur.
4. All of the COVID-19 survivors.

Question 15
A leading symptom of post-COVID syndrome is:

1. Fatigue.
2. Muscle pains.
3. Persistent cough.
4. Anxiety disorder.

Question 16

During COVID-19, allergen-specific immunotherapy (AIT) is performing:

1. Only in insect venom allergy.
2. Never.
3. In house dust mites allergies.
4. In seasonal allergies.

References

1. Khan MMA, Khan MN, Mustagir MG, Rana J, Islam MS, Kabir MI. Effects of underlying morbidities on the occurrence of deaths in COVID-19 patients: a systematic review and meta-analysis. J Glob Health. 2020;10(2):020503. https://doi.org/10.7189/jogh.10.020503.
2. Hoffmann M, Kleine-Weber H, Schroeder S, Krüger N, Herrler T, Erichsen S, et al. SARS-CoV-2 cell entry depends on ACE2 and TMPRSS2 and is blocked by a clinically proven protease inhibitor. Cell. 2020;181(2):271–80.e8. https://doi.org/10.1016/j.cell.2020.02.052.
3. Ledford H. Coronavirus reinfections: three questions scientists are asking. Nature. 2020;585:168–9. https://doi.org/10.1038/d41586-020-02506-y.
4. Wauters E, Thevissen K, Wauters C, Bosisio FM, De Smet F, Gunst J, et al. Establishing a unified COVID-19 "Immunome": integrating coronavirus pathogenesis and host immunopathology. Front Immunol. 2020;11:1642. https://doi.org/10.3389/fimmu.2020.01642.
5. Mehta P, McAuley DF, Brown M, Sanchez E, Tattersall RS, Manson JJ. COVID-19: consider cytokine storm syndromes and immunosuppression. Lancet. 2020;395(10229):1033–4. https://doi.org/10.1016/S0140-6736(20)30628-0.
6. Niles MA, Gogesch P, Kronhart S, Iannazzo SO, Kochs G, Waibler Z, Anzaghe M. Macrophages and dendritic cells are not the major source of pro-inflammatory cytokines upon SARS-CoV-2 infection. Front Immunol. 2021;12:647824. https://doi.org/10.3389/fimmu.2021.647824.
7. Larenas-Linnemann DE, Ortega-Martell JA, Brandón-Vijil MV, Rodríguez-Pérez N, Luna-Pech JA, Estrada-Cardona A, et al. Coronavirus disease 2019, allergic diseases, and allergen immunotherapy: possible favorable mechanisms of interaction. Allergy Asthma Proc. 2021;42(3):187–97. https://doi.org/10.2500/aap.2021.42.210013.
8. Lindsley AW, Schwartz JT, Rothenberg ME. Eosinophil responses during COVID-19 infections and coronavirus vaccination. J Allergy Clin Immunol. 2020;146:1–7. https://doi.org/10.1016/j.jaci.2020.04.021.
9. Rowlands M, Segal F, Hartl D. Myeloid-derived suppressor cells as a potential biomarker and therapeutic target in COVID-19. Front Immunol. 2021;12:697405. https://doi.org/10.3389/fimmu.2021.697405.
10. Islam H, Chamberlain TC, Mui AL, Little JP. Elevated interleukin-10 levels in COVID-19: potentiation of pro-inflammatory responses or impaired anti-inflammatory action? Front Immunol. 2021;12:677008. https://doi.org/10.3389/fimmu.2021.677008.
11. Shi J, Zhou J, Zhang X, Hu W, Zhao J-F, Wang S, et al. Single-cell transcriptomic profiling of MAIT cells in patients with COVID-19. Front Immunol. 2021;12:700152. https://doi.org/10.3389/fimmu.2021.700152.
12. Shah VK, Firmal P, Alam A, Ganguly D, Chattopadhyay S. Overview of immune response during SARS-CoV-2 infection: lessons from the past. Front Immunol. 2020;11:1949. https://doi.org/10.3389/fimmu.2020.01949.
13. Vabret N, Britton GJ, Gruber C, Hegde A, Kim J, Kuksin M, et al. Immunology of COVID-19: current state of the science. Immunity. 2020;52:910–41. https://doi.org/10.1016/j.immuni.2020.05.002.

14. Okba NMA, Müller MA, Li W, Wang C, Geurtsvan Kessel CH, Corman VM, et al. Severe acute respiratory syndrome coronavirus 2-specific antibody responses in coronavirus disease 2019 patients. Emerg Infect Dis. 2020;26(7):1478–88. https://doi.org/10.3201/eid2607.200841.
15. Brynjolfsson SF, Sigurgrimsdottir H, Einarsdottir ED, Bjornsdottir GA, Armannsdottir B, Baldvinsdottir GE, et al. Detailed multiplex analysis of SARS-CoV-2 specific antibodies in COVID-19 disease. Front Immunol. 2021;12:695230. https://doi.org/10.3389/fimmu.2021.695230.
16. Corey L, Beyrer C, Cohen MS, Michael NL, Bedford T, Rolland M. SARS-CoV-2 variants in patients with immunosuppression. N Engl J Med. 2021;385(6):562–6. https://doi.org/10.1056/NEJMsb2104756.
17. Copley HC, Gragert L, Leach AR, Kosmoliaptsis V. Influence of HLA class II polymorphism on predicted cellular immunity against SARS-CoV-2 at the population and individual level. Front Immunol. 2021;12:669357. https://doi.org/10.3389/fimmu.2021.669357.
18. Guihot A, Litvinova E, Autran B, Debre P, Vieillard V. Cell-mediated immune responses to COVID-19 infection. Front Immunol. 2020;11:1662. https://doi.org/10.3389/fimmu.2020.01662.
19. Centers for Disease Control and Prevention. People with certain medical conditions. 15 March 2021. https://www.cdc.gov/coronavirus/2019-ncov/need-extra-precautions/people-with-medical-conditions.html
20. Timberlake DT, Narayanan D, Ogbogu PU, et al. Severity of COVID-19 in hospitalized patients with and without atopic disease. World Allergy Organ J. 2021;14(2):100508. https://doi.org/10.1016/j.waojou.2021.100508.
21. Joshi A, Mullakary R, Iyer VN. Successful treatment of coronavirus disease 2019 in a patient with asthma. Allergy Asthma Proc. 2020;41(4):296–300. https://doi.org/10.2500/aap.2020.41.200044.
22. Jackson DJ, Busse WW, Bacharier LB, Kattan M, O'Connor GT, Wood RA, et al. Association of respiratory allergy, asthma and expression of the SARS-CoV-2 receptor, ACE-2. J Allergy Clin Immunol. 2020;146(1):203–6.e3. https://doi.org/10.1016/j.jaci.2020.04.009.
23. Bradding P, Richardson M, Hinks TSC, Howarth PH, Choy DF, Arron JR, et al. ACE2, TMPRSS2, and furin gene expression in the airways of people with asthma-implications for COVID-19. J Allergy Clin Immunol. 2020;146(1):208–11. https://doi.org/10.1016/j.jaci.2020.05.013.
24. Kimura H, Francisco D, Conway M, Martinez FD, Vercelli D, Polverino F, et al. Type 2 inflammation modulates ACE2 and TMPRSS2 in airway epithelial cells. J Allergy Clin Immunol. 2020;146(1):80–8.e8. https://doi.org/10.1016/j.jaci.2020.05.004.
25. Wark PAB, Pathinayake PS, Kaiko G, Nichol K, Ali A, Chen L, Sutanto EN, Garratt LW, Sohal SS, Lu W, Eapen MS, Oldmeadow C, Bartlett N, Reid A, Veerati P, Hsu AC, Looi K, Iosifidis T, Stick SM, Hansbro PM, Kicic A. ACE2 expression is elevated in airway epithelial cells from older and male healthy individuals but reduced in asthma. Respirology. 2021;26(5):442–51. https://doi.org/10.1111/resp.14003.
26. Kermani NZ, Song WJ, Badi Y, Versi A, Guo Y, Sun K, Bhavsar P, Howarth P, Dahlen SE, Sterk PJ, Djukanovic R, Adcock IM, Chung KF; U-BIOPRED Consortium. Sputum ACE2, TMPRSS2 and FURIN gene expression in severe neutrophilic asthma. Respir Res. 2021;22:10. https://doi.org/10.1186/s12931-020-01605-8.
27. Tanno LK, Demoly P, Martin B, Berstein J, Morais-Almeida M, Levin M, et al. Allergy and coronavirus disease (COVID-19) international survey: real-life data from the allergy community during the pandemic. World Allergy Organ J. 2021;14(2):100515. https://doi.org/10.1016/j.waojou.2021.100515.
28. Ramakrishnan RK, Al Heialy S, Hamid Q. Implications of preexisting asthma on COVID-19 pathogenesis. Am J Physiol Lung Cell Mol Physiol. 2021;320(5):L880–91. https://doi.org/10.1152/ajplung.00547.2020.
29. Skevaki C, Karsonova A, Karaulov A, Xie M, Renz H. Asthma-associated risk for COVID-19 development. J Allergy Clin Immunol. 2020;146:1295–301. https://doi.org/10.1016/j.jaci.2020.09.017.

30. Sitek AN, Ade JM, Chiarella SE, Divekar RD, Pitlick MM, Iyer VN, et al. Outcomes among patients with COVID-19 and asthma: a systematic review and meta-analysis. Allergy Asthma Proc. 2021;42:267–73. https://doi.org/10.2500/aap.2021.42.210041.
31. Mahdavinia M, Foster KJ, Jaurequi E, Moore D, Adnan D, Andy-Nweye AB, et al. Asthma prolongs incubation in COVID-19. J Allergy Clin Immunol Pract. 2020;8(7):2388–91. https://doi.org/10.1016/j.jaip.2020.05.006.
32. Guterres DS, Dos Santos AC, Laubi MAPM, Brandão V, Saito T, Lima G. COVID-19 pandemia: atopy and prospective analysis of the clinical evolution of patients infected with the SARS-CoV-2 virus. J Allergy Clin Immunol. 2021;147(2 Suppl):AB79. https://doi.org/10.1016/j.jaci.2020.12.303.
33. Wu D, Yang XO. TH17 responses in cytokine storm of COVID-19: an emerging target of JAK2 inhibitor Fedratinib. J Microbiol Immunol Infect. 2020;53:368–70. https://doi.org/10.1016/j.jmii.2020.03.005.
34. Zhu Z, Hasegawa K, Ma B, Fujiogi M, Camargo CA Jr, Liang L. Association of asthma and its genetic predisposition with the risk of severe COVID-19. J Allergy Clin Immunol. 2020;146:327–9. https://doi.org/10.1016/j.jaci.2020.06.001.
35. Ferastraoaru D, Hudes G, Jerschow E, Jariwala S, Karagic M, de Vos G, et al. Eosinophilia in asthma patients is protective against severe COVID-19 illness. J Allergy Clin Immunol Pract. 2021;9(3):1152–62. https://doi.org/10.1016/j.jaip.2020.12.045.
36. Lavoignet CE, Le Borgne P, Chabrier S, Bidoire J, Slimani H, Chevrolet-Lavoignet J, et al. White blood cell count and eosinopenia as valuable tools for the diagnosis of bacterial infections in the ED. Eur J Clin Microbiol Infect Dis. 2019;38:1523–32. https://doi.org/10.1007/s10096-019-03583-2.
37. Li X, Yin D, Yang Y, Bi C, Wang Z, Ma G, et al. Eosinophil: a nonnegligible predictor in COVID-19 re-positive patients. Front Immunol. 2021;12:690653. https://doi.org/10.3389/fimmu.2021.690653.
38. Butler MW, O'Reilly A, Dunican EM, Mallon P, Feeney ER, Keane MP, McCarthy C. Prevalence of comorbid asthma in COVID-19 patients. J Allergy Clin Immunol. 2020;146(2):334–5. https://doi.org/10.1016/j.jaci.2020.04.061.
39. Morais-Almeida M, Bousquiet J. COVID-19 and asthma: to have or not to have T2 inflammation makes a difference? Pulmonology. 2020;26(5):261–3. https://doi.org/10.1016/j.pulmoe.2020.05.003.
40. Kurtuluş A, Yesilkaya S, Topel M, Turkyulmaz S, Ercelebi DC, Oncul A, et al. COVID-19 in a patient with severe asthma using mepolizumab. Allergy Asthma Proc. 2021;42(2):e55–7. https://doi.org/10.2500/aap.2021.42.200125.
41. García-Moguel I, Díaz Campos R, Alonso Charterina S, Fernández Rodríguez C, Crespo JF. COVID-19, severe asthma, and biologics. Ann Allergy Asthma Immunol. 2020;125:357–9. https://doi.org/10.1016/j.anai.2020.06.012.
42. Izquierdo-Domínguez A, Rojas-Lechuga MJ, Alobid I. Management of allergic diseases during COVID-19 outbreak. Curr Allergy Asthma Rep. 2021;21:8. https://doi.org/10.1007/s11882-021-00989-x.
43. Guvey A. How does allergic rhinitis impact the severity of COVID-19?: a case-control study. Eur Arch Otorhinolaryngol. 2021;278(11):4367–71. https://doi.org/10.1007/s00405-021-06836-z.
44. Suzaki I, Kobayashi H. Coronavirus disease 2019 and nasal conditions: a review of current evidence. In Vivo. 2021;35:1409–17. https://doi.org/10.21873/invivo.12393.
45. Miodońska M, Bogacz A, Mróz M, Mućka S, Bożek A. The effect of SARS-CoV-2 virus infection on the course of atopic dermatitis in patients. Medicina. 2021;57:521. https://doi.org/10.3390/medicina57060521.
46. Carugno A, Raponi F, Locatelli AG, Vezzoli P, Gambini DM, Di Mercurio M, et al. No evidence of increased risk for coronavirus disease 2019 (COVID-19) in patients treated with Dupilumab for atopic dermatitis in a high-epidemic area - Bergamo, Lombardy, Italy. J Eur Acad Dermatol Venereol. 2020;34(9):e433–4. https://doi.org/10.1111/jdv.16552.

47. Nguyen C, Yale K, Casale F, Ghigi A, Zheng K, Silverberg JI, Mesinkovska NA. SARS-CoV-2 infection in patients with atopic dermatitis: a cross-sectional study. Br J Dermatol. 2021;185(3):640–1. https://doi.org/10.1111/bjd.20435.
48. Gong F, Dai Y, Zheng T, Cheng L, Zhao D, Wang H, et al. Peripheral CD4+ T cell subsets and antibody response in COVID-19 convalescent individuals. J Clin Invest. 2020;130(12):6588–99. https://doi.org/10.1172/JCI141054.
49. The Lancet. Understanding long COVID: a modern medical challenge. Lancet. 2021;398(10302):725. https://doi.org/10.1016/S0140-6736(21)01900-0.
50. Gattinger P, Borochova K, Dorofeeva Y, Henning R, Kiss R, Kratzer B, et al. Antibodies in serum of convalescent patients following mild COVID-19 do not always prevent virus-receptor binding. Allergy. 2021;76(3):878–83. https://doi.org/10.1111/all.14523.
51. Klimov VV. Adaptive immune response. In: From basic to clinical immunology. Cham: Springer; 2019. https://doi.org/10.1007/978-3-030-03323-4.
52. Fiocchi A, Jensen-Jarolim E. SARS-COV-2, can you be over it? World Allergy Organ J. 2021;14(2):100514. https://doi.org/10.1016/j.waojou.2021.100514.
53. Kared H, Redd AD, Bloch EM, Bonny TS, Sumatoh H, Kairi F, et al. SARS-CoV-2-specific CD8+ T cell responses in convalescent COVID-19 individuals. J Clin Invest. 2021;131(5):e145476. https://doi.org/10.1172/JCI145476.
54. Redd AD, Nardin A, Kared H, Bloch EM, Pekosz A, Laeyendecker O, et al. CD8+ T cell responses in COVID-19 convalescent individuals target conserved epitopes from multiple prominent SARS-CoV-2 circulating variants. Open Forum Infect Dis. 2021;8(7):ofab143. https://doi.org/10.1093/ofid/ofab143.
55. Trinkmann F, Muller M, Reif A, Kahn N, Kreuter M, Trudzinski F, et al. Residual symptoms and lower lung function in patients recovering from SARS-CoV-2 infection. Eur Respir J. 2021;57(2):2003002. https://doi.org/10.1183/13993003.03002-2020.
56. Beurnier A, Jutant E-M, Jevnikar M, Boucly A, Pichon J, Preda M, et al. Characteristics and outcomes of asthmatic patients with COVID-19 pneumonia who require hospitalisation. Eur Respir J. 2020;56(5):2001875. https://doi.org/10.1183/13993003.01875-2020.
57. Dayal AK, Sinha V. Trend of allergic rhinitis post COVID-19 pandemic: a retrospective observational study. Indian J Otolaryngol Head Neck Surg. 2020;20:1–3. https://doi.org/10.1007/s12070-020-02223-y.
58. Garcia-Pachon E, Grau-Delgado J, Soler-Sempere MJ, Zamora-Molina L, Baeza-Martinez C, Ruiz-Alcaraz S, Padilla-Navas I. Low prevalence of post-COVID-19 syndrome in patients with asthma. J Infect. 2021;82(6):276–316. https://doi.org/10.1016/j.jinf.2021.03.023.
59. Moreno-Pérez O, Merino E, Leon-Ramirez J-M, Andres M, Ramos JM, Arenas-Jiménez J, et al. Post-acute COVID-19 syndrome. Incidence and risk factors: a Mediterranean cohort study. J Infect. 2021;82(3):378–83. https://doi.org/10.1016/j.jinf.2021.01.004.
60. Matsuyama S, Kawase M, Nao N, Shirato K, Ujike M, Kamitani W, et al. The inhaled steroid ciclesonide blocks SARS-CoV-2 RNA replication by targeting the viral replication-transcription complex in cultured cells. J Virol. 2020;95(1):e01648–20. https://doi.org/10.1128/JVI.01648-20.
61. Song W-J, Hui CKM, Hull JH, Birring SS, McGarvey L, Mazzone SB, et al. Confronting COVID-19-associated cough and the post-COVID syndrome: role of viral neurotropism, neuroinflammation, and neuroimmune responses. Lancet. 2021;9:533–44. https://doi.org/10.1016/S2213-2600(21)00125-9.
62. Carlton SM. Nociceptive primary afferents: they have a mind of their own. J Physiol. 2014;592(16):3403–11. https://doi.org/10.1113/jphysiol.2013.269654.
63. Dror AA, Eisenbach N, Marshak T, Layous E, Zigon A, Shivatzki S, et al. Reduction of allergic rhinitis symptoms with face mask usage during the COVID-19 pandemic. J Allergy Clin Immunol Pract. 2020;8(10):3590–3. https://doi.org/10.1016/j.jaip.2020.08.035.

64. Patella V, Delfino G, Florio G, Spadaro G, Bianchi FC, Senna G, Di Gioacchino M. Management of the patient with allergic and immunological disorders in the pandemic COVID-19 era. Clin Mol Allergy. 2020;18:18. https://doi.org/10.1186/s12948-020-00134-5.
65. Milman O, Yelin I, Aharony N, Katz R, Herzel E, Ben-Tov A, et al. Community-level evidence for SARS-CoV-2 vaccine protection of unvaccinated individuals. Nat Med. 2021;27(8):1367–9. https://doi.org/10.1038/s41591-021-01407-5.
66. Krause PR, Fleming TR, Longini IM, Peto R, Briand S, Heymann DL, et al. SARS-CoV-2 variants and vaccines. N Engl J Med. 2021;385:179–86. https://doi.org/10.1056/NEJMsr2105280.

Afterword

In human populations, allergen tolerance is the consequence of many tolerogenic responses to environmental allergens. Most people with atopic heredity have IgE-sensitization and a high level of IgE but do not suffer from any atopic disease. The number of sufferers does not coincide with the number of practically healthy persons with atopic predisposition but without clinical symptoms who are significantly prevalent. This is a matter of allergen tolerance. The tolerogenic response to the causative allergen resembles an adaptive immune response. A tolerogenic dendritic cell exerts itself as an allergen-presenting cell, whereas a peripheral regulatory T cell is an allergen-recognizing cell. Further, there is no activation, clonal expansion, or differentiation into effector lymphocytes, but allergen-specific memory regulatory T cells are formed.

Allergens are only a small molecular group, less than 2% of all known protein families. However, people with atopic heredity sensitized with house dust mites and other allergens may fall ill with asthma, allergic rhinitis, atopic dermatitis, and even anaphylaxis. Why does anaphylaxis happen to some but not to others? This has always been a difficult question with no answer as of yet. Although genetics plays a vital role in the manifestation of most atopic diseases, epigenetics also matters much through epigenetic mechanisms like DNA methylation. Monogenic mutations associated with a single severe allergy have not been found, but separate facts about some mutations causing metabolic disturbances have accumulated. Therefore, it may be essential for the interactions between various susceptibility genes, immunologic processes, and environmental factors.

Allergen tolerance is the established evolutionary system of allergen tolerance maintenance, which consists of cells, biomolecules, and mechanisms: tolerogenic dendritic cells (tDCs), allergen-specific (peripheral) pTregs, other cells with pro-tolerogenic action, the inhibition of helper T cells via immunosuppressive cytokines and coinhibitory molecules, blocking or competing antibodies, pro-tolerogenic neurotransmitters and neuropeptides, enzymes, and tolerogenic microbiota. All allergists dream of allergen tolerance becoming lifelong in allergy patients. "Ah, stay a while! You are so lovely!" (von Goethe's Faust Part One, 1699–1702)

Allergen tolerance may be the medical purpose of a disease-modifying treatment method of atopic diseases, allergen-specific immunotherapy (AIT), invented by Dr.

V. V. Klimov, *Textbook of Allergen Tolerance*,
https://doi.org/10.1007/978-3-031-04309-3

Leonard Noon at the beginning of the twentieth century. Over 100 years, AIT has been developing and improving to help millions of people; although biologics appeared as a new approach in treating atopies, they can be used in combination with AIT. Nowadays, researchers' and clinicians' intention is to focus on oral AIT in food allergies and the development of a new generation of medications for all routes of AIT.

Answers to Quizzes

Chapter 1A

1.	4
2.	4
3.	2
4.	4
5.	1
6.	3
7.	1
8.	1
9.	3
10.	4
11.	3
12.	4
13.	4
14.	4
15.	1
16.	3

Chapter 1B

1.	3
2.	2
3.	1
4.	4
5.	1
6.	2
7.	2
8.	4
9.	1
10.	2
11.	1
12.	3
13.	2
14.	4
15.	1
16.	1

V. V. Klimov, *Textbook of Allergen Tolerance*,
https://doi.org/10.1007/978-3-031-04309-3

Chapter 2

1.	3
2.	1
3.	4
4.	2
5.	1
6.	2
7.	4
8.	2
9.	1
10.	4
11.	4
12.	4
13.	2
14.	1
15.	2
16.	4

Chapter 3A

1.	2
2.	3
3.	1
4.	4
5.	1
6.	3
7.	1
8.	1
9.	1
10.	3
11.	3
12.	3
13.	2
14.	3
15.	1
16.	3

Chapter 3B

1.	3
2.	1
3.	1
4.	3
5.	2
6.	2
7.	4
8.	1
9.	3
10.	1
11.	3
12.	1
13.	2
14.	4
15.	1
16.	4

Chapter 4A

1.	2
2.	1
3.	1
4.	2
5.	3
6.	4
7.	4
8.	1
9.	2
10.	3
11.	4
12.	2
13.	2
14.	2
15.	1
16.	3

Chapter 4B

1.	2
2.	3
3.	3
4.	1
5.	3
6.	2
7.	1
8.	2
9.	4
10.	1
11.	3
12.	4
13.	1
14.	2
15.	3
16.	3

Chapter 5A

1.	3
2.	1
3.	2
4.	1
5.	3
6.	1
7.	2
8.	1
9.	3
10.	2
11.	1
12.	3
13.	2
14.	2
15.	4
16.	1

Chapter 5B

1.	1
2.	2
3.	3
4.	2
5.	1
6.	4
7.	1
8.	3
9.	1
10.	2
11.	3
12.	4
13.	1
14.	2
15.	2
16.	4

Chapter 6

1.	2
2.	3
3.	2
4.	1
5.	2
6.	1
7.	4
8.	1
9.	3
10.	2
11.	1
12.	3
13.	2
14.	1
15.	2
16.	2

Chapter 7A

1.	3
2.	1
3.	4
4.	3
5.	1
6.	1
7.	2
8.	3
9.	2
10.	1
11.	2
12.	3
13.	2
14.	2
15.	3
16.	4

Chapter 7B

1.	2
2.	4
3.	2
4.	1
5.	2
6.	4
7.	1
8.	2
9.	3
10.	4
11.	1
12.	2
13.	3
14.	4
15.	2
16.	1

Chapter 8A

1.	3
2.	2
3.	1
4.	4
5.	4
6.	2
7.	4
8.	3
9.	4
10.	3
11.	4
12.	1
13.	4
14.	3
15.	2
16.	4

Chapter 8B

1.	3
2.	3
3.	2
4.	2
5.	4
6.	1
7.	3
8.	3
9.	2
10.	4
11.	1
12.	1
13.	4
14.	2
15.	3
16.	4

Chapter 9

1.	2
2.	2
3.	2
4.	4
5.	2
6.	3
7.	1
8.	2
9.	4
10.	3
11.	3
12.	1
13.	4
14.	1
15.	1
16.	2

Chapter 10

1.	2
2.	4
3.	2
4.	1
5.	3
6.	1
7.	3
8.	2
9.	4
10.	3
11.	1
12.	1
13.	3
14.	2
15.	3
16.	1

Index

V. V. Klimov, *Textbook of Allergen Tolerance*,
https://doi.org/10.1007/978-3-031-04309-3

Batch number: 10370712

Printed by Printforce, the Netherlands